Clinical Psychology for Trainees

Foundations of Science-Informed Practice,
Second Edition

Clinical Psychology for Trainees

Foundations of Science-Informed Practice, Second Edition

Andrew C. Page
Winthrop Professor at the School of Psychology, University of Western Australia, Perth, Australia

Werner G. K. Stritzke
Associate Professor at the School of Psychology, University of Western Australia, Perth, Australia

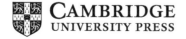

CAMBRIDGE
UNIVERSITY PRESS

University Printing House, Cambridge CB2 8BS, United Kingdom

One Liberty Plaza, 20th Floor, New York, NY 10006, USA

477 Williamstown Road, Port Melbourne, VIC 3207, Australia

4843/24, 2nd Floor, Ansari Road, Daryaganj, Delhi - 110002, India

79 Anson Road, #06-04/06, Singapore 079906

Cambridge University Press is part of the University of Cambridge.

It furthers the University's mission by disseminating knowledge in the pursuit of education, learning and research at the highest international levels of excellence.

www.cambridge.org
Information on this title: www.cambridge.org/9781107613980

© A. Page and W. Stritzke 2015

First published 2006
Second edition 2015
Reprinted 2016

A catalogue record for this publication is available from the British Library

Library of Congress Cataloging in Publication data
Clinical psychology for trainees : foundations of science-informed practice / [edited by] Andrew C. Page, Werner G. K. Stritzke. – Second edition.
    p. ; cm.
Includes bibliographical references and index.
ISBN 978-1-107-61398-0 (paperback : alk. paper)
I. Page, Andrew C. (Andrew Charles), 1964– , editor.   II. Stritzke, Werner G. K., 1956– , editor.
[DNLM: 1. Psychotherapy – methods.   2. Professional-Patient Relations.   3. Psychology, Clinical – methods. WM 420]
RC467.2
616.89–dc23   2014036110

ISBN 978-1-107-61398-0 Paperback

....

Every effort has been made in preparing this book to provide accurate and up-to-date information which is in accord with accepted standards and practice at the time of publication. Although case histories are drawn from actual cases, every effort has been made to disguise the identities of the individuals involved. Nevertheless, the authors, editors and publishers can make no warranties that the information contained herein is totally free from error, not least because clinical standards are constantly changing through research and regulation. The authors, editors and publishers therefore disclaim all liability for direct or consequential damages resulting from the use of material contained in this book. Readers are strongly advised to pay careful attention to information provided by the manufacturer of any drugs or equipment that they plan to use.

To Gilbert and Ruth (AP)
To Alfred and Ursula (WS)

Contents

Preface

The first edition laid out a model for the science-informed practice of clinical psychology. It aimed to give clinical psychology trainees a blueprint for how science can be used to influence the day-to-day practice of clinical psychology. The second edition retains that theme, but much has changed. In the intervening years our profession's knowledge base has grown and one of the key classificatory systems for mental disorders has been revised. Therefore, our book required updating. But even more fundamentally, a second edition was needed because in the past eight years there has been a seismic shift in the practice of clinical psychology. Like most change in life we were carried along with it and adapted to it as it happened. However, the starkness of the change was evident when we were confronted by the growing disparity between the health care environment in which we now live and the clinical psychology practice we described in 2006. Therefore, the second edition is not just an updating; it is in many ways a qualitatively different book. Some of the seeds that we described in 2006 have now become young saplings. The vista of clinical psychology has grown as the profession has developed greater depth and breadth. Therefore, the new edition not only incorporates new chapters on brief interventions, routine monitoring of treatment progress, and managing alliance ruptures, with around 200 new references, but it captures the profession at an exciting juncture. Today's clinical psychology trainees venture into health care environments that are increasingly interdisciplinary. Their skill set has broadened from specialist care and research expertise to incorporate a range of generalist competencies. Together, these define the unique value they add to integrated care settings. This second edition conveys the development of the profession and the excitement of the new challenges facing clinical psychology. We trust that after reading this book, not only will you feel that you have a sense of what a science-informed practice of clinical psychology might look like, but you will also share our enthusiasm for exploring the vital contributions that this science-informed brand of clinical psychology can make to the well-being of people in our society.

A science-informed model of clinical psychology practice

It has never been a better time to train as a clinical psychologist for three reasons. First, there is an increasing response to the recognition of the unmet need in mental health which is resulting in an increase in the number of clinical psychology jobs. Second, clinical psychology is enjoying a privileged position in mental health care because of its ability to provide an evidence base for the services it offers (Newnham & Page, 2010). Thus, despite the expense incurred by the provision of psychological services, we can show that their effectiveness assures savings that offset those costs. Third, the profession is facing a crossroads because the global demand for psychological services far exceeds the capacity of clinical psychologists to meet it (Schoenwald, Hoagwood, Atkins, Evans, & Ringeisen, 2010). This is the exciting challenge facing the graduates of today's programmes. How will you shape clinical psychology?

Considering the first of these points, governments across the world are realizing the need to deal effectively with mental health. Within the United Kingdom, the response has been the development of an Improving Access to Psychological Therapies (IAPT; see iapt.nhs. uk/) programme. This initiative aims to deliver interventions for people with depression and anxiety disorders that have been approved by the National Institute for Health and Care Excellence (NICE). In the United States, the Affordable Care Act (ACA) aims to improve equitable access to an improved quality of mental health care. In Australia, the Better Outcomes in Mental Health Care (health.gov.au/internet/main/publishing.nsf/Content/mental-boimhc) programme improves community access to quality primary mental health care by providing Access to Allied Psychological Services which enables General Medical Practitioners to refer consumers to allied health professionals who deliver focused psychological strategies. These initiatives are not limited to Western nations, with China's first national mental health legislation being adopted by the Standing Committee of the National People's Congress with the law that took effect in 2013. The law will prompt the need for greater community mental health care. Thus, the desire being expressed internationally (and tailored to the specific contexts of each nation) is to increase the access to mental health services. This desire is leading to an increasing demand for mental health professionals who are able to provide the treatments required.

Second, there is a common theme across the international initiatives to increase the quantity of mental health care; namely a focus on quality. Funding agencies want to ensure that they receive value for money. Consequently, funding is often limited to treatments that have a strong evidence base. Private and public funders are looking to allocate scarce health care resources into areas where there is an assurance that the treatment is effective and efficient (McHugh & Barlow, 2010). The profession of clinical psychology has enjoyed a privileged position as a result of these pressures because it has a long history of accountability (Lilienfeld, Ammirati, & David, 2012). Its professionals are trained in the critical skills required to evaluate the evidence and research methods to generate the data on both existing and new treatments (Pachana, Sofronoff, Scott, & Helmes, 2011). The status afforded to clinical psychologists, by virtue of their long history in demonstrating the accountability of their treatments, has meant that the profession as a whole benefits from the research base documenting the efficacy, effectiveness, and efficiency of psychological treatments (Barlow, 2010; McHugh & Barlow, 2010).

While these two reasons why it is great time to train as a clinical psychologist look backwards and rely on the actions of past clinical psychologists, the third reason looks forward to the future. We are at a juncture when clinical psychology will carve out the path that will affect the profession as it goes forward (Barkham, Hardy, & Mellor-Clark, 2010a). The decision facing the profession is, will science-informed practice inform the future practice of clinical psychology? The perception that psychology is scientific is not universal (Lilienfeld, 2012). Thus, will science continue to inform the future practice of clinical psychology (see Safran, Abreu, Ogilvie, & DeMaria, 2011a)? To contextualize this decision, we will take a brief digression into a discussion of the revisions of the psychiatric classification system.

Allen Frances chaired the committee responsible for the fourth revision of the American Psychiatric Association's diagnostic system: the *Diagnostic and Statistical Manual of Mental Disorders* (DSM-IV). After the publication of the fifth revision (i.e., the DSM-5) he wrote a book, *Saving Normal* (2013), in which he cogently critiqued the new taxonomy and the malign forces which he believed responsible for the errors. As a psychiatrist writing from retirement, there is a sense of his personal exclusion from the decision-making but there is another level on which the book can be read. Much of his invective is directed at the multinational pharmaceutical companies who, in his opinion, control the agenda and directly and indirectly influence the formation of the diagnostic categories and the uses to which they are put. However, what is clear is that Frances has seen (perhaps too late) the predicament that psychiatry has found itself in. In recent years the number of prescriptions for medications used to treat mental health conditions has increased to meet the rising demand. Since the number of psychiatrists has remained relatively static, general practitioners have taken over the role as the key provider of psychopharmacology. Psychiatrists have been relegated to small players in a big market and their voice, once pre-eminent, has become one among many. For example, the head of the Royal Australian and New Zealand College of Psychiatrists echoed the same sentiment in an interview (abc.net.au/pm/content/2014/s3987162. htm) where he noted that some groups in the community were increasingly more likely to seek advice from their GP rather than a psychiatrist. Thus, psychiatry is realizing that its pre-eminent position in mental health care has been eroded. As society has realized that the burden of mental health care is far larger than psychiatry can ever manage, it has sat by while other professions have stepped up to the task.

This cautionary tale provides clinical psychology with a window of opportunity. In the coming years the profession of clinical psychology will be settling itself down into the new mental health care environment. Clearly there are not enough clinical psychologists to meet the mental health care needs of the twenty-first century. Clearly, there will never be enough (Kazdin, 2011). The appropriately stringent and lengthy training of the profession will always be a limiting factor. Therefore, the exciting challenge for clinical psychologists is how to adapt themselves to this new environment. If the profession continues in the way it has been operating, it risks losing its pre-eminent role, just as psychiatry has. The remainder of the book will outline one possible future, where we will argue that clinical psychology must be a science-informed practice. By continuing to develop, evaluate, and offer evidence-based treatments; by delivering treatments in a monitored error-correcting clinical practice (Scott & Lewis, 2014); by training other mental health professionals in evidence-based treatments; and by fostering skills that complement (rather than duplicate) those of our colleagues in other professions clinical psychologists will bring to a mental health team expertise that will ensure them a continuing strong future (Barlow, 2010).

These are exciting times and the profession of clinical psychology has a bright future ahead. We are confident, because psychologists know that the best predictor of future be-haviour is past behaviour. If we consider the history of clinical psychology we can see that a science-informed approach to practice has served the profession well. Last century, Hans Eysenck (1952) threw down the gauntlet to clinical psychologists when he reviewed the 24 available studies and concluded provocatively that individuals in psychotherapy were no more likely to improve than those who did not receive treatment. Although the conclusion itself was questionable given the extant data (Lambert, 1976), the field responded assertively and effectively to these criticisms (e.g., Meltzoff & Kornreich, 1970). Perhaps the most ef-fective response came from Smith, Glass, & Miller (1980). Using meta-analytic statistical techniques to review 475 studies, they provided *quantitative* support for the conclusion that psychotherapy was superior to both no-treatment and placebo control conditions (see also Andrews & Harvey, 1981; Prioleau, Murdock, & Brody, 1983). More recently, reviewers in the US, UK, and Australia have sought to take the next step and identify criteria for em-pirically supported treatments, thereby providing listings of treatments that are 'effective' for particular disorders (e.g., Andrews, Crino, Hunt, Lampe, & Page, 1999; Chambless & Hollon, 1998; Nathan & Gorman, 2007; Roth & Fonagy, 2004; Task Force on Promotion and Dissemination of Psychological Procedures, 1995). In parallel, other reviewers have collated evidence regarding the effective components of psychotherapy relationships (e.g., Norcross, 2000, 2002; Orlinsky, Grawe, & Parks, 1994; Orlinsky, Rønnestad, & Willutzki, 2004). To-gether, these two lines of research provide a strong response to Eysenck's criticism. While people continue to debate the relative merits and contributions of the psychotherapy rela-tionship and the specifics of particular therapies (e.g., Norcross, 2000; Norcross & Wampold, 2011; Wampold, 2001), the conclusion that psychotherapy is better than no treatment, and better than a supportive caring relationship alone, is strongly supported.

Thus, Eysenck's provocative criticisms spurred a spirited and methodical response that allowed clinical psychology to clearly defend itself against general criticisms of ineffective-ness. In addition, the profession is able to identify, with increasing precision, the relational and specific therapeutic factors that mediate clinically meaningful change. Why was clinical psychology able to respond so effectively?

The scientist-practitioner model

Arguably, the manner and effectiveness of the response owes a debt to the origins of clini-cal psychology within the scientific discipline of psychology and to an early and sustained commitment to a scientist-practitioner model (Eysenck, 1949, 1950; Raimy, 1950; Shakow et al., 1947; Stewart, Stirman, & Chambless, 2012; Thorne, 1947; see Hayes, Barlow, & Nelson-Gray, 1999 and Pilgrim & Treacher, 1992 for historical reviews). From the establish-ment of the first clinical psychology clinic by Lightner Witmer, it was clear that science and practice were strategically interwoven (Norcross & Karpiak, 2012). For instance Witmer (1907) wrote:

The purpose of the clinical psychologist, as a contributor to science, is to discover the relation between cause and effect in applying the various pedagogical remedies to a child who is suffering from general or special retardation … For the methods of clinical psychology are necessarily invoked wherever the status of an individual mind is determined by observation and experiment, and pedagogical treatment applied to effect a change. (p. 9)

Although there has been much written about the scientist-practitioner model, the broad principles are that clinical psychologists, as scientist-practitioners, should be *consumers* of research findings, *evaluators* of their own interventions and programmes, and *producers* of new research who report these findings to the professional and scientific communities (Hayes et al., 1999). The commitment to an ideal of combining research and practice has infused the profession of clinical psychology to such a degree (e.g., Borkovec, 2004; Martin, 1989; McFall, 1991) that the response to Eysenck's scepticism (see also Peterson, 1968, 1976a, 1976b, 2004) was not an appeal to the authority of a psychotherapeutic guru, nor a rejection of its legitimacy followed by attempts to ignore it, but the profession produced and collated empirical data to refute the claim (Butler, Chapman, Forman, & Beck, 2006).

Despite the success of the scientist-practitioner model in shaping clinical psychology as a discipline committed to empiricism and accountability, advocates of the model have not been blind to its failure to achieve the ideal (Hayes et al., 1999; Nathan, 2000). Shakow et al. (1947) aimed to train individuals who could not only be a scientist and a practitioner, but could blend both roles in a seamless persona. They sought to achieve this goal by giving an equal weighting in training programmes to research and practice. However, ensuring the mere presence of these two equally weighted components did not by default produce an integrated scientific practice and did not win the hearts and minds of many graduates. In the words of Garfield, 'unfortunately, [psychologists in training] are not given an integrated model with which to identify, but are confronted instead by two apparently conflicting models – the scientific research model and the clinical practitioner model' (1966, p. 357; Peterson, 1991). More recently, there have been renewed efforts to provide a concrete instantiation of a scientific practice (Borkovec, 2004; Borkovec, Echemendia, Ragusea, & Ruiz, 2001; Scott & Lewis, 2014). Hayes and colleagues (1999) attributed the apparent lack of better science-practice integration to two factors: First, the 'almost universally acknowledged inadequacies of traditional research methodology to address issues important to practice', and second, the 'lack of a clear link between empiricism and professional success in the practice context' (p. 15). Our goal in the remainder of the book is not to address the first of these concerns (see Hayes et al., 1999a; Neufeldt & Nelson, 1998; Seligman, 1996a), but to speak to the second. Our goal is to articulate ways that a scientific clinical psychology can be practised.

The aim of this book

Our aim is to assist the student of clinical psychology to contemplate a scientific practice and to develop a mental model of what a scientist-practitioner actually *does* to blend state-of-the-science expertise with quality patient care. Our goal is not to describe a model of clinical practice (e.g., Asay, Lambert, Gregerson, & Goates, 2002; Borkovec, 2004; Edwards, 1987), nor to outline a broad conceptual framework for a scientist-practitioner (see Beutler & Clarkin, 1990; Beutler & Harwood, 2000; Beutler, Moliero, & Talebi, 2002; Fishman, 1999; Hershenberg, Drabick, & Vivian, 2012; Hoshmand & Polkinghorne, 1992; McHugh & Barlow, 2010; Nezu & Nezu, 1989; Schön, 1983; Spencer, Detrich, & Slocum,

2012; Stricker, 2002; Stricker & Trierweiler, 1995; Trierweiler & Stricker, 1998; Yates, 1995), or even to portray a scientifically grounded professional psychology (Peterson, 1968, 1997), since each of these has been effectively presented elsewhere. Our aim is to consider each of the core competencies that a trainee clinical psychologist will acquire with the question in mind, 'how would a scientist-practitioner think and act?' The value of the scientist-practitioner model as a sound basis for the professional identity and training of clinical psychologists lies in its emphasis on generalizable core competencies, rather than specific applications of these core competencies to each and every client problem or service setting (Shapiro, 2002). Accordingly, we will first describe our conceptual model of the core elements of science-informed practice. Then, in the remainder of the book, we will illustrate how this model allows individual practitioners to provide value for money in a competitive health care market indelibly shaped by the forces of accountability and cost-containment (see also Fishman, 2000; Kraus, Castonguay, Boswell, Nordberg, & Hayes, 2011; Woody, Detweiler-Bedell, Teachman, & O'Hearn, 2003).

A science-informed model of clinical psychology practice

The starting place of any action in clinical psychology practice is the client and his or her problems. Therefore, the discussion of a science-informed model needs to begin with the client. In addition, the meeting of client and therapist involves a relationship, so that at its heart the interaction is relational. The beginning of the relationship involves the presentation of the client's problems to the clinical psychologist. As shown in Figure 1.1, this information is conveyed to the clinician (depicted by the thin downward arrows) and some of it passes through the 'lens' of the clinical psychologist. This lens comprises the theoretical and empirical literature as well as the clinical (and non-clinical) experience and training. This lens serves to focus the information about the client. Continuing with the lens metaphor, not all the information passes through the lens (indicated by some arrows missing the lens) because clinicians will be limited by the level of current psychological knowledge, their theoretical orientation, and the extent of their experience. As with all metaphors, the notion of a lens filtering client data is limited in that it does not capture the dynamic nature of the interaction between client and clinician. The client is not analogous to a light source passively emitting illumination, but a client actively engages in an interactive dialogue with the clinician so that the information elicited is influenced by the clinician's responses, and the material the client proffers in turn influences how the clinician chooses to proceed. Thus, the interaction between client and clinician is a rich and dynamic dialogue, but while it has the potential to be a free-ranging and unconstrained discussion, the process has an 'error correcting' mechanism in that the information is focused by the clinician and channelled into diagnosis and a case formulation. The case formulation, described later, provides direction to the decisions that a clinical psychologist makes about treatment (indicated by the dotted arrows), which are then implemented and their outcomes measured, monitored, and evaluated. These processes involve feedback loops, so that information garnered at each stage feeds back to support or reject earlier hypotheses and decisions in a cycle of error correction.

Finally, there are processes associated with the public accountability of clinical practice. The results of treatment are fed forward by the clinical psychologist to modify the theoretical and empirical bases of practice. In addition, the results will be fed back to inform the person's clinical experience that will guide future clinical practice. Dissemination of

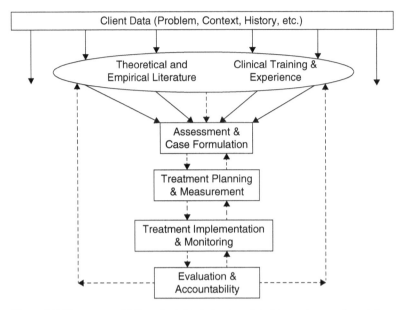

Figure 1.1 The process of linking client data to treatment decisions using case formulation.

evaluations of clinical practice outcomes serves not only to demonstrate that the practice is accountable, but also ensures the sustainability of clinical psychology. In the same way that logging forests without replanting new trees is unsustainable because it starves the timber industry of its raw material, if clinical psychology fails to replenish its resources (effective assessment and treatment), then it will be unsustainable. Other professions will step forward with potentially more efficient and effective alternatives to those which are presently available. Thus, we would agree with Miller (1969) that, 'the secrets of our trade need not be reserved for highly trained specialists. Psychological facts should be passed out freely to all who need and can use them in a practical and usable form so that what we know can be applied by ordinary people' (pp. 1070–1). We can 'give psychology away' in the sure knowledge that we are capable of generating new knowledge at least as fast as we can disseminate existing knowledge.

Stakeholders in the practice of clinical psychology

In the previous section we outlined how the foundations of science-informed practice rest on the clinical psychologist assuming three interrelated roles. Clinical psychologists are consumers of research, in that they draw on the existing theoretical and empirical literature, they are evaluators of their own practice, and they are producers of new practice-based research and knowledge. However, the style of research and type of research product varies according to the stakeholder. Three classes of stakeholders can be identified (see Figure 1.2). The first stakeholder is the *client* (included in this category are the client's family, friends, and supporters). The second class of stakeholder is the *clinician*, including the professional's immediate employment context (e.g., clinic, hospital, government department, etc.). The final class of stakeholder includes the broader *society* comprising individual members of society, government agencies, professional groups, academics, the private sector,

Client   Clinician   Society

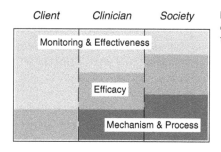

Monitoring & Effectiveness

Efficacy

Mechanism & Process

Figure 1.2 The relevance of three types of research activity in clinical psychology for three classes of stakeholder. The larger the area, the greater the relevance for a particular group.

etc. The type of research that each group will be interested in is displayed schematically in Figure 1.2

Clients have a legitimate interest in efficacy studies. Efficacy studies demonstrate in randomized controlled designs the superiority of a clinical procedure or set of procedures, presented in a replicable manner (e.g., using a treatment manual) over a control condition. The research has clearly defined inclusion and exclusion criteria, with an adequate sample size, and participants are evaluated by assessors blind to the experimental condition. Collating information across a group of efficacy studies permits identification of evidence-based or 'empirically supported treatments' (e.g., Andrews et al., 1999; Chambless & Hollon, 1998; Nathan & Gorman, 2007; Roth & Fonagy, 2004; Task Force on Promotion and Dissemination of Psychological Procedures, 1995). Clients may find this information useful in deciding which treatment has a good probability of success for carefully selected groups of individuals with problems like their own.

Clients will have an even greater interest in the effectiveness of a given treatment and ongoing monitoring of their own condition. That is, effectiveness research evaluates treatments as they are usually practised. In contrast to the treatment described in efficacy studies, clients who present for treatment may have multiple problems, may not meet all diagnostic criteria, and they will choose (rather than being randomly assigned) to receive a particular treatment whose duration is aimed to match their needs. The clinician may modify treatment based on a client's response. Within this class of research one can include studies that examine the generalizability of efficacious treatments to 'real world' settings (e.g., Peterson & Halstead, 1998), consumer surveys (e.g., Seligman 1995, 1996a, 1996b), as well as information on the outcomes of a specific clinic or clinician. Effectiveness can also be used broadly to refer to the measurement of change (e.g., pre- and post-treatment) within the client in question, the ongoing and idiographic monitoring of the client's problems (see Dyer, Hooke, & Page, 2014; Hawkins, Lambert, Vermeersch, Slade, & Tuttle, 2004; Howard, Moras, Brill, Martinovich, & Lutz, 1996; Lyons, Howard, O'Mahoney, & Lish, 1996; Newnham, Hooke, & Page, 2010a, 2010b; Sperry, Brill, Howard, & Grissom, 1996 for examples), and issues concerning service delivery. Arguably, as the data become more personal, they become more relevant to the particular client and those who may be involved in the client's care. Thus, in the left-hand box in Figure 1.2, proportionally more space is allocated to monitoring and effectiveness (light grey), than efficacy research (grey) to reflect the interests of an individual client.

Moving to the far right-hand side of Figure 1.2, the interests of society are depicted. In contrast to the individual client, society will have a general interest in knowledge about the effectiveness of treatments but will have no particular interest in monitoring the progress in treatment of a particular individual. Thus, the relevance of monitoring and effectiveness studies (light grey) is less for society in general than for the individual, indicated by the smaller proportion of the right-hand rectangle devoted to it. Society will have a greater interest in knowing the results of efficacy studies, so that governments and investors can make rational planning and funding decisions and services can be efficiently and effectively managed. Additionally, society takes an interest in a research agenda that may have little interest to individual clients, namely the research on the mechanisms and processes of disorders and treatment (dark grey). Included within this category of research endeavour are investigations of descriptive psychopathology and the aetiological mechanisms that initially cause or maintain a set of client problems as well as those mechanisms involved in client change (e.g., O'Donohue & Krasner, 1995). The category also includes research into the process of psychotherapy (e.g., Norcross, 2000, 2002); that is, research on the relationship variables critical to client improvement.

Standing between the clients on the one hand and society on the other, is the clinical psychologist. Clinical psychologists share the interests of both the client (in the monitoring and measurement of each client's particular problems and the delivery of the most efficacious treatment) and society (in understanding the fundamental mechanisms involved in each problem a client may present with and knowing which treatments are efficacious for a particular problem, and the degree to which these treatments translate into practice). For example, for the present authors, when we manage our clinic's smoking cessation (Stritzke, Chong, & Ferguson, 2009) and anxiety disorder programmes (Andrews et al., 2003; Page, 2002a) we not only want to know that the programmes are empirically supported, that they are effective outside the centres where they were tested on carefully selected samples, but we need to be able to demonstrate that the outcomes of our clinicians running our programmes are comparable to those in the published literature. Likewise, while a single case study may not be publishable, it provides an excellent way for individual practitioners to demonstrate to themselves and to a client the degree of improvement (Fishman, 2000).

Drawing together the themes discussed (and portrayed in Figures 1.1 and 1.2), the scientific practice of clinical psychology exists in a social network that ripples outward from the individual client, with a research agenda that becomes more general, theoretical, and generalizable as the conceptual distance from the client increases. Thus, there is probably not one single science-informed model of clinical psychology, but an array of ways that science informs practice and vice versa. The knowledge generated by large-scale efficacy studies (e.g., Elkin et al., 1989) exists alongside the knowledge generated by an individual clinician tracking the Subjective Units of Discomfort (SUD) of a phobic progressing through an exposure hierarchy. Both can appropriately be considered the products of a scientific practice of clinical psychology. Acknowledgement of diversity in the type of research product across different stakeholders is not to imply that there are no boundaries to a scientific clinical psychology, just that it is broader than it is often characterized.

Presenting evidence to stakeholders

It is worth noting that specification of the different stakeholders helps to clarify what information needs to be presented to which groups and by whom. Individual clients will be interested in feedback about how they have performed on psychological tests relative to appropriate normative samples and about the rate and extent of progress, both referenced against their pre-treatment scores and relevant norms (see Crawford, Cayley, Lovibond, Wilson, & Hartley, 2011; Woody et al., 2003). Further, the results of therapy may be communicated to other stakeholders in ward rounds, clinic meetings, training workshops, and other clinical settings (cf. Castonguay, 2011; Haynes, Lemsky, & Sexton-Radek, 1987; Mitchell, 2011). In contrast to the local presentation of individual client data, professional societies and funding bodies will seek information about the most cost-effective ways to treat specific disorders of all clients who present for treatment. They will require reliable answers, based on a body of research studies comprising good internal and external validity that point to answers that can be generalized to particular populations. Thus, an important skill for clinical psychologists is not only to be able to produce evidence, but to know how to generate and present research outcomes relevant to the target stakeholder.

One example of the targeted presentation of research evidence is the way that clinical psychology is responding to the increasing industrialization of health care. Health care costs began to rise dramatically during the 1980s and it became clear that both the private and public sectors needed to be more assertive in the management of health funds. Employee Assistance Programmes (EAPs) were one of the first responses, offering corporations targeted services of early identification and minimal, time-limited interventions followed, if necessary, by appropriate referral. In the US, managed (health) care organizations evolved with the development of Health Maintenance Organizations (HMOs; where individuals or companies contract an organization to provide all health services), Preferred Provider Organizations (PPOs; who reimburse a panel of providers on a fee-for-service basis, typically with some form of co-payment), and Individual Practice Association (IPAs; in which providers organize themselves to contract directly with companies to provide health services). Although the particular structure of health care varies markedly across different countries, all Western nations face the same problems of increasing costs of health care (compounded by a growing aged population) and share the same need of third-party payers (i.e., insurance companies and governments who pay the health bills) to rein in health care costs. Increasing costs have focused attention more than ever upon efficient and effective health care and thus, the need for clinical psychologists to be able to demonstrate that their assessment and treatment processes are not only effective, but they can be targeted, delivered in a timely manner, and offered in a definable and reproducible manner. Thus, in the past the rationale for a scientific-informed practice was promoted within the discipline by professional organizations (e.g., the American Psychological Association, British Psychological Society) and foresighted individuals (e.g., Thorne, 1947), but in recent times the rationale has become increasingly externally motivated, in the form of third-party payers who are demanding cost-effective health care. Whereas in the past the scientist-practitioner model could be seen as a luxury representing an ideal worthy of pursuit, in the present era of accountability it is a necessity ideally suited to demonstrate the value that can be returned for every health care dollar invested in clinical psychology services (Schoenwald et al., 2010). As consumers seek to purchase quality services at cheaper prices, there will be a market edge to those who are able to demonstrate that their products are both effective and economical.

In sum, science-informed clinical psychology does not have a single product to market, but it produces many different outputs relevant to diverse audiences (Castonguay, 2011). Clients will be interested in their personal well-being, whereas society will be interested in the broader issues of descriptive psychopathology, aetiological models of disorders, treatment processes and outcomes, as well as efficient and effective health care (Kazdin & Blase, 2011). The individual clinical psychologist requires the skills to collect and present data relevant to particular stakeholders. Not all clinical psychologists are employed in the same capacity and the stakeholders each person deals with are different, and therefore it is better to conceptualize the implementation of a science-informed model of clinical practice as not being epitomized by a particular instantiation, but as a strategic commitment to a scientific approach at the core of clinical practice. Priority of strategy over procedure is essential, because the evidence base will always be incomplete. The core competencies of a scientist-practitioner are most needed when the evidence is equivocal or lacking (Newnham & Page, 2010; Shapiro, 2002). In the remaining chapters we outline ways that a person with a commitment to the application of science to clinical practice might approach the many tasks clinical psychologists engage in. The first of these activities will be the difficult task of developing a strong therapeutic relationship.

Relating with clients

2

Imagine sitting face to face with your first client. What is the best thing to do or say? What if you open your mouth and say the wrong thing?

This is an appropriately daunting image because you want to do the best for your client and the stakes are high. Minimally, a therapist must aim to do no harm, but how is one to exert a positive influence? One common response among students is to seek technical guidance in the form of a treatment manual. There are published lists of evidence-based treatments (e.g., Nathan & Gorman, 2007) that identify the relevant treatment manuals and it makes sense to find the manual that matches the client's problem and to begin therapy. Furthermore, this seems reasonable because the practice is scientific, in that you can base your clinical decisions on the scientific literature. Other students respond to the challenge of exerting a positive influence upon clients by seeking to focus on the therapeutic relationship (Norcross, 2002). Once again, this is not an unscientific strategy since there is a substantial literature identifying aspects of the therapeutic process beneficial to outcomes (e.g., Beutler et al., 2004; Bohart & Wade, 2013; Castonguay & Beutler, 2006; Norcross, 2010; Orlinsky et al., 2004). This approach has a long history with Frank (1973) suggesting that psychotherapy is an encounter between a demoralized client and a therapist aiming to energize the client. Frank placed less emphasis on *what* was done in therapy, and more emphasis upon *how* it was done; specifically, he emphasized the therapist's ability to mobilize a client's motivation and hope.

Thus, there are sound reasons for identifying an evidence-based treatment best suited to a client, but there are also good reasons for fostering the therapeutic relationship. The clinical psychologist will begin therapy by thinking how best to manage the relationship with the client to foster change and will be constantly reviewing it, and responding to it (see Figure 2.1). This still leaves you with the apparent dilemma as a new therapist; what is the best thing to do or say? However, the dilemma is easily resolved if one understands that the two approaches are not mutually exclusive, but complement each other.

Borkovec (2004) spoke to this issue as he outlined his vision of an integrated science and clinical practice. In answer to the question, 'What is the empirical evidence for what you do with a client?', he commented that,

Certainly research on relevant empirically supported treatments (ESTs) is part of this review process, but it goes further. The professional commitment of clinical psychologists is to be *knowledgeable about, and guided by, the empirical foundation of everything they do during the therapy hour,* and the psychological literature contains far more information relevant to this potential foundation than merely (though importantly) therapy outcome studies documenting the efficacy of specific protocol manuals. (p. 212; italics added)

The empirically based choice of the best treatment programme is one component of a scientific practice of clinical psychology, but it is not the whole of it. To use a culinary metaphor,

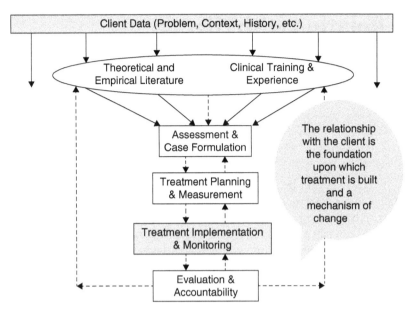

Figure 2.1 The therapeutic relationship is central to change in psychotherapy.

scientific practice is not a garnish sprinkled onto clinical psychology, but it is like salt that once added to food permeates the whole dish. The scientific practice of clinical psychology and the use of evidence-based treatments do not abdicate a clinician from the responsibility of fostering a therapeutic relationship in the best interest of the client. We will later consider some components of evidence-based treatments, but first we will review evidence-based components of the therapeutic relationship. The separation is not intended to imply that these are alternative options of conducting psychotherapy. Both aspects are integral parts of a strategic approach to provide an empirical foundation for everything that happens in a therapy hour.

Empirical foundations of the therapeutic relationship

The promulgation of treatment manuals could give the false impression that the therapist behaviour exerts little influence over and above the specific ingredients of the manualized therapy. A series of studies by Miller and colleagues highlights how this conception would be false (Miller, Taylor, & West, 1980; Miller & Baca, 1983). They found that a treatment programme for problem drinking was equally effective when delivered by therapists or in a self-help format. However, when they further explored the data, they found considerable variability within the therapist-administered treatment programme. Specifically, two thirds of the variance in drinking outcomes at six months post-treatment was predicted by the degree of therapist empathy. Even two years after the completion of therapy, still one quarter of the variance in drinking outcomes was predicted by therapist empathy. Thus, there were some therapists who administered a standard treatment programme with outcomes that far exceeded those achieved with self-help, but there were other therapists whose clients would have been better off if they had read the book by themselves. Therefore, scientist-practitioners will need to identify and cultivate those therapeutic behaviours that reliably relate to positive client outcomes (e.g., Miller & Rollnick, 2012).

One way to identify evidence-based therapeutic behaviours is to determine which be-haviours that occur during treatment are positively correlated with therapeutic outcomes. These were reviewed by a task force of Division 29 of the American Psychological Associa-tion (Ackerman et al., 2001; see also Orlinsky et al., 1994, 2004; Norcross, 2010; Norcross & Wampold, 2011). They divided the behaviours into those that were demonstrably effec-tive and those that were promising and probably effective. Of the demonstrably effective behaviours they identified the therapeutic alliance (or cohesion in the context of group therapy), empathy, and having goal consensus and a collaborative relationship. Of prom-ising and probably effective behaviours they identified establishing a relationship where there is positive regard for the client, the therapist interacts in a manner where they are genuine (i.e., their manner of presentation is congruent with who they really are), elic-its feedback about the psychologist's behaviour, repairs ruptures to alliance (an issue we will return to in subsequent chapters), occasionally and appropriately discloses infor-mation about themselves, while keeping their own issues out of therapy (i.e., manages countertransference).

From the review it is clear that process variables can be divided into three categories, namely those related to the client, the therapist, and the relationship. In addition, Norcross and Wampold (2011) noted a variety of ways that therapy can be adapted to individual clients that may enhance outcomes. Their review noted that outcomes could be improved when therapists adapted therapy in response to factors such as the resistance expressed by the client, the preferences for therapy, the client's cultural background, the client's religious beliefs and spiritual values, as well as the client's typical coping style, and where in the stages of change the person was. We will return to the methods of adapting therapy in light of the client's response to therapy and their particular attributes later in the book, but for now we will focus on the general issues concerning the client, the therapist, and their relationship. Bearing in mind the caveat that the actions of a client and therapist affect each other recipro-cally, it is possible to draw a number of lessons from this review of the literature.

First, the quality of the therapeutic relationship is strongly related to outcome and both client and therapist behaviours are involved. Thus, it is critical to consider what activities enhance the therapeutic bond. Second, clients possess a variety of qualities that are posi-tively associated with outcome. While there will be individual differences in these qualities, it behoves the therapist to maximize the extent to which these behaviours are exhibited dur-ing treatment. For instance, client conversational engagement is positively correlated with outcome and although clients will vary in terms of their levels of verbal activity, the therapist should be mindful of strategies to maximize client verbal activity. Third, a novice therapist may take some comfort from the observation that although therapist credibility is related to outcome, the size of the effect is weaker than many others. That is, even if you feel unsure when you are seeing a client, remember that this variable is not among the largest predictors of therapeutic outcome.

Thus, certain client behaviours as well as specific therapist behaviours should be maxi-mized to enhance outcome. Outcomes will be enhanced when the therapist creates an en-vironment in which the client is able to discuss their problems collaboratively in an open and easy manner. The therapist will be working hard to maximize the therapeutic bond, by showing empathic affirmation (acceptance, warmth, positive regard) of the client. In a nut-shell, the therapist will work hard to develop the therapeutic alliance.

Building a therapeutic alliance

Broadly speaking, the therapeutic alliance involves three components (Bordin, 1979). First, the client and therapist agree on therapeutic goals. Second, the therapeutic alliance involves the assignment of a task or set of tasks for the client, which can occur within the therapy session or between sessions. The final component is the development of a therapeutic bond. As Ackerman and Hilensroth (2003) noted, despite much research focusing on the relationship between the therapeutic alliance and outcome (e.g., Bohart & Wade, 2013; Martin, Garske, & Davis, 2000; Norcross & Wampold, 2011; Orlinsky et al., 1994, 2004), much less research has addressed the particular behaviours of the therapist that foster and strengthen the alliance. Based on a review of the existing literature, they identified a set of therapist attributes and techniques that are positively related to a strong therapeutic alliance. Their work suggests that in terms of personal qualities, a good alliance is associated with therapists who present with a *warm* and *friendly* manner, and who appear *confident* and *experienced*. Therapists with a good therapeutic alliance will be *interested* in and *respectful* towards their clients, and they will relate with *honesty, trustworthiness*, and *openness*. During therapy they will remain *alert* and *flexible*. In terms of providing a safe environment for clients to discuss their issues, therapists will be *supportive* and use *reflective* listening skills, *affirm* the clients' experiences, and demonstrate an *empathic understanding* of each client's situation. Therapists will *attend to the clients' experiences* and *facilitate the expression of affect*, to enable a *deep exploration* of concerns. In terms of the practice of therapy, clinicians with a positive alliance provide *accurate interpretations* of client's behaviours, are *active* in treatment, and *draw attention to past therapeutic successes* (Ackerman & Hilsenroth, 2003).

Drawing together the themes evident from the preceding reviews of therapy processes and the therapeutic alliance, a number of general conclusions can be drawn about the conduct of a therapy session. First, in terms of the therapist, it is important to be warm, empathic, and genuine. Second, the client needs to be actively engaged in therapy, with a good understanding of what is occurring. Third, the relationship between the client and therapist needs to be collaborative with a good rapport. We will now illustrate the specific behaviours that can strengthen the alliance by describing how they may be appropriate at different points in an initial session with a client.

Relating with a client to build an alliance

To begin a session it is useful to begin with a polite introduction, taking the effort to be warm and friendly. Therefore, make sure that you make eye contact as you say the client's name and permit time for the small talk that often follows an introduction (e.g., a discussion of parking difficulties or problems finding the clinic). However, the small talk must not detract from attention to the problem, so to convey a genuine interest in the client you need to shift focus swiftly to the client's main concerns. Thus, invite the client to sit down with chairs arranged so that you sit side on, but still facing the client, at a comfortable distance. Before asking the client to describe their concerns, it is important to discuss issues of confidentiality (see Chapter 10). Briefly, there are two aspects to this. On the one hand, you want to make it explicit that material raised remains confidential. On the other hand, confidentiality is not absolute and there will be occasions when you may be legally or ethically bound to inform a third party. It is prudent to draw the client's attention to these circumstances (e.g., when there is an explicit threat to harm the self or another specified person, when a child is in danger, or when subpoenaed by a court of law) verbally or in written documentation. Although it may seem a little awkward to raise these issues, it is easier to raise them at this point and it also allows clients a few moments to settle themselves.

Once the preliminaries are over, it is time to ask the client to introduce the problem. Since you are trying to be respectful and affirming, it is useful to let the client provide this introduction. On some occasions you will have referral information or prior case notes and therefore you may want to begin by indicating to the client that you would 'like to hear it from you first'. In asking about the client's difficulties you are aiming to create a sense of openness. One way to do this is to begin by asking, 'What seems to be the problem?' or 'What brought you along today?' In so doing do not impose a structure, but let the client raise the issues as they would like to (but see Chapter 7 for circumstances when it is important to impose structure right away; for example, in many medical settings, time constraints often require rapid assessment skills, and a purposeful structure is essential for eliciting as much information as possible in the limited time available). Ask questions, but permit the client to define their problems. Sometimes you will have prior information and it can be helpful to mention this. For example, 'You mentioned on the phone that you were having difficulty with "depressed mood", could you tell me about it?'

On occasions clients are reticent at the outset of therapy and it may be useful to acknowledge some of the discomfort, perhaps by saying, 'People are often concerned about seeking professional help, but I'm glad you came to see me. It is the first step in doing something about your difficulties.'

In asking a client questions, the form of questions can be closed or open. Closed questions can be answered in a few words or even with a simple 'yes' or 'no' (e.g., 'Do you live with your family?'). They are useful for focusing an interview and obtaining specific information, but used to excess they constrain the client and place the burden of directing the session upon the therapist. Open questions are those that take many words to answer and in so doing, encourage the client to provide the maximum amount of information (e.g., 'What is your relationship with your family like?'). Thus, open questions are preferable as ways to begin an initial interview with a client, but relatively more closed questions may be used to begin a session later on in therapy (e.g., 'Last week we talked about managing your tension while asserting yourself. How did you go with that?').

As the client is talking you need to reflect upon how you are coming across to the client. First, be aware of your eye contact. Make sure that you look at the client. Although you will normally look away more often when you are speaking than when you are listening and eye contact is rarely a continuous stare, you need to be able to watch the client for behavioural signs relevant to their problems (e.g., breaks in eye contact, shifting in their seat). In addition, eye gaze is an important implicit cue in communication used to signal turn taking (i.e., a speaker will restore eye contact to signal that a communication is complete) or to seek confirmation (e.g., a speaker will look to a listener when expecting a response to their communication). It is also important to be aware of cultural differences in eye contact (e.g., Australian Aboriginal people tend to avoid contact when discussing serious topics). One trap for the novice therapist to avoid is excessive note taking. The client is not a topic to be studied, but a person with whom you are relating. Therefore, jot down an occasional aid to memory rather than a transcript of the conversation. Building a warm and friendly relationship is more important to the therapeutic alliance than a comprehensive record of the session.

Second, in terms of body language scan both the client and yourself. Ensure that your proximity is comfortable to the client, so that if they move their chair forward or backward, do not adjust yours to a distance negating the client's move. Watch for changes in body posture that indicate discomfort or greater assurance. Also be alert for discrepancies between the client's body language and their verbal tone and content. For example, the client who folds her arms while saying that she is quite comfortable with her boss's decision. Likewise, ensure that your body posture does not communicate impatience (e.g., pen tapping), boredom (e.g., doodling), defensiveness (e.g., arms crossed), and discomfort (e.g., breaking eye contact). Your aim is to convey honest acceptance while supportively affirming the client. If you feel unsure how best to sit, mirroring the client's behaviour can be a good start or leading the client by modelling a relaxed and open manner (e.g., feet firmly on the floor, arms on your legs with palms open).

Third, you voice needs to convey friendly interest. Therefore, watch for signs of emotional tone in your voice and ensure that it matches any emotional content. Likewise, pay attention to the client's emotional tone. In addition to tracking the vocal tone, track the verbal content. Align your conversation with the client's interest and signal any transitions (e.g., 'I was wondering if we could switch from the problems you are presently having with your drinking and go back to when it all began, so that I can get a clearer idea of where it all came from. Is this OK with you?'). Transitions signal a change, but it is also useful to include a brief summary of the material covered most recently in the session to indicate that you have been listening to the client. The way that you respond to the client will influence the course of the interview, so track the verbal tone and content of your responses. For instance, consider how the tone of the interview and the content of the client's response would vary if you responded to the client saying, 'I've just lost my job' with (a) 'that was very careless of you', (b) 'how did that happen?', or (c) 'how do you feel about losing your job?' Another way to track the client's verbal content is to identify important words. Statements that begin with 'I' can often be relevant because they are important to a client and the use of the personal pronoun communicates the personal significance. Clients will also emphasize certain words to highlight key issues. For instance, confusion or ambivalence about impulsive behaviour may be indicated by emphasis in a sentence such as, '*WHY* do I keep drinking too much and getting together with the wrong sort of guys?'

The questions that you ask will help the client to elaborate upon their responses. For example, in an initial interview you could ask open questions to facilitate greater discussion of a topic by asking, 'Could you tell me more about that?' or 'How did you feel when that happened?' Sometimes you will need to get a client to be more specific or concrete and at such times you could ask, 'Could you give me a specific example?' or 'Tell me about a typical drinking session'.

The form of a question will also influence the type of answer. *What* questions often lead to factual answers, therefore they are the easiest to answer. *How* questions initiate a discussion of processes and an account of a sequence of events. *Why* questions bring about a discussion of possible reasons. One problem with why questions is that even though they give you an indication of the client's perceptions of causation, they can put individuals on the defensive and may produce discomfort if they imply blame. Further, Nisbett and Wilson (1977) mount a convincing case that humans do not have introspective access into the causal cognitive processes despite being happy to elaborate on what they believe to be the correct answer. This is perhaps also one reason why a frequent response by clients to a 'why' question is 'I don't know'. 'Why' questions are difficult to answer on the spot. Nonetheless, awareness of a client's perception of the cause of their problems (independent of its validity) is useful information when presenting to a client a problem formulation. An alternative to asking direct 'why' questions is to indirectly pave the way towards some causal insight by beginning with a 'what' question. For example, an answer to the question 'Why are you upset with your husband's decision?' requires considerable cognitive processing entailing deliberation and judgement. In contrast, the question 'What is it about your husband's decision that upsets you?' prompts the client to simply describe and list all the 'things' that come to mind that are upsetting to her. It is far easier for the client to look at a list of concrete exemplars, and then arrive at an overall judgement 'why' she was upset, than to ponder that question in the abstract via internal processes. Thus, 'what' questions are often better than 'why' questions when it comes to eliciting answers about the reasons for a client's behaviours, thoughts, or feelings. Finally, *could* questions (e.g., 'Could you tell me what your husband does that makes you mad?') tend to be maximally open-ended and generate many options for the client (including a refusal to answer, which can be beneficial).

However, as you ask questions, remember the goal of therapy is not just to elicit information, but to facilitate a communication. Therefore, track the client's responses to your style of interaction. If your client looks confused, check that you have not been using multiple questions (e.g., 'I wonder if you could tell me when the difficulties with your wife began, first her jealousy and then her drinking, but also tell me how you felt about each of them and how each of your children reacted to the whole situation?'). If your client looks uncomfortable, check that you are not asking an excessive number of overly probing or closed questions. In a therapy context, the clinician exerts a degree of influence over the interview that is not present in social contexts, such that clients feel obliged to answer each question. Therefore, reflect on each question and ask yourself if you need to know the information. Although the material elicited in a session is confidential, you do not wish to explore a client's private life any more than you need to. Also, if the client is reticent about answering your questions, consider if you have been using statements framed as questions. For instance, you might say, 'Don't you think it would have been more helpful if you had studied harder?' which is really a judgement about the client's effort rather than a helpful therapeutic question. In our experience, one word to watch out for in this respect is 'so'. Often a question or statement that begins with 'so' is one that is about to tell the client what you think. For instance, you might say, 'So you've been feeling pretty bad lately.' These comments are much better re-phrased as genuine questions (e.g., 'Could you tell me how you've been feeling lately?').

Fourth, non-attention and silence are potentially useful therapist responses. If a client repeatedly brings up the same topic, you may feel the need to shift attention elsewhere. The danger with this strategy is that clients may keep returning to topics when they do not believe you have understood what they are saying or how distressed they are. We will discuss reflective listening in more detail later, but if you are sure that you have heard the message and it is time for a change in topic it is sometimes useful to say, 'I hear how distressed you are' while maintaining eye contact with the client. Wait until you get a clear sense that your message has been heard by the client before moving on.

The novice therapist is sometimes worried about silence, believing that the job of the therapist is to fill the therapy hour with words. Notice in our review of the process variables that were related to outcome, the verbal output of the client, but not of the therapist was consistently related to outcome. Therefore, do not worry about silence. Sometimes saying nothing is the best support you can give. Sometimes you cannot think of what to say because there is nothing to say. Sometimes you need time to think about the best response. Either way, a receptive silence can be a useful therapeutic tool.

Encouraging, restating, and paraphrasing

So far we have considered the style of questioning and behaving. Although these techniques are important, the goal of a session is to both give and receive information. The information the client is providing will be both verbal and non-verbal. Some information will be explicitly communicated by the client. Other information will be communicated without the client's awareness or will need to be inferred by the therapist. Receiving all the client's messages, decoding them correctly, and conveying to the client that you have accurately heard and understood the rich and complex tapestry of words, emotion, and behaviours is at the heart of empathic communication.

Three strategies that assist the therapist to communicate that client messages have been received are encouraging, restating, and paraphrasing. Encouraging typically involves behaviours such as head nods, open gestures, positive facial expressions, and verbal utterances (e.g., 'Uh-huh'). Each of these therapist responses seeks to convey an encouragement to continue with a particular line of style of responding. These encouragers need to be used judiciously, since too few leave the therapist looking wooden and too many can be annoying. Remember, the responses are intended to encourage elaboration on particular points, so make sure that you use them when you wish to reinforce a particular utterance. Thus, one trap to avoid is saying 'yes' before a client has finished a sentence or idea.

Therapists can also provide encouragement by repeating key words from a client's response. For instance, if a client said, 'It happened again. I walked into the office, it went quiet, and I felt that everyone was looking at me. Suddenly I felt that rush of anxiety and started to blush' you might respond, 'Everyone was looking at you?' or 'You blushed?' Each response encourages the client to elaborate on a particular facet of the experience and the clinician will opt for a particular line of response depending on the overall agenda. The preceding responses would lead the session towards a discussion of the office workers' perceptions on the one hand or the client's physiological response on the other. Later in therapy a clinician might wish to explore recurring patterns and may wish to draw attention to the repetition by responding, 'It happened again?'

Other encouragers may be more focused. For instance, you might ask questions to establish the generality of a behaviour (e.g., 'How often do you drink each day?'), situational influences (e.g., 'Where do you drink?'), onset (e.g., 'When did it all begin?'), or course (e.g., 'Has it been the same all the time?').

Paraphrasing is a deceptively simple skill. The aim is to distil the client's explicit and implicit messages into a single utterance. The verbal and non-verbal cues, the key ideas that have been spoken and inferred concepts, are concisely summarized. Thus, the key skill in paraphrasing is not speaking, but listening. Begin by paying attention to everything the client is communicating and take time to reflect on the explicit and implicit messages. Consider any themes or important features, evaluate the discrepancies between verbal and non-verbal communications, and formulate a response. Although we will now turn to ways that a summary can be expressed, we cannot emphasize enough the extent to which the key to a successful summary is the thought that occurs before you open your mouth. Providing a good summary can also be facilitated by collecting relevant information. Asking the client how they react to their problems and how others respond can provide you with key elements to include in a summary.

A summary often begins with a stem, such as 'It looks to me...' or 'What I'm hearing is ...' or 'Putting these ideas together...' The summary brings together the main points of the issue from a client perspective. To convey clients' perspectives, try to use their language. For instance, if clients have used the terms 'sadness' and 'grief' to describe their experiences, use their words rather than another such as 'depression'. Try to clearly express the main elements of the problem. Often clients will be confused and ambivalent so the therapist can assist by highlighting key themes or drawing together seemingly unrelated symptoms into a coherent picture. Finally, after presenting a clear, succinct, and meaningful summary, request explicit feedback to check your understanding. You might ask, 'Am I hearing you right?' In addition, check that your coverage has been sufficient. We prefer questions such as 'What have I missed out?' rather than 'Have I missed anything out?' because the former presumes incompleteness and inaccuracies and therefore implicitly encourages correction.

Putting together these three skills of encouraging, restating, and paraphrasing, imagine how you would respond to a client who said, 'I'm really concerned about my teenage daughter. She used to talk to me and now she has become sullen and withdrawn, so we don't talk. I'm so worried that she's getting into something bad. She's got all these new friends and she won't tell me what they get up to. I don't know what to say, but if she's been using drugs then she can just leave home as far as I'm concerned!'

An encourager might be to respond, 'You don't talk?' A restatement might be, 'You are terribly concerned about your daughter'. Finally, a paraphrase might be, 'I'm hearing a few themes emerge in what you say. One theme is that you seem concerned; concerned about the loss of communication with your daughter and concerned about the possibility of harm, so much so that you'd consider asking her to leave. Another theme seems to be one of loss; you describe a sense of loss of communication, closeness, and influence. Have I heard you right?' In the paraphrase, some elements are reflections back of what the client said, but others are inferences based on the client's comments. That is, the client did not discuss her feelings about a loss of influence and control over her daughter as she becomes more independent. However, the therapist knows this is a common issue between parents and teenage children, so speculated that this unspoken theme was present, and therefore presented it as a hypothesis. It is wise to check that a paraphrase is correct, but essential to do so when an inference or speculative interpretation is being presented.

These three communication skills are useful steps in developing an empathic understanding between you and your client; however, empathy goes deeper than communication. Empathy is the ability to see the world from the perspective of another person and communicate this understanding. Behaviourally, it is possible to define verbal and non-verbal actions and attending skills that are associated with empathy, but at its heart empathy is a relational construct. It involves putting yourself into another person's shoes so that you can share a deeper relationship (Egan, 2002). The deep relationship involves positive regard. Positive regard involves selectively attending to the positive aspects of a client's communication. It stems from a humanistic worldview that people are inherently moving forward and growing in positive way (i.e., self-actualizing). Highlighting these positive aspects identifies positive assets a client can build upon and conveys a sense of warmth and acceptance. Empathic communication also conveys respect and warmth. Clients may not have told others about the issues that they raise in therapy and thus it is important to convey respect for the client. Show that you know that they are doing their best to deal with their issues. Transmit appreciation for the person's worth as a human being and communicate warmth by smiling or using facial expressions conveying empathic concern when responding to a client's emotions.

The empathic therapist also needs to demonstrate congruence (having a minimal discrepancy between their perceived and actual self), genuineness, and authenticity. Possession of these attributes ensures congruence between verbal and non-verbal behaviours which ultimately facilitates communication with clients. Clients are the focus of any session and therefore the therapist's issues must not clutter the therapy process. Therapists who are not fully accepting of their clients may exhibit incongruence between their verbal and non-verbal behaviours which clients may pick up on.

Like reflecting the verbal content of a communication, reflecting an emotion begins with a sentence stem followed by a feeling label. The emotional word or phrase aims to use the minimum number of concepts to reflect the affect in the correct tense. For example, match your tense to that used by the client, so that if a client says, 'I felt down' it would be better to use the past tense, than to say, 'Your mood seems low'. Once again, conclude with a check to ensure that your reflection of feeling is accurate.

One facet of a session that is easy to omit is an assessment of the client's skills, strengths, and resources. It is a common trap to fall into because clients want to discuss their problems. However, clients are first and foremost people, who also happen to have some problems. Therefore, spend time explicitly considering clients' coping mechanisms and supports. You might ask, 'With whom do you talk most often?' and then discuss what they enjoy talking about. Evaluate if they use other people for distraction, dependence, encouragement and motivation, or clarification. You can also ask the client about interests, social activities, and religious/spiritual practices.

When coming to the end of a session summarize the issues covered and draw the themes together. Typically clients will have identified a set of concerns, thus you could say, 'Have I got it right, it seems that the main issues for you are…let us try to rank them into a "step-ladder" of concerns beginning with the least problematic and stepping up to the more concerning.' This hierarchy can help set an agenda and identify a tentative treatment plan. Also check that nothing has been omitted by saying, 'You have talked about your checking and the intrusive thoughts as well as your depressed mood. Are there any issues we haven't talked about that you'd like to discuss?' or 'Is there anything else you would like to tell me?' Finally, at the end of a session, conclude with a clear statement about what is going to happen next. This may involve psychological testing or scheduling a referral or another appointment. The goal is to leave clients with a sense of closure and clarity about the next step.

Troubleshooting

One of the attributes of a strong alliance is flexibility. Therefore, as a clinician it is important to be able to bend with clients. A planned session structure may need to be put on hold or reorganized depending on what clients raise. The uncertainty created may instil a degree of discomfort which the therapist needs to learn to tolerate in order to be responsive. Having said this, there are common issues clients raise for which it is good to have some considered answers.

First, clients often ask, 'Do you think you can help me?' Therapists must avoid being overly optimistic, especially if clients raise the issue at the outset of an initial session. If you have not collected sufficient information to answer the question, then indicate that you would prefer to return to it at the end of the session. If you say this, then make sure you do return to the issue (perhaps putting a reminder at the end of your notes). On the other hand, if you have a clear idea about the probable treatment response and a client asks 'Can you cure me?', then emphasize that you will be working with the client to help them to learn strategies to better manage troubling situations, relationships, behaviours, and emotions.

Sometimes describing a stress-diathesis model is helpful in communicating to the client their role in dealing with their problem. For instance, a sunscreen metaphor can be of assistance, where you explain that a person with fair skin will burn more easily in the sun. They might not be able to change their tendency to burn, but they can learn to put sunscreen on to cope better with the potentially damaging rays of the sun.

Second, some clients (especially those with anxiety) may worry that they are going crazy. Silence can be damning at this point, as clients will watch you for signs of hesitation and interpret these as indications of your true beliefs. Therefore, respond quickly and convincingly. Typically, people (with anxiety) are worried that they have schizophrenia and comparing and contrasting their symptoms with those of a psychotic disorder can be helpful.

Third, clients will often cry during a session. Ensure that tissues are on hand (and it is wise to routinely check they are within a client's easy reach before the session begins). In addition, use non-verbal cues to convey support and sympathy. Lean forward in your chair (but do not touch the client) and allow silence. Do not rush in and provide reassurance, but allow the client's crying to reach a natural conclusion. Be satisfied with silence until the client uses verbal or non-verbal cues to signal they are seeking a response. Clients often end a period of crying by apologizing or saying 'that was silly'. Rather than engaging with these sentiments, it is more useful to redirect attention to the trigger and its response by saying something like, 'It seems this situation upsets you a great deal'.

Fourth, clients can be agitated in the session. When you notice increasing agitation, it is most helpful to break off from the current line of enquiry and focus on it directly by saying, 'You seem uncomfortable today, what is wrong?'

Fifth, although novice therapists often worry they will not be able to fill the therapy hour (and hence over-prepare), a more common problem is a talkative client. It is particularly a problem for novice therapists because if you have worried that you will not fill the session, or are concerned that you might say the wrong thing, a talkative client is a seeming godsend since you do not have to say another word. However, silence is not always the best response. The client may need your guidance, so start to use closed questions. You also may need to be more intrusive and interrupt the client to impose some order. For instance, you might say, 'You have raised many issues, which one is the most important?'

Sixth, clients can ask you for your advice (e.g., 'What do you think I should do?') or invite you to take sides (e.g., 'You agree with me don't you? No one should have to put up with that sort of behaviour'). In each of these situations, it is helpful to draw attention to the collaborative nature of the session. As a therapist you are there to work with the client, but at the end of the day, they are the ones who must live their lives. Therefore, you might respond, 'I don't want to talk about what I would do, because we are talking about the problems you are facing. However, I am going to work with you to see if we can find some solutions to these problems.'

Seventh, clients (and therapists) may wander off topic and it becomes necessary to refocus the interview. Sometimes is it useful to say, 'I'd like to get back to your main concerns' or 'I'm wondering if it might be more productive to focus on you current situation for the time being'. Clients may also depart from the therapist's schedule by wanting to move too rapidly into treatment. This is understandable, since clients seek resolution of their problems, but it may be necessary to cover other material in the session first. The clinician might say, 'I need to know more about your current problems before we can work out a plan of action'. The client may also want to focus on a domain (e.g., childhood relationships) before fully explaining the problem. Thus, the therapist might say, 'I would like to know more about your upbringing, but first I need to understand more about your current difficulties. Is this OK with you?'

Finally, clients can ask you for information that you deem to be personal and off limits. The therapeutic relationship is not the same relationship that exists between friends, acquaintances, or even doctor and patient. Rather, it is friendly, in that it is truthful, honest, caring, and attentive. Thus, there is empathy, but also a degree of disengagement. Clients come to discuss their problems; you are not there to discuss yours. Clients are there to discuss their lives; you are not there to elaborate on yours. That being said, it can be discourteous and unhelpful to refuse to respond to any requests. Clients may reasonably desire to have some idea of the person they are sharing intimate details with. Therefore, consider before therapy begins, the nature and extent of material you are willing to divulge. For instance, clients can ask if you have had a problem like theirs. Therefore, consider if you have, how you will respond and equally, if you have not, how you will respond. Additionally, clients may ask about your personal life (e.g., 'Do you have children?') since this may establish your credibility to them. How will you respond comfortably in a genuine and truthful way and what will be most beneficial to the client? Refusing to answer questions point blank can disrupt the relationship and evasive and disingenuous answers are often annoying to clients. Further, in some settings (e.g., rural and remote locations) the issue of therapist confidentiality is a moot point. Since you live in the community in which you work and socialize with the people who are potential clients, the boundaries need to be made explicit with clients (see Chapter 14). Even therapists in urban areas need to reflect on the possibility of meeting a client in a non-therapy setting. For example, the authors have met their clients in the changing room of a gym, at parties, at airports, and even on a remote wilderness track! Therefore, consider how you are going to respond when you meet your clients outside of therapy and if this is likely, then it may be wise to raise it explicitly.

Destroying the therapeutic alliance

The novice psychologist can often be daunted by the prospect of building a therapeutic alliance and may worry, 'Am I doing the right thing?' To this end, it can be helpful to reflect on the therapeutic behaviours that can undermine a good relationship with your client. Being cognizant of these factors can provide a sense of the 'boundary conditions' of a good therapeutic alliance.

Norcross and Wampold (2011; Norcross, 2010) in their review identified a series of factors that damage the alliance. The authors warned psychologists to avoid confrontation and criticism of clients. Miller, Wilbourne, and Hettema (2003) demonstrated that confrontation tended to lead to adverse therapy outcomes, whereas rolling with the resistance was associated with positive outcomes (Lundahl & Burke, 2009). Therefore, avoid comments that are pejorative, critical, blaming, invalidating, or rejecting. Norcross and Wampold also cautioned against being therapist-centric and assuming omniscience. The client's perspective predicts outcomes better than the therapist's perspective (Orlinsky et al., 2004) and psychologists are not good judges of poor progress (Lambert, 2010). This raises the question, how can a psychologist know the client's perspective on therapy and be sure of their progress? Subsequent chapters will consider how best to obtain the client's perspective, but at this stage it is sufficient to say that using the listening skills described can provide a good foundation. We will move on to consider how to complement this information with a measurement system to collect objective data to supplement your clinical impressions which will assist this process (see Lambert, 2010; Newnham & Page, 2007, 2010; Nordberg, Castonguay, Fisher, Boswell, & Kraus, 2014; Scott & Lewis, 2014).

Summary

In conclusion, a science-informed clinical psychologist needs to be cognizant of the empirical literature relevant to the therapeutic relationship. Empirically supported treatments may include specific components that bring about change in the client's behaviour, but the therapeutic relationship is a way of bringing the client into contact with the therapy. Deciding upon a treatment requires careful consideration of many client-related factors and making this decision requires careful assessment of the client as a person and their presenting problems. Assessing clients is the topic to which we now turn.

Assessing clients

Picture yourself conducting a clinical interview. A 32-year-old married woman has presented to the service where you are working with difficulties getting to sleep and so you have prepared by reading about insomnia. You open the interview by asking the client to elaborate on her problem. She describes lying in bed, unable to sleep because concerns and worries spin around her mind. In addition to the symptoms you expected, the client tells you that she is overly irritable during the day, has extreme difficulty concentrating, is chronically indecisive, and feels immense fatigue. Suddenly, the seemingly simple problem of insomnia has expanded as the client describes other problems that could be part of the sleep difficulties, but could represent another problem altogether. As a clinician you are faced with a number of dilemmas:

- Are the problems related in any way? If so, which problem do you treat first?
- Are the problems manifestations of one underlying cause or multiple causes?
- What treatment is best for which problem or constellation of problems?

Clinical psychologists tackle these dilemmas with every new client. From Figure 3.1 it is apparent that the assessment process involves an objective psychometric assessment, the gathering of relevant background information during an intake interview, and an examination of the client's mental state based on observations made during the interview. Together, these data permit a description of the particular profile of symptoms, along with a formulation of the predisposing, precipitating, and maintaining factors of symptom presentation.

Diagnostic manuals represent the distillation of clinical experience and research into a format that identifies which problems tend to group into meaningful clusters. These clusters can assist therapists to plan potentially effective treatments because as scientist-practitioners they are then able to refer to and use the psychological literature that bears on the relevant diagnoses. In this chapter we will first consider current diagnostic practices and their limitations, as well as structured ways to conduct diagnostic interviews and a mental state examination. However, before considering diagnostic systems, it is necessary to define 'mental disorder'.

What is a mental disorder?

In its Tenth Revision of the International Classification of Diseases and Related Health Problems (ICD-10, WHO, 1992), the World Health Organization does not define a mental disorder. Rather, the authors note in the section on classification of mental and behavioural disorders that although they use the term disorder (in preference to 'disease' and 'illness'), it

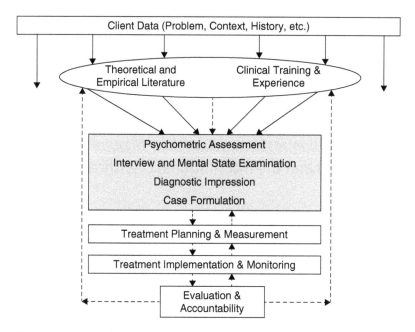

Figure 3.1 The complementary processes of testing, interviewing, and examining mental state as precursors to diagnosis, case formulation, and treatment planning.

is 'not an exact term, but is used here to imply the existing of a clinically recognizable set of symptoms or behavior associated in most cases with distress and interference with personal functions' (WHO, 1992, p. 5). In contrast, the American Psychiatric Association's (APA) *Diagnostic and Statistical Manual of Mental Disorders* (DSM-5, APA, 2013) does attempt to define a mental disorder. A mental disorder is a

clinically significant disturbance in an individual's cognition, emotion regulation, or behavior that reflects dysfunction in the psychological, biological, or developmental processes underlying mental functioning. Mental disorders are typically associated with significant distress or disability in social, occupational, or other important activities. An expectable or culturally approved response... socially deviant behavior and conflicts that are primarily between the individual and the society are not mental disorders unless the deviance or conflict results from a dysfunction in the individual. (p. 20)

In addition, the authors note that the definition does not include an expectable and culturally sanctioned response to a particular event (e.g., bereavement). Further, they note that the 'behavioral, psychological, or biological dysfunction' must lie within the individual, thereby excluding behaviour that is deviant (e.g., political, religious, or sexual) or conflicts with society (see Blashfield, 1998; Rounsaville et al., 2002).

Current diagnostic practices

The many different instances of psychopathology present a complex array of phenomena to be organized. Clinicians need to organize the various manifestations of psychopathology for a number of reasons. First, it is necessary to have an agreed nomenclature so that mental health professionals can share a common language. Second, a common language is needed so that information about particular psychopathologies can be retrieved. Third, classification is a fundamental human activity that is necessary to organize the world within which we live. Presently, there are two main diagnostic systems, the American Psychiatric Association's DSM-5 (APA, 2013) and the World Health Organization's ICD-10 (1992, 1993). Both of these diagnostic systems classify disorders (rather than clients; Spitzer & Williams, 1987) and thereby assist clinicians as they try to plan treatment in a systematic, rational, and scientific way.

Diagnostic systems: the *Diagnostic and Statistical Manual of Mental Disorders* (DSM) and the International Classification of Diseases (ICD)

The DSM

The opening section of the DSM-5 (APA, 2013) provides a comprehensive discussion of how to use the manual. Importantly, the manual acknowledges that in addition to a mental disorder diagnosis, it is necessary to construct a clinical case formulation to identify factors that may have contributed to developing the mental disorder. Case formulation will be discussed in a later chapter but for now we will focus on diagnostic issues and postpone consideration of how to manage the complexity of moving from a description of the presenting problem to a treatment plan using a conceptual formulation of the causes of the client's presentation.

The psychological disorders that may be the reason for treatment that the DSM-5 lists are: (i) Neurodevelopmental Disorders, (ii) Schizophrenia Spectrum and Other Psychotic Disorders, (iii) Bipolar and Related Disorders, (iv) Depressive Disorders, (v) Anxiety Disorders, (vi) Obsessive-Compulsive and Related Disorders, (vii) Trauma- and Stress-Related Disorders, (viii) Dissociative Disorders, (ix) Somatic Symptom and Related Disorders, (x) Feeding and Eating Disorders, (xi) Elimination Disorders, (xii) Sleep–Wake Disorders, (xiii) Sexual Dysfunctions, (xiv) Gender Dysphoria, (xv) Disruptive, Impulse-Control, and Conduct Disorders, (xvi) Substance-Related and Addictive Disorders, (xvii) Neurocognitive Disorders, (xviii) Personality Disorders, (xix) Other Mental Disorders, (xx) Medication-Induced Movement Disorders and Other Adverse Effects of Medication, and (xxi) Other Conditions That May Be a Focus of Clinical Attention.

Each section in the DSM-5 follows a similar format. The title of the disorder (accompanied by a DSM code and a corresponding ICD code) is followed by the diagnostic criteria and a verbal description of the diagnostic features. This final section provides clarification of the diagnostic criteria and includes examples. It complements the somewhat stark listing of the diagnostic criteria, in that it provides a rich verbal picture of the disorder, thereby giving the clinical psychologist the context within which the symptoms occur and the manner in which the disorder may present. It develops a sense of the 'flavour' of each disorder, over and above a list of the criteria, and in addition to the DSM material, case studies are a useful complementary source of information. Some particularly good examples include Barnhill (2013), Meyer & Weaver (2012), Oltmans, Neale, & Davison (2003), Oltmans, Martin, Neale, & Davison (2012), Sattler, Shabatay, & Kramer (1998), and Spitzer, Gibbon, Skodol, Williams, & First (2001).

Following this section, the DSM-5 provides information on the subtypes of the disorder, associated features, specific cultural, age, and gender features, and the prevalence, course, familial patterns, and differential diagnosis (i.e., distinguishing from similar or related disorders). By way of illustration, a Major Depressive Disorder is characterized by a period of at least two weeks with depressed mood or a loss of interest in pleasure. In addition to one or both of these symptoms, to meet diagnostic criteria, a client must also report or exhibit a total of five of the following: significant weight or appetite change, insomnia/hypersomnia, psychomotor agitation or retardation, fatigue/energy loss, feelings of worthlessness or excessive/inappropriate guilt, decreased thinking ability or concentration, or indecision, recurrent thoughts of death, suicidal ideation without plan, or suicide attempt or plan. Subsequent criteria require the clinician to ensure that the distress or impairment in social, occupational, or other important areas of functioning is 'clinically significant' and to rule out other possible diagnoses (e.g., a medical condition or the effects of a substance). The criteria for clinical significance rely upon clinical judgement and may use information from friends, family, and other third parties.

The clinician is then asked to specify the severity and other features of the disorder. The severity of a disorder is coded as mild if few, or no, symptoms in excess of those required to make the diagnosis are present (in this case five), and symptoms produce minor impairment in social or occupational functioning. It is coded as severe if many symptoms in excess of those needed to make a diagnosis are present, and severity is moderate if number of symptoms falls between 'mild' and 'severe' categories. For instance, a client with severe repeated episodes of depression would receive a diagnosis of 'Major Depressive Disorder, severe, Recurrent Episode'. The DSM diagnostic code would be 296.33 and the corresponding ICD code would be F33.2. The clinician also needs to consider a variety of specifiers that describe the course of the disorder (e.g., chronic), its recurrence, and the features that are present. By way of example, one set of features is melancholia, in which the depression involves loss of pleasure in activities and lack of reactivity to usually pleasurable stimuli in the presence of other symptoms such as 'empty mood', a depression that is worse in the morning, involves early morning wakening, psychomotor agitation or retardation, significant weight loss, and excessive or inappropriate guilt.

The previous edition of the DSM permitted the clinician to code significant psychosocial and environmental problems that have occurred in the preceding year, in part acknowledging that such factors may moderate the treatment and prognosis of mental disorders. Environmental problems included negative life events, environmental difficulties or deficiencies. Psychosocial problems included relationship difficulties and the associated interpersonal stress, as well as insufficient social support or personal resources. Both psychosocial and environmental problems are relevant as they may be causally related to the onset of problems, but can also be a consequence of mental health problems. However, the DSM-5 has decided not to develop its own listing of such problems, and encourages clinicians to use the WHO's taxonomy, ICD 9's V codes (or Z codes in the ICD 10). A listing of the codes can be found in the DSM-5. Consider once more the previous example of the woman who plunged into a deep depression following her forced idle state due to a medical condition preventing her from lifting heavy objects. The situation was exacerbated by her also losing her part-time job as a carer working with disabled adults, where heavy lifting of patients was part of her daily job routine. Thus, noting the concomitant job loss as an 'Other problem related to employment' provides insight into the pervasiveness of her recent role transition from active provider for the family to 'being a burden' to her family.

The previous edition of the DSM provided the clinician's Global Assessment of the individual's Functioning (GAF). Although the measure has been criticized in terms of both reliability and validity, the information is useful in planning treatment and measuring its impact, and in predicting outcome. Functional impairment is not the same construct as subjective distress, even though impairment and distress are frequently confounded in the concept of 'problem severity'. Separating the constructs is important because impairment is negatively related to improvement during treatment (McClellan, Woody, Luborsky, O'Brien, & Druley, 1983), clients with a high degree of impairment appear to improve to a greater degree with longer and more intensive treatment (Shapiro et al., 1994), and impairment is a predictor of relapse (e.g., Brown & Barlow, 1995). Functioning can be measured with the full 36-item or the 12-item short version of the World Health Organization Disability Assessment Schedule (WHODAS; www.who.int/classifications/icf/whodasii/en/). The scale measures the extent to which there is disability in six areas: cognition, mobility, self-care, interacting with others, life activities, and participation in society.

From the perspective of a clinical psychologist, arguably the most progressive step forward in the DSM system is a tentative move towards dimensional assessments. While medical approaches have tended to favour discrete categories, psychologists have typically viewed many constructs dimensionally. That is, while we are happy to speak casually about a person being 'intelligent', we understand intelligence to be a construct that is distributed (approximately) normally across the population. We may identify cut-points in the distribution for clinical purposes, but we tend to think about the meaning of a person's location on a distribution.

Section III of the DSM-5 lists 'emerging measures and models' and contains a set of tools to assist the clinical decision-making process. The cross-cutting symptom measures (www.psychiatry.org/practice/dsm/dsm5/online-assessment-measures) provide dimensional assessments of constructs such as anxiety, depression, mania, memory, somatic symptoms, suicidal ideation, psychosis, sleep problems, memory, repetitive thoughts and behaviours, dissociation, personality function, and substance use. These measures can help the clinical psychologist not only in forming a diagnosis, but also by providing a richer picture of the symptom profile than a diagnostic label can achieve.

ICD-10

Despite the popularity of the DSM in many countries, the official coding system for international comparisons is the International Classification of Diseases, Tenth Revision, (ICD-10; WHO, 1992). The ICD diagnoses are presented in two volumes. The first volume includes the clinical descriptions and the diagnostic guidelines. Like the DSM-5, the ICD-10 organizes the disorders into various categories which are (i) Organic, including symptomatic, mental disorders (e.g., dementia in Alzheimer's disease), (ii) Mental and behavioural disorders due to psychoactive substance use (e.g., harmful use of alcohol), (iii) Schizophrenia, schizotypal, and delusional disorders, (iv) Mood (affective) disorders, (v) Neurotic, stress-related, and somatoform disorders (e.g., generalized anxiety disorder), (vi) Behavioural syndromes associated with physiological disturbances and physical factors (e.g., eating disorders), (vii) Disorders of adult personality and behaviour (e.g., transsexualism), (viii) Mental retardation, (ix) Disorders of psychological development (e.g., childhood autism), and (x) Behavioural and emotional disorders with onset usually occurring in childhood and adolescence (e.g., conduct disorders).

Each disorder under each of these broad categories is listed, beginning with a description of the main clinical and important associated features, followed by diagnostic guidelines. In contrast to the DSM-5, the ICD-10 does not list explicit criteria for each diagnosis. That is, there are no verbal descriptions that indicate the quantity and balance of symptoms required before a diagnosis can be made. Therefore, the ICD provides a degree of flexibility that is less evident in the DSM system, because sometimes clinical decisions need to be made 'before the clinical picture is entirely clear or information is complete' (WHO, 1992, p. 1). The companion volume within the ICD-10 (WHO, 1993) lists the research diagnostic criteria, and the format is much more similar to the DSM in that particular criteria are specified for each disorder.

By way of comparison and contrast, the ICD identifies three varieties of a depressive episode, ranging from mild to severe. In contrast to the DSM, where a client with a mild diagnosis must first meet the two diagnostic criteria for a Major Depressive Episode plus at least five additional criteria, a mild depressive episode in ICD would require only two symptoms from a list including depressed mood, loss of pleasure, reduced energy and fatigue, and two symptoms from tiredness, reduced concentration and attention, reduced self-esteem and self-confidence, ideas of guilt and unworthiness, bleak views of the future, ideas or acts of self-harm or suicide, disturbed sleep, and diminished appetite. The diagnostic specifiers used in DSM-5 are incorporated into the ICD by asking the clinician to code the particular category. Therefore, a client with repeated mild episodes of depression may receive a diagnosis of 'F33.0 Recurrent depressive disorder, current episode mild'. Note that the diagnostic codes are equivalent, yet the quantity and type of diagnostic criteria are not identical (see Rounsaville et al., 2002).

Both diagnostic systems acknowledge the need for cultural sensitivity when assigning diagnoses. This will be achieved by explicitly considering the client's ethnic or cultural reference groups and possible cultural explanations of a client's symptoms. For instance, the mode of expression may vary across cultures (e.g., greater somatic presentations of mood disorders in some cultures), and so too can the meaning of symptoms and causal models used by clients to explain their symptoms. Although some disorders appear culture-specific, the more usual situation facing the clinician requires sensitivity to the ways in which cultural and other social factors influence the presentation and impact of a disorder, as well as the way they are communicated to and understood by the clinician.

Conducting a diagnostic interview

Independent of the diagnostic system used, one product of an initial interview (when possible) is a diagnosis. Eliciting symptom information is a necessary, but not sufficient component of a diagnostic interview. In addition to determining which symptoms a client possesses and which they do not, the clinician aims to develop a clear picture of the client, the problem(s), and the personal, social, and environmental context within which these issues occur. The exact nature of the interview will be tailored to the client and to the problem, but a useful conceptual structure for an interview is outlined below.

The way that you meet the client will frame the dialogue. Since your aim is to assist a client discuss potentially sensitive issues, a good rapport is required. Therefore, communicate a sense of goodwill by being courteous. As discussed in Chapter 2, questioning at the outset of the interview should be open and designed to help the client talk while the clinician listens. One possible obstacle to an open dialogue is note taking. This occurs when the clinician focuses excessively on the notes at the expense of the client. Spend time building rapport with the client and respond to what the client says in a way that communicates that you understand not only what the client has said, but how the client felt. Therefore, try to take sufficient but brief notes and in a manner that does not interfere with the flow of the interview.

Usually, a diagnostic interview will quickly move to the presenting problem(s) and the aim will be to identify the problem that the client has brought to therapy. While there may be times when tact and sensitivity dictate a more gradual introduction, clients typically arrive at a consultation prepared to tell their story. Thus, it may be helpful to encourage the client to phrase the problem in their own words. For instance, you may ask, 'I wonder if you could tell me what brought you here today?' As the client begins to respond to this question, ensure that you model good listening behaviour. Respond with verbal and non-verbal indications that you have heard and understood both the content of the speech, but also the broader emotional and social context that the person is in.

For example, a clinician might interview a client with Generalized Anxiety Disorder (GAD) in the following manner.

THERAPIST: Your referral suggests that you are having trouble with sleeping. Could you tell me a bit about the troubles you've been having?

CLIENT: Well, I just can't get off to sleep at night because these worrying thoughts keep popping into my head. They just go around and around, so that I can't fall asleep. I'm now so tired that I feel that if I could just get a good night's sleep everything will be OK again.

THERAPIST: These worries seem to be having a huge impact on you.

CLIENT: They are. In fact, they seem to be the main problem.

THERAPIST: What sort of things do you worry about?

CLIENT: About anything and everything. I worry about my children's health, I worry about not having enough money, I worry about the house burning down, I worry about work…I even worry that I worry about worrying.

THERAPIST: Can you tell me about this 'worry about worrying'?

CLIENT: I feel I *need* to worry. If I don't, then I worry that something terrible will happen. Like when my children go out at night, I'm never sure that they'll be safe, but if I worry then I feel that things are better because I've done everything I can.

THERAPIST: Do these worries occur at times other than when you are trying to go to sleep?

CLIENT: Yes, they happen all the time. Right now I'm worrying that you might not be able to help me because I'm not being clear enough. This has been going on for years now and I don't know if I have a problem or if it's just the way I am.

THERAPIST: When people worry a lot for a long time, there can be effects in the rest of their life. Have you noticed any impact of the worry?

CLIENT: As well as the sleep, I notice that I get really tense. The muscles around my neck tighten up so much that I'm in pain.

THERAPIST: That must be exhausting as well as painful.

CLIENT: You're right. I am so tired from all the worry and tension, but I still don't seem to be able to sleep. It doesn't make sense.

THERAPIST: We'll talk about trying to make sense of your experience a little later, but for the time being I'd like to continue to get a clear idea in my head of the problems you are facing. When other people experience excessive worry and uncontrollable tension, they sometimes notice that they are more irritable or feel on edge and tense. Have you felt like this?

CLIENT: Always on edge and … erm … what was the other thing?

THERAPIST: Irritable?

CLIENT: Yes, often irritable at home, but never at work.

THERAPIST: How about difficulties with concentration?

CLIENT: I don't seem to have trouble concentrating, just that I concentrate on my worries.

THERAPIST: When you are trying to concentrate on your work, do your worries break into that concentration?

CLIENT: Yes, but it's not that I can't concentrate. I concentrate on the wrong thing.

A number of issues are evident in the preceding conversation. First, if you consult the DSM-5 criteria for Generalized Anxiety Disorder you can see that the clinician is asking the client about symptoms relevant to the disorder. At the beginning, the clinician begins with open questions, but towards the end of the section, the questioning becomes closed and more focused as the clinician moves to check that material was omitted because the symptoms are indeed absent, rather than the client just failing to report material even though the symptoms are present. Second, you will see that the client becomes confused when multiple symptoms are included in a single question. Try to avoid questions that contain multiple issues and requests. Third, you will see that the client and clinician do not have a shared understanding of the word 'concentration'. For the client, concentration refers more to the cognitive process, whereas the clinician is referring to the ability to focus on a particular thought. In the preceding conversation, the client took the initiative in clarifying the issue, but had the client not done this, the clinician could have been more explicit in questions. Finally, at the end of this section, the clinician would be in a position to speculate that the client may be suffering from GAD. Further questioning would clarify this but it would appear that the client has been experiencing excessive worry about a number of events more days than not for some years (DSM-5 Criterion A). There is difficulty controlling the worry (Criterion B), the worry is associated with feeling keyed up or on edge, easily fatigued, irritability, muscle tension, and sleep disturbance (Criterion C), and there is clinically significant distress and impairment (Criterion D). Criteria E and F require the clinician to determine that the worries are not better explained by another disorder. Thus, the clinician will need not only to explore GAD, but it will be necessary to entertain the possibility that the symptoms are a manifestation of other disorders (e.g., primary insomnia, major depression, and substance abuse) and hence a differential diagnosis is required to determine the best label to describe the client's problems. It is also possible that the client exhibits comorbidity, and hence two disorders (e.g., GAD and depression) are present simultaneously. Further interviewing is required and for each disorder, the DSM-5 provides details about how to make a differential diagnosis.

After the client has begun to describe the problem, the clinician is confronted with a choice of direction. On the one hand, the clinician could choose to remain with a discussion of the presenting problem and elicit personal and historical information later. The advantages of this strategy are that the interview continues to flow naturally and the client keeps relating the details of the presenting problem. However, the disadvantage is that the clinician does not have a good picture of the client as a person, the social and historical background to the problems, a sense of other psychological problems, and so on. Instead, the clinician could signal a change of direction by saying, 'Thank you. You have given me an idea of the difficulties that you are having. I would like to pursue them in more detail, but before we talk about these difficulties I was wondering if I could get some idea about you as a person?' The interviewer could then proceed to ask questions about the social and personal background. The advantages of this strategy are that the psychological problems are then unveiled in the context of the whole person. The main disadvantages are that the clinician may not know what aspects of the personal history are relevant until the problem is explicated and the interview may need to be cut short because insufficient time remains to discuss the client's difficulties before the session ends.

Assuming that the clinician has decided in this instance to remain with a discussion of the presenting problem, this could be signalled with a comment such as, 'I wonder if we could discuss the difficulty you have been mentioning in some detail. When did you first notice that something was not right?' This will direct the client to discuss the evolution of the problem; acknowledging the fact that psychological difficulties exist in a dynamically evolving system. However, within the complexity, the clinician will be focused on trying to highlight the key milestones in the problem development. This history will lead the client towards the present, at which time it will be possible to get a clearer description of the difficulties and any associated behaviours. As a mental checklist, the clinician will be aiming to identify (i) what the problem is, (ii) when it occurs, (iii) where it happens, (iv) how frequently the problem takes place, (v) with whom these difficulties arise, (vi) how distressing and (vii) impairing the problem is. In collecting this information, the clinician will also identify distal factors associated with the problem. These will be identifiable from a discussion of the environment, context, and lifestyle present when the problem began, other predisposing and triggering factors, the consequences of the problem's onset, the way the problem has changed over time and factors associated with these changes (both increases and decreases in severity and frequency). The interview will evolve from a historical discussion to consideration of the problem in its current form. The clinician might ask, 'Could you please tell me about a typical day or occurrence of the problem?' and then explore some of the maintaining factors. The clinician will also ask about the variability in the problem and factors associated with the fluctuations (i.e., moderating variables).

As far as the diagnostic aspect of an interview is concerned, the clinician will elicit a comprehensive description of the problem and its various manifestations. Clients may often focus on one aspect of the problem because it is salient to them, but remember to explicitly consider the behaviour and actions, consciously available thoughts and other cognitive processes, as well as physiological changes. The clinician also needs to ask about the frequency, intensity, topography (typical and unusual patterns), duration, and temporal sequence of symptoms. In addition, the consequences of any behaviour need to be thoroughly assessed (see Chapter 5).

After the clinician has a good sense of the presenting problem, its present manifestation, and its history, the interview can expand to provide a more complete picture of the person. The clinician might say, 'You have given me a good idea of the problems you are struggling with, but I don't think I have got a good idea about you as a person. Could you tell me something about you, apart from these difficulties?' The aim of this process is to be able to put yourself in the client's shoes and imagine what it must be like to experience the life the client has had. Therefore, it may be relevant to ask about family history (details of parents, other significant figures, brothers and sisters, as well as the childhood environment of family, school, and peers), a personal history (birth date and any significant issues, general adjustment in childhood, lifelong traits or behavioural patterns and tendencies, significant life events), schooling (duration and significant events), work history and present duties, relationships (current status, history and problems), leisure activities, living arrangements, social relationships, prior significant accidents, diseases and mental health problems, and personality (and particularly any changes).

An important aspect of a diagnostic interview is to identify the coping resources that a client can bring to bear in seeking to overcome their problems. Therefore, enquire about coping resources and other personal strengths the individual possesses. Within this context, motivation for change is a critical dimension (see Miller & Rollnick, 2012 for an excellent discussion). The clinician will not only attempt to identify the motivations intrinsic to the person, but identify any extrinsic motivators that are present or have been successful in the past. The clinician can also try to identify the 'stage of change' that the client is in. Prochaska, Norcross, and DiClemente (1995; Prochaska & Norcross, 1998) have suggested that clients move through a series of stages. In the first instance, individuals are pre-contemplators – they have their problem, but have not yet got to the point of desiring to modify their behaviour. As a person begins to notice the impairment or becomes increasingly concerned about the distress being triggered, they move into the contemplation phase, in which they

Annotated Initial Interview Pro Forma

Interview Date: ____/____/____

Name: _____.
Sex: M/F
Date of Birth: _____

Presenting Problem

What has brought you here today?

Relevant Background/Personal History

Family history
Personal history
Birth
Childhood adjustment
Schooling
Work
Relationships
Leisure
Significant illnesses/disorders
Accidents
Physical illnesses
Mental disorders/problems.
Personality

Problem History

Evolution
Distal Factors
Context of problem
Circumstances of onset
Consequences of onset
Change over time/Milestones
Variables assoc. with severity

Figure 3.2 Annotated pro forma of initial interview.

Current Problem Presentation

Proximal factors
Typical presentation
Variations in presentation
Maintaining factors?
1. Antecedents
2. Behaviour
3. Consequences
Motivation for change
Stages of change
Mental Status Examination

Summary

Test Results

DSM /ICD Diagnosis:

Formulation

Presenting problems
Predisposing factors
Precipitating variables
Perpetuating cognitions and consequences
Provisional conceptualization
Prescribed interventions
Potential problems and client strengths

Action Plan

1. Treat
2. Refer
3. Other

Figure 3.2 (*cont.*)

are considering the pros and cons of dealing with the problem. From contemplation, a client will move into preparation and action, after which time they will either relapse into any of the preceding stages or continue to manage the problem successfully.

At the end of the interview, summarize and synthesize the material covered. Often it is useful to present this summary in a provisional manner by saying, 'I will try to draw together some of the themes we have been discussing. If I miss something out or if I get a point wrong, please let me know.' It is also prudent to ask the client if there are any problems or issues which you have not asked them about or which there has not been time to discuss. This increases confidence that the main problems have been covered and also provides an opportunity for clients to raise other significant issues now they feel more at ease.

A pro forma (Figure 3.2) may assist you with note taking and structuring an interview. The text in the right hand column is a series of prompts and can function as a checklist.

Adapting diagnostic interviews for different client groups (children and the elderly)

The diagnostic interview will need to be adapted in a flexible manner to be suitable for each client. However, some general points can be made about certain client groups. One important group to consider is children. When interviewing children the clinician needs to contextualize the information in the normative developmental process. Deviations from normal childhood development need to be understood both in terms of the normative processes, but also in terms of the typical variability (see Sattler, 2008, 2014). Assessments of children may also require the collection of information from parents, teachers, other family members, and professionals. Collection of data from multiple sources provides a rich picture of the problem as well as insight into the way the problematic behaviours are observed and interpreted by individuals prominent in the child's life (see Sattler, 2008, 2014).

When interviewing the elderly, there are a variety of considerations when arriving at a diagnosis. Medical conditions, cognitive impairment, and pharmacological issues may all have a bearing on the client's presentation (Edelstein, Koven, Spira, & Shreve-Neiger, 2002). The same disorder does not always present itself in the same way in older adults as it does in younger adults. For instance, depression is more likely to present with somatic symptoms and with less dysphoria (Fiske, Kasl-Godley, & Gatz, 1998). Further, the clinician will need to entertain differential diagnostic possibilities among older adults that are less common with younger clients. For instance, depression and dementia can co-occur at times, and need to be distinguished (see Edelstein, 1998; Kaszniak & Christenson, 1994).

Screening for psychological symptoms

A large amount of information needs to be collected during a diagnostic interview and there is a risk that key issues will be missed. One way to complement the information gleaned from a diagnostic interview is to collect information from screening tests. Screening is the 'presumptive identification of unrecognized disease or defect by the application of tests, examinations or other procedures which can be applied rapidly to sort out apparently well persons who probably have a disease from those who probably do not' (Commission on Chronic Illness, 1957, p. 45). Therefore, when administered before a diagnostic interview, tests provide the clinician with an efficient means of collecting and collating symptom information, as well as giving an indication of the extent to which a client's symptom profile deviates from statistical norms.

SCL-90-R & BSI

The Revised Symptom Checklist 90 (SCL-90-R, Derogatis, 1994) is a broad symptom measure that covers nine dimensions (Somatization, Obsessive-compulsive, Interpersonal sensitivity, Depression, Anxiety, Hostility, Phobic anxiety, Paranoid ideation, and Psychoticism). Three global indices of distress can be derived from the dimensional scores. The 90 items (a briefer version is available in the form of the Brief Symptom Index; BSI, Derogratis & Spencer, 1982) are scores referring to the past seven days, including today, and the checklist takes clients about 15 minutes to complete. Responses can be interpreted in terms of the global indices, the nine dimensions, or the items themselves, and the chief advantage is that the clinician is provided with a broad range of symptom information in a very efficient manner.

General Health Questionnaire (GHQ)

Developed by Goldberg (1972), the GHQ is a 60-item scale that identifies four factor-analytically derived subscales describing Somatic Symptoms, Anxiety and Insomnia, Social Dysfunction, and Severe Depression. Briefer forms (GHQ-30 and GHQ-12) are available and the scale has been validated for use among many different samples (including geriatric, traumatically injured, and medically ill patients).

Center for Epidemiological Studies – Depression Scale (CES-D)

The CES-D is a 20-item self-report scale that assesses mood and functioning over the past seven days (Radloff, 1977). It identifies Depressed affect, Positive affect, Somatic problems, and Interpersonal problems. The scale can be abbreviated to a five-item version and has been validated in community, medical, and clinical samples.

Beck Depression Inventory (BDI)

The BDI (Beck, Ward, Mendelson, Mock, & Erbaugh, 1961) is a 21-item scale designed to assess the present severity of depression by assessing attitudes and symptoms related to depression, with the latest revision aiming to assess the existence and severity of the DSM's symptoms of depression (Beck, Steer, & Brown, 1996). Cut-off scores of 0–13 indicate minimal depression, 14–19 mild depression, 20–28 moderate depression, and 29–63 severe depression. A number of studies have supported the reliability and validity of the BDI and it is useful for measuring depressive symptoms, indicating the severity of present symptoms, and quantifying the extent of treatment changes (Beck, Steer, & Garbin, 1988; Sundberg, 1987).

Behaviour and Symptom Identification Index (BASIS-32)

Another brief screening instrument is the BASIS-32 (Eisen & Grob, 1989). This 32-item self-report inventory assesses over a one-week interval the major symptom domains and current function that required inpatient psychiatric treatment. The subscales measure relation to self and others, daily living and role functioning, anxiety and depression, impulsive and addictive behaviour, and psychosis.

Hamilton Anxiety Scale (HAS) and the Hamilton Rating Scale for Depression (HAM-D)

The Hamilton Anxiety Scale (Hamilton, 1959) is a 14-item clinician-rated scale assessing the symptoms of anxiety. The subscales are psychic and somatic anxiety. The Hamilton Rating Scale for Depression (Hamilton, 1967) is a 21-item clinician-rated scale. Both of these tests have been used with a wide variety of client groups; they are commonly used, and they have good psychometric properties.

The United Kingdom's National Health Service has introduced a good series of measures as part of its Improving Access to Psychological Therapies (IAPT; www.iapt.nhs.uk/data/measuring-outcomes/). The IAPT lists a series of outcome measures and recommends particular measures to be used for specific problems. Details can be found in the *IAPT Data Handbook*, but for present purposes one example will be highlighted.

All patients seen through the IAPT system are to be assessed in terms of depression (using the 9-item Patient Health Questionnaire; PHQ-9), general anxiety (using the 7-item Generalized Anxiety Disorder scale; GAD-7), phobias (using the IAPT Phobia Scales), functioning (using the Worker and Social Adjustment Scale), and the IAPT patient choice and experience questionnaire. In addition, specific instruments are recommended for particular clinical presentations. Each of the scales is provided with relevant psychometric information and clinical cut-offs. For instance, the PHQ-9 can be used to monitor change in symptoms of depression over time and the clinical cut-point of 9 identifies 'caseness', such that any person who scores 10 or higher is judged to be experiencing clinically significant symptoms of depression. Clinical psychologists can use these scales not only to be accountable in their own practice, but they can also use these scores to discuss progress with their clients. In summary, each of the preceding scales provides a good screening for psychopathology. They can assist the clinician in recognizing a disorder by making the clinician aware of particular symptoms, as well as their levels and patterns. However, none of the screening instruments reviewed can indicate that a client has met diagnostic criteria for a particular disorder. Structured and semi-structured diagnostic interviews serve this function.

Structured and semi-structured diagnostic interviews: adults

Any diagnostic method must be both reliable and valid. However, the validity of a diagnostic interview and a diagnostic system are not identical. The validity of a diagnostic interview is judged by the extent to which the outcome of the interview matches onto the disorder in the diagnostic taxonomy. The validity of a diagnostic system is judged by the degree to which the disorders describe clinically meaningful clusters of symptoms. Although reliability does not guarantee validity, validity requires reliability. In the past, diagnoses were notoriously unreliable, but the decision to introduce specific diagnostic criteria for each disorder into the DSM-III (APA, 1980) successfully increased the reliability of diagnoses. Although some have suggested that the validity of the diagnoses themselves was sacrificed in the pursuit of reliability (see Rounsaville et al., 2002), another source of unreliability is the diagnostic interview itself. Clinicians may omit key questions, fail to consider all diagnostic possibilities, or be overly influenced by dramatic symptoms and hence arrive at a diagnosis that would not be obtained by a second interviewer, or even by the same clinician on a separate occasion. One way to increase diagnostic reliability in generating DSM and ICD diagnoses is to use structured and semi-structured diagnostic interviews (Summerfeldt & Antony, 2002).

Structured diagnostic interviews are particularly helpful in research (where replicability is essential), in training (where the structure can assist a novice clinician), and in practice (where use of a standardized instrument can increase the confidence in a diagnosis). A variety of instruments are available and they will be reviewed next. There are a set of dimensions along which the instruments vary (e.g., diagnostic breadth and depth, duration of the interview, extent to which clinical skill is required, target population) and thus the individual electing to use a structured diagnostic interview will need to consider the purpose of the interview. Specifically, the clinician will need to evaluate the instrument in terms of (i) coverage and content, (ii) the target population, (iii) the psychometric features of the instrument, (iv) practical issues (e.g., duration, training), (v) administration requirements and support (e.g., scoring algorithms, standardized manual; see Page, 1991a; Summerfeldt & Antony, 2002). With the release of DSM-5 new versions of structured interviews will be developed, but many of the instruments and much of the psychometric data relate to the previous editions of the DSM. Therefore, caution needs to be exercised when evaluating the generalizability to the most recent diagnostic system.

Anxiety Disorders Interview Schedule for DSM-IV (ADIS-IV)

The ADIS-IV (Brown, Di Nardo, & Barlow, 1994) is a semi-structured interview that follows a structure similar to a clinical interview and relies on the clinician to ask additional questions to follow up issues of relevance. Although its primary focus is the DSM-IV Anxiety Disorders, it also assesses Mood, Substance Use, and Somatoform Disorders due to their high rates of comorbidity with anxiety. The relatively narrow coverage can be offset by the detailed information provided by the interview about conditions, aetiology, and dimensional symptom ratings. The whole interview assessing current and lifetime disorders takes 2–4 hours in clinical samples. The reliability of the instrument is acceptable and the limited validity data upon its predecessor are supportive (e.g., Rapee, Brown, Antony, & Barlow, 1992). In addition to its use in research, the ADIS-IV is suitable as a primary diagnostic measure when used by trained mental health professionals.

Diagnostic Interview Schedule (DIS) and the Composite International Diagnostic Interview (CIDI)

The DIS-IV (Robins, Cottler, Bucholz, & Compton, 1995) is a structured diagnostic interview that is suitable for use by lay interviewers as well as mental health professionals. The diagnostic coverage is broad and is even broader in the more extensive version; the CIDI (Robins et al., 1988). The most recent version of the CIDI is compatible with both DSM-IV and ICD-10 and therefore is suitable for international comparisons (Andrews & Peters, 1998). Due to their similarity, they will be considered together. The instruments are organized in a modular format to permit customization of the interview and the structured format has permitted computerization. The administration time is 2–3 hours with clinical samples and they yield both current and lifetime diagnoses. The instruments are useful in large-scale epidemiological studies, but the level of agreement with clinical diagnoses is poor and therefore it is recommended that the findings are supplemented with other sources of data (Segal & Falk, 1997). Consequently, they are not suitable as primary diagnostic instruments in psychiatric settings.

Mini-International Neuropsychiatric Interview (MINI)

The MINI (Sheehan et al., 1999; https://medical-outcomes.com/index/mini) is a clinician-administered structured diagnostic interview that assesses both DSM-IV and ICD-10 criteria. Being designed to provide a valid structured interview for clinical and research contexts, it covers a broad range of disorders, but does so in around 15 minutes. The reliability and validity of this instrument are promising (Sheehan et al., 1998).

Primary Care Evaluation of Mental Disorders (PRIME-MD)

In contrast to the preceding interviews, which provide an extensive assessment of many disorders present currently and over the lifetime, the PRIME-MD is a brief (10–20 minutes; or 3 minutes using the more recent Patient Health Questionnaire; Spitzer, Kroenke, & Williams, 1999) clinician-administered interview to permit primary care physicians to rapidly identify the mental disorders commonly seen in medical practice (Spitzer et al., 1995). Comprising a 25-item, self-report questionnaire asking about general physical and mental health issues and a semi-structured interview to follow up on items that the patient has endorsed, the instrument provides a quick assessment of DSM-IV mood, anxiety, somatoform, eating, and alcohol-related disorders. Little reliability data exist and in terms of validity, its sensitivity and specificity are good, although the correspondence with DSM-IV is only moderate. Although the speed comes at the cost of breadth and depth, and the diagnoses obtained do not map directly onto DSM-IV categories, as a quick standardized identification of psychiatric cases, the instrument performs well. Another instrument that is suitable for use by physicians in primary care is the Symptom-Driven Diagnostic System for Primary Care (SDDS-PC; Broadhead et al., 1995).

Schedule for Affective Disorders and Schizophrenia (SADS)

The SADS (Endicott & Spitzer, 1978) is a clinician-administered semi-structured interview developed to assess the research diagnostic criteria (found in the second volume of the ICD-10). The instrument assesses current and past symptoms, with other versions assessing symptoms across the whole lifetime (SADS-L; Lifetime), and changes in symptoms (SADS-C; Change). The SADS has a broad coverage of psychological disorders and the SADS-LA-IV (SADS Lifetime Anxiety for DSM-IV; Fyer, Endicott, Mannuza, & Klein, 1995 cited in Summerfeldt & Antony, 2002) also assesses DSM-IV criteria in addition to expanded coverage of anxiety disorders. A SADS interview takes an hour with non-clinical samples, and this short duration, relative to its breadth of coverage, is achieved by a structure that permits clinicians to skip sections that are not relevant because the respondent fails to endorse screening questions or they are not germane to the interview purpose. The reliability of the SADS is excellent, when compared with the other structured diagnostic interviews (Rogers, 1995) and the validity is very good (see Conoley & Impara, 1995), particularly in the area of mood disorders, making it well-suited as a primary diagnostic screening measure.

Structured Clinical Interview for DSM-IV Axis-I Disorders (SCID)

The SCID is available in a brief clinical (SCID-CV; First, Spitzer, Gibbon, & Williams, 1997) and a more extensive research (SCID-I; First, Spitzer, Gibbon, & Williams, 1996) version. According to the website (www.scid4.org/) a revision for DSM-5 is anticipated in the near future. Importantly, versions are also available for Personality Disorders. The SCID-CV is a relatively brief interview that provides coverage of the disorders commonly seen in a mental health practice. The SCID-I comes in a variety of forms and the version designed for individuals already identified as psychiatric patients (SCID-I/P) has the most extensive coverage of mental health disorders of all available instruments, with interviews taking at least an hour. The reliability is good (Segal, Hersen & van Hasselt, 1994) and validity studies of previous versions have also been supportive of the instrument (Rogers, 1995; 2001).

Schedule for Clinical Assessment in Neuropsychiatry (SCAN)

The SCAN (WHO, 1998; http://whoscan.org/) is quite different from other structured interviews. Whereas other instruments focus on diagnostic categories, the SCAN seeks to describe key symptoms. The instrument comprises a semi-structured clinical interview, a glossary to rate the experiences endorsed by respondents, a checklist to rate information provided by third parties, and a schedule to assess the respondent's clinical, social, and developmental history. The data can be scored to generate DSM-IV and ICD-10 diagnoses.

Structured and semi-structured diagnostic interviews: children and adolescents

Child and Adolescent Psychiatric Assessment (CAPA)

The CAPA (Angold et al., 1995) is a structured diagnostic interview suitable for children and adolescents aged 9–17. It assesses the onset, duration, frequency, and intensity of symptoms present in the three months prior to the interview, and permits diagnoses in both DSM-IV and ICD-10 to be made. It has a modular format that permits clinicians to use it flexibly, with the patient report version taking around an hour. The reliability and validity data are good (Angold & Costello, 2000).

Diagnostic Interview Schedule for Children (DISC)
A version of the DIS is available for children and adolescents aged 6–18 (DISC; see Shaffer, Fisher, Lucas, Dulcan & Schwab-Stone, 2000). Modelled on the DIS's highly structured format, it assesses the common psychiatric diagnoses found in children and adolescents. It has good test–retest reliability (appearing to improve with age), but validity studies have been disappointing.

Children's Interview for Psychiatric Syndromes (ChIPS)
The ChIPS (Weller, Weller, Teare, & Fristead, 1999) is a structured interview for use with children and adolescents aged 6–18, and is available in both child and parent versions. Responses to stem questions determine whether the interviewer will proceed to follow a particular line of questioning. Psychometric data on this instrument are promising (Weller, Weller, Fristead, Rooney, & Schechter, 2000).

Child Assessment Schedule (CAS)
The CAS (Hodges, Kline, Stern, Cytyrn, & McKnew, 1982) is a semi-structured diagnostic interview suitable for children aged 7 and above. Symptoms are assessed in a semi-structured interview with the child and by the interviewer's observations. Taking around an hour to complete, the psychometric data are good (Broggs, Griffin, & Gross, 2002).

Interview Schedule for Children and Adolescents (ISCA)
The ISCA (Kovacs, 1997) is a semi-structured diagnostic interview suitable for children and adolescents aged 8–17 years. The instrument provides diagnoses in DSM-IV categories and takes around three hours to complete. Psychometric data are promising (Sherrill & Kovacs, 2000).

Schedule for Affective Disorders and Schizophrenia for School-Age Children (K-SADS)
The K-SADS is a version of the adult SADS that is designed for children of age 6 and above to yield DSM-IV diagnoses. Parent and child response versions are available, and the reliability data are good and validity data are acceptable (Ambrosini, 2000).

Structured and semi-structured diagnostic interviews: older adults
Structured diagnostic interviews have not yet been developed specifically for use with older adults and the instruments already discussed can be used. However, mental state can be assessed using the Geriatric Mental State Schedule (GSM; Copeland et al., 1976) and the GMS Schedule – Depression Scale (Ravindran, Welburn, & Hardesty, 1994) is a brief semi-structured interview for discriminating between depressed and non-depressed older adults. Other instruments, such as the Comprehensive Assessment and Referral Evaluation (CARE; Gurland et al., 1977; Gurland, Goldon, Teresi, & Challop, 1984) and the Cambridge Mental Disorders of the Elderly Examination (CAMDEX; Roth et al., 1986) provide assessments of a client's mental state. The mental state of clients is an important component of an assessment

and diagnosis with older adults, but is also relevant with clients of any age. Therefore, the assessment of mental state will be considered in some detail.

Mental Status Examination (MSE)

A Mental Status Examination (MSE) provides a template that assists a clinical psychologist in the collation and subsequent conceptual organization of clinical information about a client's emotional and cognitive functioning. By systematically basing observations on verbal and non-verbal behaviour, the aim is to increase the reliability of the data upon which subsequent diagnoses and case formulation are made. The particular perspective of the interview and the use to which the data are put will vary depending upon whether the goal is psychiatric (see Daniel & Crider, 2003; Treatment Protocol Project, 1997) or neurological (see Strub & Black, 2000), but the domains covered by the clinician are similar. Reporting an MSE also requires the clinician to be familiar with the descriptors of various symptoms, such as those found in the glossary of the DSM-5 (APA, 2000; see also Kaplan & Sadock, 2004).

Broadly speaking (and following Daniel & Crider, 2003), an MSE collates information about the client's (i) physical, (ii) emotional, and (iii) cognitive state. Under each of these domains fall a number of topic areas which are summarized in Table 3.1.

The summary of an MSE will not note every detail under each heading, but draws attention to the key features that describe the client and frame the presenting problem within a context of who the client is. Typically the description begins with a statement about their age, gender, relationship status, referrer, and presenting problem (i.e., the reason for presentation at the service on the particular occasion). For instance, the description may begin by saying, 'Gill, a 35-year old single woman, was referred by her medical practitioner, who had suggested treatment for her obesity that was contributing to hypertension.'

Physical

The description will draw attention to noteworthy aspects of the client's physical state.

Appearance

A concise summary of the client's physical presentation is given to paint a clear mental portrait. The description may refer to dress, grooming, facial expression, posture, eye contact, as well as any relevant noteworthy aspects of appearance. For instance, a clinician might note that the client 'wore an expensive, but crumpled suit. He sat slumped in the chair and was unshaven, with dark circles under his eyes.' Importantly, the aim is to describe what is observed rather than your interpretation (e.g., 'he was exhausted').

Behaviour

A description of behaviour may make reference to the client's level of consciousness extending from alert, through drowsy, a clouding of consciousness, stupor (lack of reaction to environmental stimuli) and delirium (bewildered, confused, restless, and disoriented), to coma (unconsciousness). It may also include reference to the degree of arousal (e.g., hypervigilance to environmental cues and hyperarousal such as observed in anxious and manic states) and mannerisms (e.g., tics and compulsions).

Table 3.1 An outline for a Mental Status Examination

PHYSICAL	
Appearance	Motor activity
Behaviour	
EMOTIONAL	
Attitude	Mood and affect
COGNITIVE	
Orientation	Attention and concentration
Memory	Speech and language
Thought (form and content)	Perception
Insight and judgement	Intelligence and abstraction

Motor activity

An account of the observed motor activity aims to describe both the quality and the types of actions observed. Reductions in movement can be variously described as a reduction in the level of movement (psychomotor retardation), slowed movement (bradykinesia), decreased movement (hypokinesia), or even an absence of movement (akinesia). Increases in the overall level of movement are referred to as psychomotor agitation, but it is also important to note minor increases in movement such as a tremor.

Attitude

The clinician will also consider the way in which the client participates in the interview, as a way of gauging their manner and outlook. These judgements will be based on the client's response both to the context of the interview, but also to the interviewer. Identifiers may be open, friendly, cooperative, willing, and responsive, or alternatively, they may be closed, guarded, hostile, suspicious, and passive. These terms will be used to describe complex sets of behaviours including attentiveness, responses to questions, expression, posture, eye contact, tone of voice, and so on.

Emotional

Moving from the physical domain, the clinician will portray the person's emotional state, once again drawing upon the verbal and non-verbal behaviour of the client.

Mood and affect

Although affect (an external expression of an emotional state) is potentially observable, mood (the internal emotional experience that influences both perception of the world and the individual's behavioural responses) is less apparent and will require the clinician to depend to a greater degree on the client's introspections. Descriptors of mood include euphoric, dysphoric (sad and depressed), hostile, apprehensive, fearful, anxious, and suspicious. The stability of mood can also be noted, with the alternation between extreme emotional states being referred to as emotional lability. The range, intensity, and variability of affect can be variously portrayed, but some important expressions are restricted (i.e., low intensity or range of emotional expression), blunted (i.e., severe declines in the range and intensity of emotional range and expression), flat (i.e., a virtual absence of emotional expression, often with an immobile face and a monotonous voice), and exaggerated (i.e., an overly strong emotional reaction) affect. The clinician will also consider the appropriateness of the affect (and note if the emotional expression is incongruent with verbal descriptions and behaviour) as well as the client's general responsiveness.

Cognitive

The cognitive components in an MSE will be familiar to clinical psychologists, since many components are assessed more comprehensively and within memory tests. However, during the MSE, the aim is to provide a general screening which requires interpretation using clinical judgement with one outcome being to recommend further formal testing.

Orientation

A person's orientation refers to their awareness of time, place, and person. Orientation for time refers to a client's ability to indicate the current day and date (with acceptance of an error of a couple of days). Orientation for place can be assessed by asking clients where they have presented. Behaviour should also be consistent with that expected in the setting in which they have arrived. Orientation for person refers to the ability to know who you are, which can be assessed by asking the client their name or names of friends and family which you can verify.

Attention and concentration

'Working memory' (Baddeley, 1986, 1990) is the term now used in psychology to refer to the constructs called attention and concentration. The aim is to describe the extent to which a client is able to focus their cognitive processes upon a given target and not be distracted by non-target stimuli. Digit span (the ability to recall in forward or reverse order increasingly long series of numbers presented at a rate of one per second) is a common way to assess these working memory functions, and normal individuals will recall around 6–8 numbers in digits forward and 5–6 numbers in digits backwards. Another method used is 'serial sevens' in which seven is sequentially subtracted from 100. Typically people will make only a couple of errors in 14 trials.

Memory

An MSE will typically assess memory using the categories of short- and long-term memory. Although these categories do not map neatly onto models of memory in recent cognitive psychology (Andrade, 2001), the aim of the MSE is to provide a concise description of a person's behaviour and screen them in a manner that can guide further assessment. Therefore, more sophisticated assessments and analyses may follow. To assess recent or short-term memory, clients can be asked about a recent topical event or who the President or Prime Minister is. Clients can also be asked to listen to three words, repeat them, and then recall them some time later in the interview. Most people will usually report 2–3 words after a 20-minute interval. Visual short-term memory can also be assessed by asking clients to copy and then reproduce from memory complex geometrical figures (such as those in the Rey Auditory Verbal Learning Test). Long-term memory can be assessed by asking about childhood events.

Thought – form and content

During an MSE the clinician will address the client's thought processes, inferred typically from speech. Disturbances in the form of thought are evident in terms of (i) the quantity and speed of thought production. The client may jump from idea to idea (flight of ideas) or show a poverty of ideas. Thought may be disordered in terms of (ii) the continuity of ideas. The client may leave a topic of conversation and perhaps return to it much later (circumstantiality), or maybe never return (tangentiality) on the one hand or may perseverate with the same idea, word, or phrase. They may show a loosening of associations, where the logical connections between thoughts are esoteric or bizarre.

Problems in the content of thought also need to be noted by a clinician. Delusions are profound disturbances in thought content in which the client continues to hold to a false belief despite objective contradictory evidence, despite other members of their culture not sharing the same belief. Delusions vary on dimensions of plausibility, from the plausible (e.g., the CIA is spying on me) to the bizarre (e.g., the newspaper contains coded messages for me), and systematization, from those that are unstable and non-systematized to stable and systematized. The content of delusions can be persecutory (others are deliberately trying to wrong, harm, or conspire against one), grandiose (an exaggerated sense of one's own importance, power, or significance), somatic (physical sensations or medical problems), reference (belief that otherwise innocuous events or actions refer specifically to the individual), or relate to control, influence, and passivity (belief that thoughts, feelings, impulses, and actions are controlled by an external agency or force). Clients can also have delusions that are nihilistic (belief that self or part of self, others, or the world does not exist), jealous (unreasonable belief that a partner is unfaithful), or religious (false belief that the person has a special link with God). The clinician needs to consider cultural factors as well as other clinical issues in identifying delusions. For example, belief in the sovereignty of God is not a delusion of control, because this is shared by others within a culture. Also, oversensitivity to the opinions of others is not a delusion of jealousy, since clients will typically not hold the belief in the face of contradictory evidence (behavioural experiment reference) and can concede that it is conceivable that the belief is wrong. Although the distinction between strongly held false beliefs and delusions is sometimes difficult to draw, the clinician will find it easier if the focus remains on the chain of reasoning whereby a person comes to believe a particular false belief rather than solely relying upon the content of the belief.

In addition to these extreme forms of thought disturbance, there are more frequent issues such as phobias (excessive and irrational fears), obsessions (repetitive, and intrusive thoughts, images, or impulses), and preoccupations (e.g., with illness or symptoms).

Perception

Hallucinations are a perceptual disturbance in which people have an internally generated sensory experience, so that they hear, see (visual), feel (tactile), taste (gustatory), or smell (olfactory) something that is not present or detectable by others. The most frequent hallucinations are auditory and typically involve hearing voices, calling, commanding, commenting, insulting, or criticizing. Hallucinations can also occur when falling asleep (hypnogogic) or when awaking (hypnopompic).

Other perceptual disturbances include a sense that the external world is unreal, different, or unfamiliar (derealization), an experience that the self is different or unreal in that the individual may feel unreal, that the body is distorted or being perceived from a distance (depersonalization). Perceptions can also be dulled, in that perceptions are flat and uninteresting, or heightened, in that each perception is vivid.

Insight and judgement

Insight is a dimension that describes the extent to which clients are aware that they have a problem. A strong lack of insight can be an important indicator of unwillingness to accept treatment. Insight refers also to an awareness of the nature and extent of the problem, the effects of the problem on others, and how it is a departure from normal. For instance, clients may deny the presence of a problem altogether, or may recognize the problem, but judge the cause to lie within others.

Judgement is another issue that the clinician will consider during an MSE. The ability to make sound decisions can be compromised for a number of reasons. The clinician will try to ascertain if poor decisions are the result of problems in the cognitive processes involved in the decision-making process, motivational issues, or failures to execute a planned course of action.

Speech and language

A client's speech can be described in terms of its rate (e.g., slow, rapid), intonation (e.g., monotonous), spontaneity, articulation, volume, as well as the quantity of information conveyed. At one end of the dimension of information conveyed is mutism (i.e., a total absence of speech), extending through poverty of speech (i.e., reduced spontaneous speech) to pressured speech (i.e., extremely rapid speech that is hard to interrupt and understand).

Speech is a subset within the broader domain of language. Language also includes reading, writing, and comprehension. Cognitive dysfunctions can be indicated by language disturbances (see Lezak, Howieson, & Loring, 2004 for an extended discussion) such as aphasia. Aphasia can be non-fluent, in which speech is slow, faltering, or effortful, or fluent. Fluent aphasia involves speech that is normal in terms of its form (rhythm, quantity, and intonation), but is meaningless perhaps including novel words (i.e., neologisms).

Intelligence and abstraction

A general indication of intelligence can be gained from the amount of schooling a person has had, with a failure to complete high school indicating below average intelligence, completion of high school indicating average intelligence, and college or university education indicating high intelligence.

Abstraction is the ability to recognize and comprehend abstract relationships – to extract common characteristics from a group of objects (e.g., in what way are an apple/banana or music/sculpture alike?), interpretation (e.g., explaining a proverb such as 'a stitch in time saves nine'). However, care needs to be exercised interpreting responses to abstract questions, since they may reflect the degree to which the person's cultural group has permitted exposure to the content of the sayings.

Summary

An MSE provides a useful conceptual organization for the clinician and a mental checklist to consider a client's functioning across broad domains. During a diagnostic interview it would be rare to systemically work through each area, but relevant questions are included as judged appropriate. Brief, formal versions with standard scoring of the MSE are available in the

Mini Mental State Exam (Folstein, Folstein, & McHugh, 1975; see also Treatment Protocol Project, 1997). This is an 11-item scale to measure orientation, registration, attention and calculation, recall, language, and praxis. Score ranges from 0–30 and lower scores indicate greater impairment. The chief problem is that it is less sensitive for cases with milder impairment and scores are influenced by educational level of the subject. Some other options are the Cognitive Capacity Screening Examination (CCSE; Jacobs, Berhard, Delgado, & Strain, 1977); a 30-item screener to detect diffuse organic disorders, especially delirium, that is more appropriate for cognitively intact individuals, the High Sensitivity Cognitive Screen (HSCS; Faust & Fogel, 1989); a 15-item scale that is a valid and reliable indicator of the presence of cognitive impairment, the Mental Status Questionnaire (MSQ; Kahn, Goldfarb, Pollack, & Peck, 1960); a 10-item scale that shares the same weaknesses as the MMSE and omits some key domains of function (e.g., retention and registration), and the Short Portable Mental Status Questionnaire (SPMSQ; Pfeiffer, 1975); a 10-item scale for use with community or institutional residents that is a reliable indicator of brain injury.

Limitations of diagnosis and future directions

Diagnosis is important because without it, the social processes required for delivery of mental health services could not be justified, research would be hampered, and communication among professionals and information retrieval would be difficult. However, this is not to say that current diagnostic systems are without fault. Rather, the clinician needs to be cognizant of these weaknesses and use diagnoses accordingly.

First, following the introduction of specific criteria and a focus on observable (rather than inferred) symptoms, the reliability of diagnoses has increased. Notwithstanding the improvements in reliability, the outcomes of the DSM-5 field trials have been questioned and attention has been drawn to the low reliability of some diagnostic categories (Greenberg, 2013). Additionally, the validity of some diagnoses has been called into question. A problem with the diagnostic system is that the confidence in the validity of each diagnosis is not specified, yet not all diagnostic categories are equally valid. Second, generally there are no identifiable psychometric assessments that relate to particular diagnoses. Thus, the clinician will need to evaluate the available psychological tests and determine which tests, and which normative groups and cut-offs, are relevant for supplementing a diagnosis. Third, the diagnostic system is focused upon existing disorders and makes no reference to precursors to particular disorders. With the increasing focus on prevention and early intervention, the clinical psychologist needs to remember that there may be good reasons for intervening in specific problem behaviours, even though they may not be listed in DSM-5 or ICD-10. Fourth, many psychological models of psychopathology are dimensional and the aetiological processes are found in both normal and abnormal populations, but to varying degrees. The DSM and ICD systems are both categorical systems that identify the presence of a disorder rather than locating an individual upon a dimension. Within the area of personality disorders, there is increasing awareness of the need to consider psychopathology in a dimensional manner. For the clinical psychologist, this is relevant, as the clinician will not solely be searching for qualitatively different processes, but trying to identify the extent to which behaviour, cognition, and physiology are disturbed. Fifth, it is critical for clinical psychologists to remember that many problems worthy of intervention and treatment are not listed as clinical disorders within diagnostic systems. Relational disorders (First et al., 2002), such as couple distress, are just one example of the disorders that do not fit within the focus of current diagnostic taxonomies upon the individual, rather than a dyad, family system, or other social groups.

Finally, perhaps the most serious criticism of the diagnoses arrived at using current diagnostic systems is that they are limited predictors of treatment outcome (Acierno, Hersen & van Hasselt, 1997). Ultimately, diagnostic systems are valuable if they can predict treatment response. Symptoms are one factor that determines outcome, but not the sole predictor; however, the DSM-5, the ICD-10, and the empirical literature tend to focus almost exclusively upon this dimension. Further, the assignment of a DSM or ICD diagnosis does not regularly imply that a specific intervention is indicated (see Nathan & Gorman, 2002, 2007). From the perspective of a clinical psychologist, the absence of indices other than symptoms is disturbing. Most psychological models of psychopathology acknowledge the important aetiological role of stressful life events (Miller, 1996), yet these factors are absent from diagnoses. Alternative systems have been proposed, including suggestions to measure (i) symptoms of behaviour, cognition, and physiology through behavioural observation, self-report, and physiological monitoring (Bellack & Hersen, 1998), (ii) maintaining factors through a functional analysis of contingencies of reinforcement and other contextual factors, and (iii) aetiology (see Acierno et al., 1997). Even though the current revision to the DSM-5 represented an attempt to form aetiological diagnostic systems (primarily based on neuroscience; see Charney et al., 2002) the goal seems unlikely to be achieved for two reasons. First, neuroscience presently remains too imprecise to provide a sufficiently solid foundation to achieve the 'goal to translate basic and clinical neuroscience research relating brain structure, brain function, and behavior into a classification system of psychiatric disorders based on etiology and pathophysiology' (Charney et al., 2002, p. 70; e.g., there is still no biological marker for any psychiatric diagnosis), and second, it fails to acknowledge that there are social and psychological factors that exert important and complicated effects. For instance, Gil, Wagner, and Vega (2000) have shown that higher rates of alcohol use by US-born Latino adolescents compared with recent immigrants are associated with the reduction over time in familism, cohesion, and social control. Thus, it seems unlikely that diagnostic taxonomies in the near future will incorporate factors such as a comprehensive symptom assessment, a systematic examination of maintaining factors, personality, and consideration of various aspects of aetiology. Nonetheless, there is room within a clinical intervention to address these important factors and this will be the focus of the next chapter.

Additional assessment and testing

Reviewing our model (Figure 3.3), it is apparent that assessment may begin concurrently with diagnosis, but it extends far beyond. The clinical psychologist (i) distils information into a case formulation, (ii) assists treatment planning in which interventions are matched to clients, and (iii) measures the degree of success. The process of assessment is indicated by the shaded area and the process is divided into matching, measurement, and monitoring which are located within an overall management structure.

- *Management* of outcomes involves the ongoing assessment and evaluation of clinical and administrative processes involved in the delivery of care.
- *Matching* refers to the process of matching the client to the appropriate treatment option. This process begins with *screening and problem description* which have been discussed earlier. Problem description is followed by treatment planning or *matching* (in which specific information is collected that aids the clinical decision-making

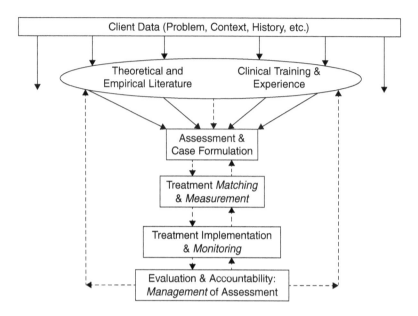

Figure 3.3 The centrality of assessment processes and techniques to the scientific practice of clinical psychology.

process). Once the problem has been accurately identified the psychologist can give thought to the most appropriate treatment (Beutler & Clarkin, 1990; Beutler & Harwood, 2000; Castonguay & Beutler, 2006). Sometimes the relevant treatment will be evident by examining a list of empirically validated treatments (e.g., Nathan & Gorman, 2007). However, at other times the picture will be more complicated, due to patterns of comorbidity and involved presentations. At these times case formulation can be used to identify potential treatments that are linked to the causal mechanisms involved.

- *Measurement* involves the pre-, post-, and follow-up assessments of a variable(s) to determine the amount of change that has occurred as a result of an intervention.
- *Monitoring* refers to the periodic assessment of intervention outcomes to permit inferences about what has produced observed changes. *Progress monitoring* determines deviations from the expected course of improvement; whereas *outcomes monitoring* focuses upon the aspects of the intervention process that bring about change.

Thus, these four activities all occur within a context of evidence-based and evidence-supported assessment. Although the concept of measurement will be familiar to a psychologist, ongoing monitoring may be less familiar (Newnham & Page, 2010). Lutz, Martinovich, and Howard (1999; see also Asay et al., 2002; Lutz, Martinovich, Howard, & Leon, 2002) distinguished treatment-focused research from patient-focused research. Patient-focused research, what we have called monitoring, asks the question, 'Is this particular client's problem responding to the treatment that is being applied?' (Lutz et al., 1999). Thus, with the move from treatment- to patient-focused research the spotlight shifts from the average client to the particular individual currently being treated.

Before describing some general principles of monitoring, a scientist-practitioner needs to consider the empirical evidence regarding monitoring. Monitoring will take time and effort on the client's part and the clinician will need to collect, score, store, collate, interpret, and feed back all data to the client. Therefore, the clinician needs to be able to justify to the client, themselves, and their employer the 'costs' incurred. To this end, work by Lambert et al., (2001) is useful. They assigned clients to treatment as usual or a condition in which their clinician received weekly feedback on their symptom change relative to expected progress. The sample was then divided into clients who were predicted to have good versus poor outcomes, based on initial assessment. For clients who were predicted to have poor outcomes, treatment duration increased and the outcomes were improved, such that twice as many clients achieved clinically significant (Jacobson & Truax, 1991) change. For clients who were expected to have a positive response to treatment, the outcomes were no better, but the number of sessions was reduced. Therefore, the provision of monitoring data to the clinicians allowed them to target therapy time to clients where it was most needed and in so doing, maximized the overall benefit.

Monitoring of clients highlights the various phases of treatment. Lutz et al. (1999, 2002) identify three phases to therapy. The client passes through *remoralization*, as subjective well-being improves, *remediation*, as symptoms begin to reduce, and *rehabilitation*, as the improvements in well-being and symptoms spread to domains of life functioning. The process of symptom amelioration will follow a log linear curve for the average client (Howard, Kopta, Krause, & Orlinsky, 1986), such that the greatest change occurs in the initial sessions, with improvement gradually flattening out. If assessments are collected during treatment (e.g., Howard, Brill, Lueger, O'Mahoney, & Grissom, 1995; Sperry et al., 1996), it is possible to plot an expected course of recovery using a variety of predictor variables. For instance, Lutz et al. (1999) used archival data on subjective well-being, current symptoms, current life functioning, global assessment of functioning, past use of therapy, problem duration, and treatment expectations to generate an expected treatment trajectory. Using a client's pre-treatment scores it is then possible to plot an expected course of improvement for each particular client, over which can be overlaid actual progress, placing boundaries around the expected trajectory of improvement so that a lower range is set by the failure boundary (e.g., scores of clients in the 25th percentile) and an upper range (e.g., mean scores of non-clinical sample). As a result, it is possible to display a graphical depiction of a client's progress through therapy relative to their expected course. Further, as the client's actual scores approach the normal range, the clinician will receive feedback that treatment is progressing optimally. On the other hand, if a client's scores approach the failure boundary, the clinician will be alerted that the treatment outcome is not optimal and an alternative treatment plan may need to be set (see Lambert et al., 2001; Mintz & Kiesler, 1982, and the next chapter for a discussion of individualized outcome measures in psychotherapy).

Thus, repeating testing during an intervention can provide an indication of the extent to which a person is changing according to expectations. Sometimes this is talked about as a 'glide path'. In the same way that an airplane approaches a runway along a glide path and deviations from the expected trajectory signal time for corrective action, the place where an individual is along a treatment trajectory provides useful information. Deviations from the expected path of improvements may signal a problem. The expected changes in symptom severity, social function, and occupational performance can all be monitored against normative references to identify if remedial action is appropriate.

Although these approaches to monitoring are more recent than efficacy and effectiveness research, the client-focused research approach typified by monitoring has great potential to bridge the gap between science and practice. Science, by its nature, is concerned with generalizable results, whereas clinical practice is concerned with the instance. By increasing the relevance of data collection to the individual client, monitoring strategies will allow clinical psychologists to collect client-relevant data that can be integrated with data available from treatment-relevant efficacy and effectiveness research. Furthermore, monitoring permits a science-informed practitioner to test and evaluate hypotheses about each client. How to monitor client progress is the topic of the next chapter.

Monitoring client progress

Clinical psychologists are referred clients who are in distress; the problems have profound impacts on their lives and the psychologist's intention is that, after some intervention, the client will leave treatment no longer distressed and with their problems resolved. One way to guide the selection of treatments to achieve this desired outcome is by using evidence-based practice. In so doing, it is possible to make inferences about the progress of the average client. Evidence-based practice draws upon efficacy studies that contrast active treatments with appropriate comparisons under controlled conditions and permit an estimate of the effect size of treatment to be made. Effectiveness studies can then examine the degree to which the effect sizes observed under controlled conditions are reproduced in clinical settings. The reduced control over the types of clients, the extent of comorbidity, and the training of therapists can all affect the extent to which effect sizes observed in efficacy studies may fail to generalize. Lambert (2013) has documented that the effect sizes tend to be smaller in clinical practice than in efficacy studies, but nonetheless, as a scientist-practitioner, it is possible to know that a given evidence-based treatment will have a particular effect size and to infer that the average client treated will experience a similar benefit. The present chapter, while not arguing against the application of evidence-based treatments, will present the case that the blind application of evidence-based treatments is not optimal clinical practice.

Monitoring and feedback is a specific therapeutic intervention

Evidence-based practice is not incompatible with practice-based evidence (Castonguay, Barkham, Lutz, & McAleavey, 2013). In evidence-based practice, we use interventions and practices that have a reliable and valid foundation in empirical findings. However, practice-based evidence allows clinicians to monitor client progress during treatment and adapt therapy accordingly. Therapists adapt treatment but they do so by allowing the clinical judgements to be guided by evidence and to be responsive to the data collected. Before describing how this can be done, let us review the evidence showing that clinical outcomes are improved by using practice-based evidence.

The pioneering research in patient monitoring and feedback was conducted by Mike Lambert and colleagues. They have published many randomized controlled trials evaluating the effectiveness of providing individualized feedback to clinicians (Harmon, Hawkins, Lambert, Slade, & Whipple, 2005; Hawkins, Lambert, Vermeersch, Slade, & Tuttle, 2004; Lambert et al., 2001; Lambert et al., 2002; Whipple et al., 2003). Conducted in routine clinical settings, each of the studies was assigned to 'treatment as usual' or to a condition in which therapists were given feedback about the progress of each client during treatment. Broadly speaking, the client data collected each session provided the therapists with feedback that could be distilled into information as to whether the client was progressing as expected (i.e., was 'on track') or was not progressing as expected (i.e., was 'not on track'). Therapists were not given any additional treatments, but were free to use their clinical experience to adapt the treatments in light of the feedback. The clear result was that when patients drifted off track, providing therapists with that information led to improvements in patient outcomes (Shimokawa, Lambert, & Smart, 2010). Specifically, the effect size was moderate (even though this was over and above the benefits of treatment) and the deterioration rate was halved.

Expressing this differently: an efficacy study provides information that the average client will improve by a particular amount. However, some people will improve more than the mean and others will improve less than the average. Just using evidence-based practice does not provide information about what to do with clients who improve less than the average. Practice-based evidence, on the other hand, complements evidence-based practice and uses data collected during therapy to allow clinicians to target those who are falling behind and then potentially avert negative outcomes. Not surprisingly, the outcomes for patients who are 'on track' are less affected by feedback. Presumably, when a clinical psychologist uses an evidence-based treatment and learns that the client is responding as expected, the therapy will not require a modification to standard practice.

Lambert's group uses the 45-item Outcomes Questionnaire (Lambert, Gregersen, & Burlingame, 2004) to measure outcomes and to provide feedback to therapists. They have amassed an impressive evidence base for their outcomes monitoring system (www.oqmeasures.com). However, other researchers have replicated the same beneficial effects using different assessment measures (e.g., Lutz, Martinovich, Howard, & Leon, 2002; Miller, Duncan, & Hubble, 2005a; Miller, Duncan, Sorrell, & Brown, 2005b) with different age groups and diagnoses (Kelley & Bickman, 2009; Kelley, Bickman, & Norwood, 2010), and across different treatment settings (Byrne, Hooke, Newnham, & Page, 2012; Newnham, Hooke, & Page, 2010b). Innovative research from Wolfgang Lutz's clinical research group has carefully studied the behaviours of clinicians and one important finding has relevance for clinical psychology trainees (Castonguay et al., 2013). They compared experienced psychologists with trainees, and found that when trainees encountered a client who was not proceeding as expected, they were more likely to seek supervision. Thus, it is clear that the provision of feedback is a specific treatment intervention that has beneficial effects on clients who are not progressing well and as such, science-informed practice should include such a system. For clinical psychology trainees, the system provides a complement to training. It does this by signalling when extra supervision could be needed and thus, timely and focused help can be sought. While there are many commercially available patient monitoring systems, the remainder of the chapter will outline the key principles of a system by describing a freely available version and then cover some reasons why feedback and monitoring might be beneficial. Trainees can then experiment with a system and use it to seek targeted help from supervisors.

A monitoring and feedback system

Think of a monitoring system like a thermometer. In physical medicine, a thermometer provides a quick measure of temperature and allows staff to compare the reading against an expected distribution with a threshold distinguishing normal from abnormal levels. An elevated temperature does not tell the doctor or nurse what is wrong, but signals that something is not right. Further investigations then guide clinical decisions about how to modify treatment.

Extending this logic to mental health, it means that we need a quick, repeatable measure of mental health and a way to identify when scores are 'normal' and 'abnormal'.

There are a number of instruments that can serve as 'mental health thermometers'. The 45-item Outcome Questionnaire (OQ-45; Lambert & Finch, 1999; Lambert et al., 2004) has been the most widely used instrument and it has been shown to be acceptable in both out-patient and some inpatient settings. Sophisticated software is available to provide clinicians with a comprehensive suite of tools to monitor outcomes and to provide feedback to clients. Added benefits are that comparable instruments have been developed for use among children and adolescents (Cannon, Warren, Nelson, & Burlingame, 2010; McClendon et al., 2011; Nelson, Warren, Gleave, & Burlingame, 2013) and the scale has been translated into many languages with the beneficial outcomes being replicated in countries other than the US (e.g., de Jong et al., 2008; de Jong, van Sluis, Nugter, Heiser, & Spinhoven, 2012; Wennberg, Philips, & de Jong, 2010). The Outcome Rating Scale (ORS; Miller et al., 2005b) is a popular measure in counselling psychology, since the system provides indications about the quality of the therapeutic relationship as well as distress. Another instrument, developed by Bickman and colleagues (Bickman, Kelley, Breda, de Andrade, & Riemer, 2011) permits assessments of youths' symptoms and functioning. Its strength is that it draws on a theoretical foundation about feedback developed within industrial and organizational psychology (Sapyta, Riemer, & Bickman, 2005) and its use has also been shown in a randomized controlled trial to improve outcomes (Bickman et al., 2011). Within the United Kingdom, the Clinical Outcomes in Routine Evaluation 10-item scale (CORE; Barkham et al., 2013; Barkham et al., 2010b; Connell et al., 2007) has proved to be popular and its strength is that it is accompanied by a whole suite of associated indices (www.coreims.co.uk/). Yet all of these different outcome monitoring systems share a common methodology in which an instrument is used to provide the practice-based evidence upon which clinical decisions are made.

By way of illustration we will describe an outcome monitoring system that we have developed. Since the instruments and the tools are in the public domain it means that you can use them in your clinical training. To capture both mental health as well as psychological distress, we have developed two companion measures. The first instrument we use is the World Health Organization's Well-Being Index (WHO-5; Bech, Gudex, & Johansen, 1996). The WHO-5 has good internal consistency in medical settings ($\alpha = 0.91$; Löwe et al., 2004) and psychiatric samples ($\alpha = 0.89$; Newnham, Hooke, & Page, 2010a). The instrument consists of five items rated on a six-point Likert-type scale measuring frequency from 'All of the time' (scores as 0) to 'At no time' (scored as 5). Participants endorse the appropriate option for the previous 24 hours (adaptation by Newnham et al., 2010a) with high scores indicating increased well-being. The items ask patients the amount of the time that they have felt (i) cheerful and in good spirits, (ii) calm and relaxed, (iii) active and vigorous, (iv) woke up feeling fresh and rested, and (v) that their daily life has been filled with things that interest them. Similar to other research groups, we demonstrated in a controlled trial that providing feedback about progress to staff and patients reduced depressive symptoms in patients at risk of poor outcomes post-treatment (Newnham et al., 2010b). A companion symptom measure assessing psychological distress is the 5-item Daily Index (DI-5; Dyer, Hooke, & Page, 2014). Items assess a variety of symptom domains, including thoughts about suicide. It has strong reliability ($\alpha = 0.88$) and has good sensitivity to treatment change. It also shows good validity, with strong correlations with other longer symptom measures, and in a recent controlled trial it was apparent that combining symptom and well-being feedback leads to even greater benefits for 'not on track' patients.

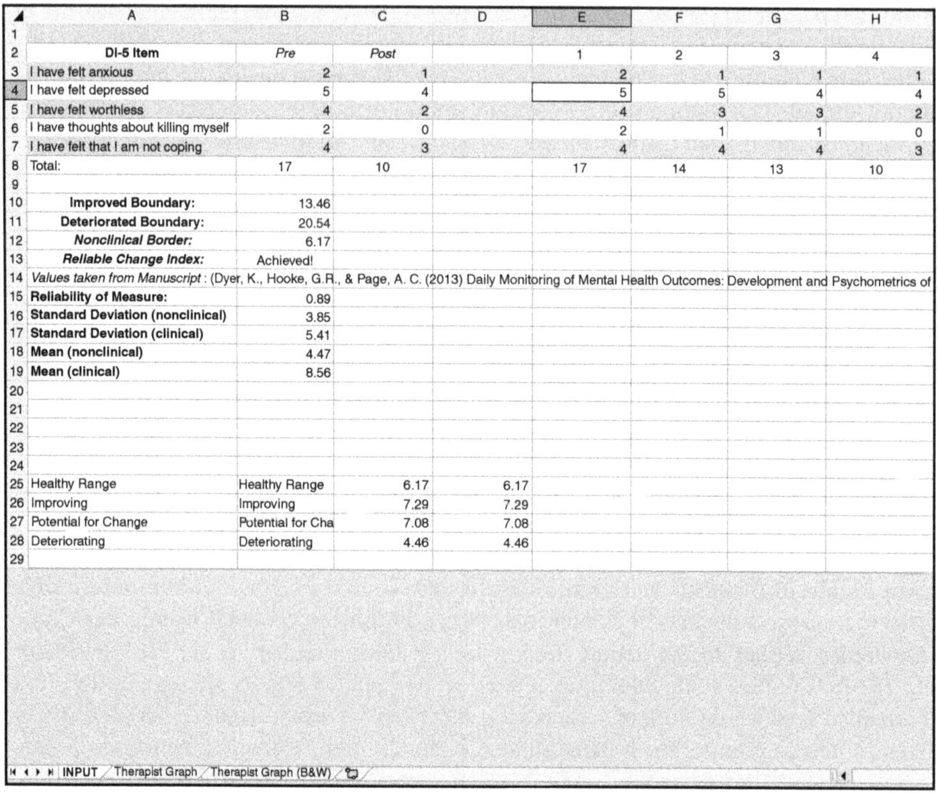

	A	B	C	D	E	F	G	H
1								
2	DI-5 Item	Pre	Post		1	2	3	4
3	I have felt anxious	2	1		2	1	1	1
4	I have felt depressed	5	4		5	5	4	4
5	I have felt worthless	4	2		4	3	3	2
6	I have thoughts about killing myself	2	0		2	1	1	0
7	I have felt that I am not coping	4	3		4	4	4	3
8	Total:	17	10		17	14	13	10
9								
10	Improved Boundary:	13.46						
11	Deteriorated Boundary:	20.54						
12	Nonclinical Border:	6.17						
13	Reliable Change Index:	Achieved!						
14	Values taken from Manuscript : (Dyer, K., Hooke, G.R., & Page, A. C. (2013) Daily Monitoring of Mental Health Outcomes: Development and Psychometrics of							
15	Reliability of Measure:	0.89						
16	Standard Deviation (nonclinical)	3.85						
17	Standard Deviation (clinical)	5.41						
18	Mean (nonclinical)	4.47						
19	Mean (clinical)	8.56						
20								
21								
22								
23								
24								
25	Healthy Range	Healthy Range	6.17	6.17				
26	Improving	Improving	7.29	7.29				
27	Potential for Change	Potential for Cha	7.08	7.08				
28	Deteriorating	Deteriorating	4.46	4.46				
29								

INPUT / Therapist Graph / Therapist Graph (B&W)

Figure 4.1 Screenshot of input for symptom monitoring using the Daily Index-5 (Dyer et al., 2014).

The DI-5 (Dyer et al., 2014) asks patients to rate five items on a 6-point Likert-type scale (0 = At no time; 1 = Some of the time; 2 = less than half of the time; 3 = more than half of the time; 4 = most of the time; 5 = all of the time). The items are 'Over the last day I have' (i) felt anxious, (ii) felt depressed, (iii) felt worthless, (iv) thought about killing myself, (v) felt that I am not coping. Each scale is scored by summing items to create a score that ranges from 0 to 25. Scores on the DI-5 and WHO-5 scales will be negatively correlated because high scores on the DI-5 represent elevated symptoms whereas higher scores on the WHO-5 reflect greater well-being. Calculation can be performed by hand, but spreadsheets were developed by Kale Dyer and are available for the DI-5 (www.researchgate.net/publication/258246782_Development_and_psychometrics_of_the_five_item_daily_index_in_a_psychiatric_sample_-_calculator?3ev=prf_pub) and the WHO-5 (www.researchgate.net/publication/259192434_WHO_5_Monitoring_Spreadsheet_for_scoring_and_interpretation?ev=prf_pub) that not only add up the relevant scores, but assist with interpretation.

The two spreadsheets are similar so we will illustrate only the DI-5. The three tabs at the foot of the page (see Figure 4.1) are labelled (i) INPUT, (ii) Therapist Graph, and (iii) Therapist Graph (B&W). The Input screen is shown for a patient who has attended four sessions. The clinical psychologist has entered data into columns E–H and the program has provided totals. The first data set is identified as the pre-treatment session (Column B) and the last and most recent data set as the post-treatment (Column C). Were data from another session

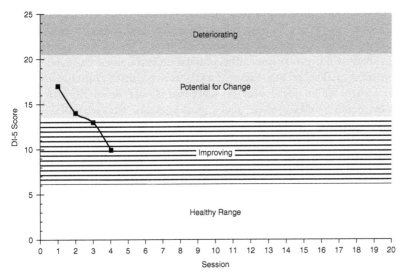

Figure 4.2 Screenshot of output for symptom monitoring using the Daily Index-5 (Dyer et al., 2014).

to be added, this would now be identified as the post-treatment. The information below the table relates to the calculation of clinical significance. Before discussing this, the Therapist Graphs on the two tabs will be reviewed.

The Therapist Graphs have identical content, but one is coloured. They plot the client's scores in a graphical manner so that progress can be evaluated. The x-axis is the number of sessions and the y-axis is the extent of psychological distress (or well-being) rated 0–25. The lines depicting the client's data are overlaid on a series of horizontal bands. In the colour version of the graph, the top red band (labelled 'deteriorating') reflects that relative to the pre-treatment score, the client has significantly worsened. The green band (titled 'improving') indicates significant improvement and the blue band (titled 'healthy range') shows that the client has improved significantly and the post-treatment score is now in the healthy range. The amber ('potential for change') band is anchored to the client's pre-treatment score and movement within this area is not yet statistically significant. Therefore, the client depicted in Figure 4.2 has psychological distress that improved non-significantly between the first and second sessions, but the change by session three was significantly different to the pre-treatment score. The client is thus now in the 'improving' range, but has not yet exhibited a reduction in psychological distress that is in the healthy range.

Clinical significance

It is important to understand the logic that underpins the categorization because the principles are those that tend to be used by the majority of outcome monitoring systems. 'Clinical significance' has been developed because statistical significance alone does not reflect the 'meaningfulness' of clinical change (Ogles, Lunnen, & Bonesteel, 2001). Even with large effect sizes, it is impossible to conclude that any participant is asymptomatic. To redress this deficiency, 'clinical significance' was developed (Jacobson & Truax, 1991). While there are a variety of calculation methods (Ronk, Hooke, & Page, 2012) and approaches available (Lambert, Hansen, & Bauer, 2008), the most common illustrative approach is the Jacobson and Truax method. It comprises two components, the first of which is the Reliable Change Index (RCI). The RCI expresses the pre- to post- difference in standardized units and identifies if pre-post change is reliable (i.e., exceeds measurement error). The second component assumes client scores are drawn from an 'unhealthy' population and non-client scores from a 'healthy' one. A cut-off is established to estimate if a client's score moves into the healthy range. Consequently, a client with a post-treatment score that is not reliably different from their pre-treatment score will be classified as 'unchanged'. Someone who has reliably improved, but failed to move into the healthy range is 'improved' whereas someone who has reliably improved and moved into the health range is 'recovered'. Finally, clients who exhibit a reliable change in the opposite direction will be classified as 'deteriorated'.

The Jacobson and Truax (Jacobson, Follette, & Revenstorf, 1984; Jacobson & Truax, 1991) method identifies a cut-off between 'functional' and 'dysfunctional' populations. There are three ways to identify a cut-off, but the optimal method is possible when both normative and clinical data are available. The resulting cut-off (i.e., criterion C) is calculated using the formula below:

$$C = \frac{S_{pop}M_{pre} - S_{pre}M_{pop}}{S_{pop} + S_{pre}}$$

where S_{pop} and S_{pre} are standard deviations of functional and dysfunctional (pre-treatment) groups respectively, and M_{pop} and M_{pre} are the means of functional and dysfunctional (pre-treatment) groups respectively. For the DI-5, the result of applying these calculations (to obtain the value of 6.17) can be seen in the Input worksheet (Figure 4.1) in the row called 'non-clinical border' and the values entered into the equation are listed in the rows above.

The second step calculates the Reliable Change Index (RCI). This expresses each individual's pre- to post-treatment change score in standard error units of measurement and signals that a reliable change has occurred when this value exceeds an increase or decrease of 1.96. The formula used is:

$$RCI = \frac{X_{post} - X_{pre}}{\sqrt{2(S_{pre}\sqrt{1 - R_{xx}})^2}}$$

where X_{post} and X_{pre} are the individual's raw scores post- and pre-treatment respectively and r_{xx} is the reliability of the measure (e.g., test–retest reliability, Cronbach's alpha). Thus, the equation expresses the difference between pre- and post- values as a standard score, and asks the question 'is the difference larger than that to obtain a probability value less than 0.05?' Since change can be both positive and negative, there are two values. One is the 'deteriorated boundary' (i.e., 20.54) and the other is the 'improved boundary' (i.e., 13.46) which are the pre-treatment score plus or minus the RCI. The categorization of 'Achieved' in Figure 4.1 is included because the change for this particular individual from the first to fourth sessions has exceeded the value necessary for reliable change.

By combining the cut-off with the RCI it is possible to create the four categories depicted in the spreadsheet. While the calculations are relatively straightforward, the spreadsheet performs the operations for you. However, understanding the logic is necessary for the informed use of the categories. The interested reader may also consider the literature about clinical significance because there are other calculation methods and approaches (Ronk et al., 2012).

The clinical psychologist can then use a monitoring tool such as the DI-5 and WHO-5 to provide feedback to clients about their progress. Since we know that the average client will respond favourably to an evidence-based treatment, the expectation would be that a client who is responding appropriately to the treatment will move from the pre-treatment levels into the 'improving' or even the healthy range. Furthermore, Howard and colleagues demonstrated that the typical trajectory of improvement follows a negatively accelerating curve. That is, the reduction in symptoms (or growth in well-being) is maximal in the first few sessions of therapy with the improvement gradually plateauing, until the amount of improvement after each subsequent session is marginal. Importantly, the degree of change in the first few sessions is predictive of later improvement. Clients who make rapid gains early in therapy go on to have the best outcomes, whereas clients who make rapid early losses will tend to have the worst outcomes (Lambert, Harmon, Slade, Whipple, & Hawkins, 2005). This information is clinically useful because the clinical psychologist does not have to wait until post-treatment to know which clients are going to fare badly. In fact, the amount of progress (or lack thereof) by three sessions into therapy is sufficient to predict end-state. The implication is that monitoring the progress allows the clinical psychologist to use this practice-based evidence to guide and inform clinical decisions about treatment progress.

If a client is not progressing as expected, the clinical psychologist can review possible obstacles. It may be that the treatment is not being appropriately applied or that elements have been omitted. It is possible that the problem has not been appropriately conceptualized. Alternatively, it may be that client is not ready for change, social support may be inadequate, the therapeutic alliance has not been established or it may have been ruptured, or life stresses or comorbid conditions may be impeding progress. The clinician can evaluate these options using relevant psychometric assessments and then implement treatment options that are appropriate (Harmon, Hawkins, Lambert, Slade, & Whipple, 2005; Lambert, Harmon, Slade, Whipple, & Hawkins, 2005). There is growing evidence that when such clinical support tools are used in the context of an outcome monitoring system, the benefits to clients are even greater still (Shimokawa et al., 2010).

The reasons why feedback works

Before leaving the discussion of outcomes monitoring it is worth considering explanations of why the provision of feedback would be beneficial. After all, don't therapists already ask clients how they are progressing? Don't clinical psychologists already know when a client is not on track and use their clinical judgement accordingly?

Clearly we must answer in the affirmative to these questions and this probably explains why the majority of clients do not deteriorate and that even without a formal monitoring system, therapists are able to turn around the negative progress of many clients who get worse during treatment (Lambert, 2010, 2013). However, the observation remains that when monitoring systems are implemented and the results fed back to therapists, the client outcomes improve. Why is this?

One part of the answer is that statistical predictions of outcome tend to be more accurate than clinical judgements (Grove, Zald, Lebow, Snitz, & Nelson, 2000). Specifically, when clinical and statistical methods for prediction of treatment failure were contrasted, clinicians tended to vastly underestimate the probability that a treatment failure would occur (Hannan et al., 2005). The authors found that even though clinicians could identify which patients were worse off during a particular session, they did not use that information to modify their

treatment. If a feedback system is in operation, it is much harder to maintain an overly positive (potentially self-serving) cognitive bias in the face of data that the client's actual treatment progress is not proceeding according to plan and it is harder to ignore the objective
evidence of potential treatment failure (Newnham & Page, 2010). Furthermore, not all patients follow the same trajectory through treatment (Nordberg, Castonguay, Fisher, Boswell,
& Kraus, 2014) and algorithms can be used to identify which group a client is a member of
and this in turn can guide treatment (Lutz, Stulz, & Kock, 2009). The identification of a particular client's therapeutic trajectory is hard for a clinician to identify, but computers can do
this more easily and this information can feed into the clinician's decision-making process.

Another part of the answer may also be that client recollections of progress may not
always be accurate. Page and Hooke (2009) found that increasing the amount of psychological therapy was associated with increased gains in self-reported pre- to post- treatment outcomes. However, when patients reflected on their treatment gains, those who had received
more therapy and improved to a greater degree recalled less improvement and were less
satisfied with treatment. Thus, retrospective self-report is not completely valid. Therefore,
by collecting data in real time and presenting it in an objective manner to therapists clinical
decisions can be made on a more rational basis (Schulte & Eifert, 2002).

How to give feedback to clients

Given that client recollections are not perfect, that clinicians tend to underestimate negative
outcomes, and that even when clinicians are aware of evidence of poor progress they do not
always use the information to modify practice it is not surprising that supplementing clinical judgement with practice-based evidence can improve outcomes. Having described the
empirical justification for progress monitoring and illustrated a method for doing so, the
remaining issue is the process of providing feedback to clients. In our experience there are a
few concerns that clinicians first need to address.

The first issue is a concern clinicians have about the possible risks of sharing the progress
graph and its meaning with a client. One worry is that it may be demoralizing to clients to
see a lack of progress. In this context it is important to remember that the graphs are a depiction of information that the client has provided. Therefore, it is typically more newsworthy
for the clinician than for the client. Concerns about a lack of progress will already have been
in the client's mind. The graph allows the topic to be put on the clinician's agenda. It is in
the open and available for discussion. The depiction legitimizes both progress and lack of
progress as a topic for collaborative consideration. The conversation can be guided by the
data and therapist and client can consider the best way to progress. However, do not be
surprised to find the graphs challenge your perception of progress more than they challenge
your client's view.

A second issue relates to the value of the self-report. It is possible that the self-report fails
to capture the nuances of the client's problems. We do not see this as a fatal flaw, but it is a reason for the clinical psychologist to interpret the meaning of the score. This interpretation will
be guided by an understanding of both the construct validity of the scales and the meaning of
the clinical significance categories. The two scales are a 'thermometer' and just as a doctor will
take a patient's temperature but will also use a plethora of other tests, the clinical psychologist
should be no different. Each test is interpreted with a view to its strengths and weaknesses.

A third concern raised by clinical psychology trainees is the view that formal feedback is
not needed, because routine clinical practice already involves therapists asking clients about

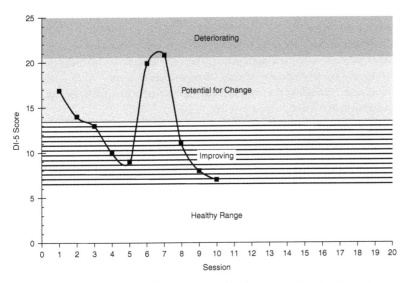

Figure 4.3 A graph depicting a client's progress with a lapse around sessions 6 and 7.

their progress. In response to this concern, it is useful to remember that the controlled trials involved 'treatment as usual' conditions. The therapists who used feedback had better outcomes than therapists who did not. One important methodological detail of the studies (see Shimokawa et al., 2010) is that it was often the *therapists* who were randomly assigned to conditions. That is, one therapist had feedback graphs on one client, but not on another. Hence, the benefits were not attributable to the normal behaviours of particular therapists, but an effect of giving a therapist access to the graphs and the opportunity to discuss them with a client which led to improvements with that person but not the next client (for whom the graph might not be available). The exact mechanisms underpinning the benefits will need to be revealed by future research, but for the time being it is sufficient to know that progress monitoring and feedback is beneficial.

With these concerns addressed, the clinical psychologist who collects data on session-to-session progress will be in a position to start to provide feedback once three sessions of data are collected. Take for example the data from a client with agoraphobia that is depicted in Figure 4.3. The client had been on antidepressant medications before coming to see the psychologist and there had been no changes in medication. The psychologist had begun a programme of cognitive behaviour therapy. The session with the client might have an interaction such as follows:

THERAPIST: Thank you for completing the questionnaires so reliably. Since the last time we reviewed the graph at the fifth session you can see that the amount of psychological distress that you reported increased. I wonder if you could tell me what you think might have been going on then?

CLIENT: I think that was when I had to start confronting the situations that I was afraid of. I found it all too much and I was about to give up.

T: But you didn't give up and what happened then?

C: My distress has come right down.

T: That's right. It has come back into the improving range which is great to see and the distress has continued to decline. To what extent does this match with your experience?

C: When things were deteriorating I was a mess and that fits, but I don't feel close to the healthy range. There are still so many normal things that I cannot do.

T: You have a sense that the questions that make up the scale aren't fully capturing the agoraphobia?

C: I guess so. They ask me about recent anxiety and stuff, but my anxiety really depends on what I've got to do. How depressed I'm feeling also seems to depend on whether I have panic attacks or not.

T: That's an interesting observation. Throughout this whole time your medication has been stable, yet your mood has been going up and down in response to events in your life.

C: I feel the medication takes the edge off my depression.

T: So, if the medication is stable and taking the edge off some of the feelings, what might explain the fluctuations?

C: When things go badly, then I get depressed.

T: When things go badly, what does it mean to you?

C: Isn't that obvious? When I get a panic, then I feel like I'm never going to get over this anxiety.

T: Can I check I've understood what happens. When you have a panic, you think, 'Oh no, I'll never recover' and then you start to feel more depressed.

C: That's right.

In the preceding interaction you can see that the clinical psychologist was able to use the graph to elicit thoughts from the client that could be used if the therapist was going to engage in cognitive restructuring. The therapist was also able to challenge the view that the medication was responsible for all mood improvements, with a view to ultimately helping the client to perceive their role as an active manager of their own mood, rather than as a passive responder. The client seemed comfortable both with an idiographic interpretation, comparing their own scores with earlier data points, and also with normative comparisons when the bands were used to interpret. One outstanding issue the clinical psychologist would need to return to was the point that the scale did not capture the agoraphobia. The clinician would need to address this point by noting that the scale is a 'mental health thermometer' and is not intended to measure all symptoms, but to capture psychological distress. Maybe it would be time to suggest some more pertinent assessments that focus on panic and agoraphobia and the scores on these instruments could be compared with the pre-treatment levels.

In summary, the monitoring of progress through treatment is possible with the repeated administration of appropriate scales. Using this practice-based evidence it is possible to identify potential treatment failures and to more accurately target treatment and reduce deterioration.

Linking assessment to treatment: case formulation

5

Case formulation is a

> hypothesis about the causes, precipitants, and maintaining influences of a person's psychological, interpersonal, and behavioral problems. A case formulation helps organize information about a person, particularly when that information contains contradictions or inconsistencies in behavior, emotion, and thought content. Ideally, it contains structures that permit the therapist to understand these contradictions and to categorize important classes of information with a sufficiently encompassing view of the patient. A case formulation also serves as a blueprint guiding treatment and as a marker for change. It should also help the therapist experience greater empathy for the patient and anticipate possible ruptures in the therapy alliance. (Eells, 2007a, p. 4)

The above quote by Eells highlights that a case formulation links the client and his or her problems with the treatment. It captures both the strengths and the weaknesses of the client, thereby placing the problem and the potential resolution in the context of the whole person. To use a metaphor, if the treatment is the locomotive and the client's problems are the carriages, then the case formulation is the coupling that holds the two together. Without the coupling, a treatment might chug along nicely but it will fail to bring about any movement in the problems. In addition, case formulation enhances the therapeutic relationship by fostering a deeper understanding of and responsiveness to the client.

Clients present to a professional psychologist with a large quantity of information. There is information specific to the presenting problem, but there is also historical, familial, demographic, cultural, medical, educational, and social information. Some of this ancillary information will have direct bearing on the presenting problem, some will provide a background and context to the problem, and other information will be largely irrelevant to the problem. In addition to this descriptive information, psychologists will aim to identify the personal meaning of the information. They will try to understand the client's experience of events and the way that they interpret them. The psychologist's task is to distil the relevant information quickly and efficiently into a treatment plan. It is the case formulation that provides the link. As shown in Figure 5.1, information about a client passes through the 'lens' of the theoretical and empirical literature and is channelled into a case formulation. The case formulation provides the coupling between diagnostic and assessment information and clinical decisions about treatment planning. Case formulation itself can be broken down into the eight steps illustrated in the callout box in the figure and described later in this chapter. As indicated by the two-way arrows, case formulation is not a one-off event. The process of assessment, formulation, and treatment planning continues to cycle throughout therapy as a client's progress is measured and monitored.

While there are a variety of psychotherapy case formulations, they typically share much common ground (see Eells, 1997b, 2007b). We will begin with a behavioural functional

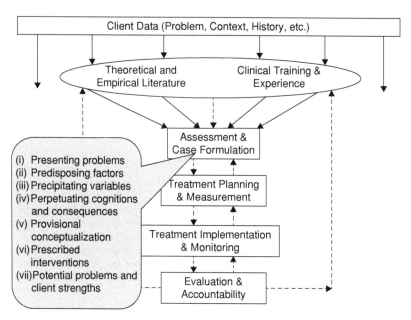

Figure 5.1 The process of linking client data to treatment decisions using case formulation.

analysis, extend this model to include cognitions, and then considered case formulations from an interpersonal psychotherapy perspective as these specifically include interpersonal aspects in the formulation.

Behavioural case formulation: functional analysis

One area where the core elements of a behavioural case formulation have been used with great success is in the area of developmental disabilities. Behavioural case formulation uses hypothesis-driven approaches to identify the function of a given behaviour and then uses this understanding in planning treatment (Repp, Karsh, Munk, & Dahlquist, 1995; Turkat, 1985). This approach has received empirical support, such as from Carr, Robinson, and Palumbo (1990), who noted that the success with non-aversive treatments was higher when the treatment was based upon an assessment of the functional relationship between environmental variables and the problem behaviours (see also Schulte, 1997). This analysis of functional relationships is called a 'functional analysis'. *A functional analysis involves the identification of important, controllable, causal functional relationships applicable to a specified set of target behaviours for an individual client* (Haynes & O'Brien, 1990). Let us examine each component of the definition in turn.

The causal variables must be important and controllable. In other words, those that explain a relatively large proportion of the variance are probably going to be more useful in treatment. They must also be controllable. For instance, a history of child abuse may be an important causal variable in the psychopathology of an adult client, but because it is no longer controllable (for this particular individual) it is not going to be an appropriate target for intervention. The aim of a functional analysis is not to 'explain' behaviour in terms of identifying all of the important causal variables, but the aim is to identify those that can be

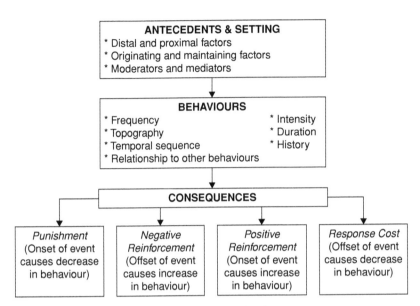

Figure 5.2 The three main components of a functional analysis.

manipulated (i.e., those under control of client and/or therapist). The purpose of identifying causal variables is so that you know which ones to modify.

Thus, the focus is upon the effects treatment has on the target behaviour. This target behaviour will exist within a broader array of behaviours. Ultimately, these behaviours exist within social systems and therefore, a functional analysis will require a consideration of the action of any changes on other aspects of the system and the bidirectional effects that these will have upon the target behaviour.

In practice, the chief elements of a functional analysis involve identifying three sets of variables; A for Antecedents, B for Behaviours, and C for Consequences (see Figure 5.2). The first set of variables in the functional analysis comprises the *antecedents*. The antecedents are those variables which are both *proximal* in time and those which are more *distal* to the behaviour. Identification of the antecedents also separates the variables that were important in the *origin* of the problem as distinct from those which are involved in the *maintenance* of the problem. Antecedents can also be divided into those which are moderators or mediators. Moderators have a direct effect on the behaviour in question, whereas mediators serve to influence a relationship between two variables. For example, a stressor such as a threatened assault might have a direct (or moderating) effect upon anxiety, whereas cognitions about being helpless in the face of possible death during the threat would have an indirect, or mediating effect on anxiety. The worrying thoughts would mediate the relationship between the threat and anxiety, by amplifying the influence of the threat upon the anxiety response.

The second set of variables examined in a functional analysis is the *behaviour* itself. The behaviour can be described in terms of its frequency, duration, intensity, and topography (such as the typical and more unusual patterns). Behaviours can also be examined in terms of their temporal sequence, their history, and their relationships with other behaviours. While the term 'behaviour' may conjure up images of actions, the term is typically used broadly to include physiological responses and cognitions.

BEHAVIOUR

		Increases	Decreases
	Onset	Positive Reinforcement	Punishment
EVENT			
	Offset	Negative Reinforcement	Response Cost

Figure 5.3 Four categories of behavioural consequences.

The final components of a functional analysis are the *consequences* of any behaviour. Traditionally, consequences have been divided into four categories based upon whether the event is turned on or off, and whether the behaviour increases or decreases (see Figure 5.3).

When the onset of an event causes an increase in a behaviour, the event is said to be a *positive reinforcer*. For instance, if a teacher responds with attention each time an otherwise disruptive child sits in his seat, the likelihood of 'in seat' behaviour will be increased. Positive reinforcers do not necessarily need to be pleasant; however, many pleasant events do make effective positive reinforcers.

When the onset of an event causes a decrease in behaviour, the event is called a *punisher*. For example, if a parent responds with criticism and ridicule every time a child plays a wrong note on a musical instrument, the probability of the child continuing to play the instrument is reduced and the ridicule and criticism would be defined as 'punishment'. Once again, just as positive reinforcers do not necessarily need to be pleasant, punishers do not need to be aversive, but many aversive events make effective punishers.

When the offset of an event causes an increase in behaviour, the event is said to be a *negative reinforcer*. For example, drinking alcohol in the early morning to alleviate the 'hangover' effects of a previous night's excessive drinking increases the probability of future early morning drinking.

Finally, when the offset of an event causes a decrease in some behaviour, this is called *response cost*. An example of a response cost is when the frequency of a child's shouting in class is reduced as a consequence of not permitting her to play during the lunch hour. The removal of the break was the cost incurred each time the child made the undesirable response and hence the behaviour would decline.

These four categories of behavioural consequences appear straightforward, but warrant careful reflection. Consider your response if you heard on breakfast radio that you could win $1,000 if you were the first caller to correctly identify the number of Australian prime ministers to date. You might well feel inclined to call up and have a guess, even if you were not sure; after all you have nothing to lose and $1,000 to gain.

Now compare how you might respond if you opened a letter from a radio station which contained $1,000 for you to keep and the accompanying letter asked you to call the station and let them know how many British prime ministers or American presidents there have been to date. The letter noted that if you were incorrect, then you would be required to return the money. Presumably, you would put the money into your wallet and not risk losing the money by calling the radio station and giving the wrong answer.

The first example was an instance of positive reinforcement and the second was an instance of response cost. If your reactions were similar to those described you would agree that in this context, the positive reinforcer encouraged (guessing) behaviour, whereas response cost inhibited (guessing) behaviour. Therefore, if you were identifying consequences that might be beneficial for a socially anxious girl and an impulsive boy, you might well choose to implement positive reinforcement as a way to draw out the girl and use response cost to curb the impulsiveness of the boy.

These concepts have been applied in the area of developmental disabilities to understand the existence of many problem behavioural excesses, such as self-injurious behaviour. In identifying the reasons for a behaviour three variables have been identified as important when making case formulations. These three variables are (i) positive reinforcement, (ii) negative reinforcement, and (iii) automatic reinforcement (Iwata, Vollmer, & Zarcone, 1990b; also called 'stimulation' by Carr, 1977). The third category of automatic reinforcement refers to the strengthening of behaviour by the consequences directly produced by a behaviour. Examples of this behaviour include rocking and rhythmic or repetitive behaviours. Technically, these behaviours could be explained in terms of the four types of reinforcement outlined in Figure 5.3, but the term is useful for describing situations where there does not appear to be any reinforcement being derived from the external environment. In the instances described, the sensory feedback itself appears to be reinforcing, so that when the sensory feedback is removed, the behaviour is extinguished (e.g., Rincover, 1978).

To identify the function of behaviour one can use three methods of assessment. First, the psychologist can use *indirect assessments*. Indirect assessments depend on questioning an observer about the occurrence and non-occurrence of the behaviour in question. These can be done with unstructured interviews or with the use of structured questionnaires (e.g., O'Neill, Horner, Albin, Storey, & Sprague, 1990; Durand & Crimmins, 1988). Second, the psychologist can use *analogue assessments*, in which artificial conditions are constructed to test hypotheses about the hypothesized reinforcers. For instance, a control condition can be contrasted with situations involving negative reinforcement, positive reinforcement, and automatic reinforcement, and the influence upon the behaviour of the schedules of reinforcement can be measured. The results of such an assessment might identify the reinforcer controlling a given behaviour (e.g., Iwata, Dorsey, Slifer, Bauman, & Richman, 1982). Third, the psychologist may identify the reinforcement contingencies that are in operation by conducting *naturalistic assessments*. That is, the behaviour is observed in its natural setting, and changes in the frequency and topography are measured as different contingencies occur (or are established).

A case example

This adaptation of functional analysis applied in the context of developmental disabilities can be illustrated by considering the presence of problem behaviours in a child with self-injurious behaviour. A 7-year-old boy, Sebastian, with severe mental retardation came to the attention of the psychologist following referral by the teacher. Sebastian would engage in tantrums that involved screaming and self-injury. The psychologist began with an interview with the teacher to obtain a description of the problem behaviour. The teacher described that he would suddenly begin to scratch at his face and forearms, beginning by pinching and squeezing the skin, which could escalate into banging his head and face with his hands. Thus, the psychologist had developed a description of the problem behaviour and thus, it was necessary to identify the antecedents of the problem behaviour. To this end, the teacher had reported that these outbursts occurred infrequently during class time, but were most common during breaks and lunchtime. However, she was unclear what consequences were maintaining the behaviour. Therefore, the psychologist collected baseline data, recording the events that occurred during each break (since this was the time with the most likelihood of observing the behaviour) and then calculating the probability of the behaviour's occurrence and non-occurrence in a one-minute interval. These formal assessments revealed that the self-injurious behaviour was more probable (i.e., 62%) when the supervising teacher was attending to another child. The probability of self-injurious behaviour was lower (i.e., 38%) when the supervising teacher was only observing the other children or attending to Sebastian. Thus, a working hypothesis was formed that there was a relationship between the self-injurious behaviour and the perceived withdrawal of attention. To test this working hypothesis, an additional teacher was assigned at one break, who then spent the time ensuring that his attention was allocated to Sebastian. When this occurred, the probability of self-injurious behaviour dropped to 0%, thus giving the psychologist confidence in the working hypothesis. This last component of the functional analysis, when the psychologist tests the working hypothesis by manipulating contingencies, is referred to as 'clinical experimentation' by Turkat and Maisto (1985). This step can often be overlooked since it takes time and effort to test a working hypothesis; however, it represents a sound step for clinical practice. Without testing in a potentially accountable manner, the risk is that a treatment strategy will be embarked upon that is misguided and potentially ineffective. If the psychologist waits for the outcome of treatment to gauge validity of the formulation, then it may well be too late, as the client has decided that therapy is ineffective and dropped out or changed psychologists.

In summary, a functional analytic strategy identifies the Antecedents of a Behaviour and its Consequences. The consequences are divided into four categories, namely punishment, negative reinforcement, positive reinforcement, and response cost. A working hypothesis is then developed and tested, which identifies which particular contingency is related to the problem behaviour. At this point a treatment will be developed which will aim to modify the contingencies that are controlling the problem behaviour. Functional analyses have been useful in the domain of developmental disabilities, but their usefulness is much broader (e.g., see a discussion by Ward, Nathan, Drake, Lee, & Pathé, 2000 of formulation-based treatments for sexual offenders). Although a very powerful clinical tool (Wolpe & Turkat, 1985), one limitation of a functional analysis is that it does not make reference to the cognitions that may occur between the antecedent and the consequence.

Cognitive behavioural case formulation

Persons and Tomkins (2007) outline an approach to case formulation that extends upon the functional analysis described in a number of ways. The most obvious extension is that it includes an assessment of cognitive beliefs and attitudes (see Beck, 1995; Freeman, 1992;

Muran & Segal, 1992; Turkat & Maisto, 1985 for other examples). We will first review their model and indicate where it overlaps with or complements a functional analytic strategy. Following identifications of some limitations of their approach, we will outline ways to address these limitations.

Problem list

Persons and Tompkins (2007) suggest that a cognitive behavioural case formulation begins with obtaining a comprehensive problem list. This is a comprehensive, descriptive, concrete list of the presenting problem(s) and any other difficulties that the client may have. The emphasis is upon the comprehensive nature of the list, in order to ensure that no difficulty is omitted or overlooked. In the language of the functional analysis introduced earlier, the problem list is analogous to the Behaviour of the ABC.

Assign a DSM diagnosis

Psychologists are next invited to consider the diagnoses that may be applicable and appropriate. In keeping with the functional analytic principles outlined by Haynes and O'Brien (1990) in which attention is focused on variables that are important, causal, and controllable, they suggest that the principle of parsimony means that the diagnosis selected is the one that accounts for the largest number of items on the problem list (i.e., is 'important' and 'causal') and is a target for change (i.e., controllable). The diagnosis provides a link to the literature on evidence-based theories and treatments, but on its own a diagnosis is limited. A diagnosis is a description of a clustering of signs and symptoms and it lacks a theory to explain their co-occurrence.

Select a nomothetic formulation of the anchoring diagnosis

The psychologist then investigates the literature surrounding the anchoring diagnosis, searching for an evidence-based nomothetic formulation. That is, since 'nomothetic' describes the study of groups of individuals, a nomothetic formulation is an explanation of the type typically found in the literature that serves to provide an account of all people who have a diagnosis. It complements a diagnostic description, by giving a causal explanation of why the symptoms occur and how they are related. By extension, the targets for treatment become evident. An example would be Rapee and Heimberg's (1997) model of social anxiety disorder or Clark's (1986) model of panic disorder. Importantly, the nomothetic formulation is not an end point. Rather, it provides a template for the development of an idiographic, or individualized, formulation.

Individualize the template

The psychologist collects additional information concerning cognitive, behavioural, emotional, and somatic aspects of the problem. The relationships between the variables are examined. The goal is to take the nomothetic explanation and apply it to the particular client. For example, Rapee and Heimberg's model makes no reference to alcohol problems or depression, both of which are commonly comorbid with social anxiety disorder. Therefore, to provide a complete account of a client who may also have depression and alcohol problems that are intimately related to the social phobia, a more complete explanation is needed. By individualizing the nomothetic template a comprehensive account is possible.

Propose hypotheses about the origins of the mechanisms

The psychologist then aims to generate hypotheses about (i) how the client has developed the cognitive schemata that underlie the problems, (ii) how the dysfunctional behaviours were learned, (iii) how functional behaviours were not acquired, (iv) how emotional regulation deficits were acquired, and (v) the origins of any genetic or biological vulnerability.

Describe precipitants of the current episode or symptom exacerbation

The clinical psychologist will enquire about the activating situations and precipitating events. The client can be asked, but family members can also provide insights into the relevant factors. Precipitants are analogous to the Antecedents within functional analysis. That is, precipitants are the events or stimuli that case the particular problem in a particular context. Activating situations are also antecedents, but refer to those that explain the problem more generally and explain the consistency across situations.

The strengths of Persons and Tompkins' (2007) approach are that (i) the process of diagnostic assignment is assigned a key role and (ii) the nomothetic formulations are linked explicitly with idiographic accounts. The chief weaknesses are that (i) it fails to describe how the hypotheses are linked to particular treatments or treatment plans and (ii) there is no encouragement to identify potential obstacles to treatment.

A model of case formulation

Thus, our preference is to organize case formulation under a modified set of headings: (i) Presenting problems, (ii) Predisposing factors, (iii) Precipitating variables, (iv) Perpetuating cognitions and consequences, (v) Provisional conceptualization, (vi) Prescribed interventions, and (vii) Potential problems and client strengths. In the course of the initial assessment interview(s), the psychologist will identify the main problem and any ancillary concerns (i.e., the *Presenting problems*), identify any experiences, social, familial or cultural issues, and temperamental factors that may set the stage for the emergence of the problem or that may influence the manifestation of the problem (i.e., *Predisposing factors*). The proximal and distal *Precipitants* of the origin problem will be identified, as well as the precipitants of the problem behaviours in the current episode. The next step will be to identify the cognitive and behavioural factors that *Perpetuate* the problem and then link the preceding information into a *Problem conceptualization* that will look backwards (and explain the origins of the problem), look around (and understand the current problem), and look forward (and make a prognosis, *Prescribe treatment* options, and identify *Potential problems* to treatment and client strengths) (see Figure 5.4).

A case example

To illustrate these various components of a cognitive behavioural case formulation, an annotated case illustration will be presented next. An example of how the worksheet (Figure 5.4) can be completed follows the case example of a client with panic disorder with agoraphobia.

Presenting problems

THERAPIST: What's brought you here today?

CLIENT: I've been suffocating, all of a sudden for no reason. My doctor tells me there's nothing wrong but she's never done a test when it's happening.

Cognitive Behavioural Case Formulation Worksheet

Presenting problems

1. _____ 2. _____

3. _____ 4. _____

5. _____ 6. _____

Predisposing factors

1. _____ 2. _____

3. _____ 4. _____

Precipitating variables

1. _____ 2. _____

3. _____ 4. _____

Perpetuating cognitions and consequences

Cognitions   Behavioural Consequences

_____   _____

_____   _____

_____   _____

Problem conceptualization

Prescribed interventions

1. _____ 2. _____

3. _____ 4. _____

Potential problems and Client Strengths

1. _____ 2. _____

3. _____ 4. _____

Figure 5.4 Cognitive Behavioural Case Formulation Worksheet.

T: What's it like when you start suffocating?

C: Well I can be sort of normal one minute and then, bang, it's like the panic button gets pushed and I've just got to get out of there to get some air. I start to choke and my throat closes over like I'm going to suffocate. If I don't get some air I'm sure I'll pass out, die, or something like that.

T: This lack of air is so great it's as if you are going to die.

C: That's right. No one seems to understand and they all say that I'm not going to suffocate, that there is plenty of air, that my lungs are OK, but it doesn't help. I know there's plenty of air, but no one seems to understand that the air isn't getting where it should. I don't need anyone to tell me that these problems are in my head. I can feel these sensations in my body. My heart pounds, I feel dizzy, my legs go to jelly. I even get tingling in my hands. Try to tell me that's not a sign of suffocation!

T: It's a pretty serious problem to have all these signs of suffocation. I'd be quite worried if I started suffocating out of the blue.

C: Out of the blue, that's how it is. I'll be walking along one minute and then my body just packs up and there's no air.

The psychologist is starting to build up a picture of the client's presenting problem. The problem for the psychologist is trying to balance the need to collect information on the symptoms and the need to establish a good rapport that will provide a foundation for the rest of the assessment and intervention. The client is making it clear that she feels a lack of understanding about her problems and is trying to convince the psychologist of the reality of the problems. Therefore, while additional material would be gleaned later in the interview about the problem, the psychologist has enough information to start building a profile of the problem. Specifically, the client is describing an experience that involves the sudden unexpected distressing bodily sensations (heart pounding, dizziness, choking, shortness of breath, and tingling in the extremities) that the client believes, despite reassurance to the contrary, are signs of possibly life-threatening suffocation.

Precipitating variables

Following a discussion of the problem, the psychologist decided that the interview would flow best if the precipitating variables were considered next.

T: Thanks for telling me about how you feel during one of the suffocating episodes. I'd like to talk some more about what they are like and the effect they are having on your life a little later, but, if it's OK with you, for the time being I'd like to concentrate on what triggers the suffocation. Could you tell me about the most recent time you felt you might suffocate?

C: I was out to dinner with some friends; a hen's night actually. I was a bit worried that I might not feel well and have to leave. Since it was Claire's hen's night I felt that I really couldn't walk out on her, so I was extra worried. Before I got to the restaurant, I got hot and flustered because I couldn't find a parking spot. I was driving round and around thinking, 'If I don't get a spot quickly, then I'll be late and all the seats near the door will be gone.'

T: And if they were all gone?

C: I wouldn't be able to get out for some air without everyone noticing. And that's just what happened. I walk in all hot and bothered only to find that the only seat left is the one at the end of the table, right down the back of the restaurant.

T: So what did you do?

C: I just felt like leaving right then and there, but I didn't. I took a couple of deep big breaths and took my seat. The moment I sat down I knew it was all over. My throat tightened up and my chest started to hurt. I started to breathe faster to get some air, but the air in the restaurant was too hot. It wouldn't get into my lungs no matter how hard I breathed – perhaps it was the spices in the cooking – but whatever it was, I knew I just had to get out.

T: What if you didn't get out?

C: I'd probably pass out or die. I don't know exactly, because I gave some excuse about having forgotten to put some money in the parking meter and I left. Just like that. I got up, walked out, and never went back.

After discussing these situations the psychologist continues:

T: Have you always had these episodes of suffocation?

C: When I was young I used to have asthma attacks, but they've stopped. Anyway, the asthma attacks were different. I can't really describe it in words, but I know an asthma attack and these feelings of suffocation are different. They're not wheezy, like asthma.

T: After the asthma attacks stopped was there a time before these episodes of suffocation began?

C: Yes, the asthma stopped in my teens and the suffocation didn't start until my mid-20s.

T: Was there anything going on around the time they started?

C: It was a pretty horrible time in my life. Things were pretty stressed at work. There were lots of people being made redundant and there was a new round of redundancies in the wind. I went to a party and everyone was smoking dope. I hadn't smoked before because of my asthma, but I figured that since it was gone I deserved a bit of relaxation. The first few puffs were OK, but then I started to feel short of breath, my throat started to close up, and I started to think I was having an asthma attack. I stopped smoking and ran outside to get some fresh air.

From this section of the interview you will notice that the psychologist is asking about precipitating events, but the client's answers are blurring into the next section, namely the perpetuating cognitions and consequences. This is not a problem and your job is to use the case formulation as a template to filter and organize information. Even if you are asking about one domain and the client gives information about another, you can keep that information in mind for later. Nonetheless, a series of precipitants were evident.

The psychologist covers both the precipitants of the present attacks and those of the first panic. This is important because the initial precipitants will assist the psychologist in presenting a formulation that covers both the initial onset as well as the maintenance of the problem. In terms of the current precipitants a number of elements can be gleaned from the interview. First, it is clear that the client is apprehensive about the event even before she arrives. This anticipatory anxiety is setting the stage for a panic attack. Second, building on this foundation of anticipatory anxiety is the failure to find a parking spot, which increases the worry and encourages her to rush, which in turn generates a number of bodily sensations – becoming hot and breathing rapidly. Third, upon entering the restaurant she takes a series of big deep breaths, effectively hyperventilating. Hyperventilation produces a number of bodily sensations which are able to exacerbate the sensations of panic (Andrews et al., 2003; Hazlett-Stevens, & Craske, 2009); these sensations include feelings of choking and smothering among others. Finally, the atmosphere of the restaurant appears to have exacerbated the feelings. It appears to have been hot and this could have increased feelings of discomfort given that the client was already reporting feeling hot and bothered from driving around looking for a parking spot. However, in addition to all these triggers is it clear that the client is not just a passive recipient of environmental stimuli; she is actively processing the information. Thus, the clinician can expand upon these cognitions and identify the consequences (e.g., punishment, negative reinforcement, positive reinforcement, or response cost) of any actions the client takes.

Perpetuating cognitions and consequences

T: You have told me about a lot of things that seemed to trigger these sensations of suffocation, but I wonder if you could tell me more about what you were thinking. What is the last thought you remember before the feelings of suffocation were at their worst?

C: When they were at their worst I don't think I was thinking anything. I just go blank.

T: What was the last thought you remember before going blank?

C: I thought, 'I've just got to get out.'

T: Why did you need to get out?

C: I needed fresh air. I've found that when I'm suffocating, getting out and into the fresh air sometimes helps.

T: What if you hadn't been able to get out?

C: That was what I was worried about. I was sure that I was going to run out of air. The restaurant was full of people, the door was closed, and there was an open fire in the kitchen out the back.

T: An open fire?

C: You know a BBQ type of thing where they were cooking the steaks. I could see the flames coming up and I know that flames use oxygen to burn.

T: So, the fire was using up the oxygen in the room?

C: And because the door was closed and the restaurant was full, the oxygen was getting used up. If I had been able to sit closer to the door I might have been able to get more oxygen, but being close to the kitchen meant that I had less oxygen.

T: Had anyone else noticed the lack of oxygen?

C: No. I think I've got some sort of allergy that makes me sensitive to the absence of air. I've read about this disease called Undine's Curse where babies die because they aren't sensitive to oxygen or carbon dioxide or something so they don't breathe enough. I've worried I might have that, but all the doctors say my heart and lungs are fine.

T: Does their reassurance help?

C: For a while, but once the suffocation comes back again I think, 'What do they know. If they had done their tests while I was suffocating, the readings would be different.'

T: You can't remember what you were thinking when the feelings of suffocation were at their worst, but do you remember how you were feeling?

C: Really panicky, freaked out. My heart was beating so fast and I was really scared I was going to die.

T: And then what happened to these feelings when you left?

C: Once I got out into the cool air, they melted away. I walked away from the restaurant and after a few minutes of letting myself breathe the rich air I started to feel the oxygen flooding through me. I didn't have to breathe so quickly and I knew that I was going to be OK. Well, sort of OK.

T: Sort of OK?

C: Well, I wasn't going to suffocate, but then I started to think about my friends. They would all be sitting there waiting for me to come back, but there was no way I was going back. By the time I got back to the car I had tears running down my face. They were tears of relief that I had got out alive as well as tears of shame that I couldn't even sit in a restaurant without leaving. Why can't I be normal?

In terms of the cognitions associated with the situation, the client was interpreting the sensations as consistent with fears that she was going to suffocate. The environment was scanned to provide information (e.g., the fire was consuming the oxygen) to justify the belief that the sensations of choking and chest pain were signals of imminent death through suffocation. However, it is more plausible that the physical sensations were a normal consequence of worry and anxiety, combined with sensations generated by exertion, and exacerbated by hyperventilation (Andrews et al., 2003; Page, 2002b; Taylor, 2000).

It is also apparent that there was a clear contingency between the client's actions and the intensity of the panicky feelings. After the client had fled the situation, the unpleasant experience of anxiety and panic reduced (albeit to be replaced by feelings of shame, embarrassment, and distress), increasing the probability of future avoidance. Thus, their avoidance would be maintained by negative reinforcement. In addition, it is clear that the client would not be able to test the validity (or otherwise) of her beliefs about the lack of oxygen. Had she remained, she would have been able to attest to the fact that the oxygen would not have run out, she would not have suffocated and died. However, the client escaped without ever finding out if the threat would prove fatal.

Predisposing factors

So far the sections of the interview that have been reproduced do not reveal the background to the problem. Thus, to help the psychologist to contextualize the problem, it is important to consider the variables that may have predisposed the client to the attacks of panic.

> T: You have described some pretty terrifying experiences, all of which seem to involve intense feelings of suffocation. Feeling you are about to suffocate leads you to do the only sensible thing, which is to get out and get to a place where there is more air. I wonder if you have thought about where this all has come from?
>
> C: I don't really know, but my mother was pretty highly strung and worried about everything. When I was a child she worried a lot about my asthma. There were certainly lots of kids at school who were worse than me, but she kept insisting that we went to the doctor or emergency room to get me checked out. It seemed to make her feel better when they said I was OK.
>
> T: How's you asthma now?
>
> C: The doctors say they can't find a trace of it but sometimes I think I've taken on the role of my mother, looking after my health.
>
> T: You described your mother as 'highly strung'. Are you like your mother in this respect?
>
> C: I've always been a nervous person. I've worried about my health for as long as I can remember.

From this interaction, the psychologist was able to establish a couple of hints about predisposing variables. First, it seems it could be that the mother was high on trait anxiety or neuroticism and this family trait has passed on to her daughter, perhaps through inheritance or learning. Second, the health behaviour of her mother regarding her asthma could well have established a pattern for dealing with these sensations. That is, there is a similar pattern of concern about symptoms of suffocation, followed by an escape response that reduces the distressing emotion. Thus, the psychologist is in a position to start to develop a formulation and present this to the client for feedback.

Provisional conceptualization

In this instance, the psychologist suggested that the client's personality was likely to reveal elevations on neuroticism, which set the stage for the development of an anxiety disorder. The experience of management of asthma attacks provided a template for health behaviour that involved worry about symptoms and escape and reassurance seeking as ways to reduce the distress associated with possible illnesses. Against this backdrop, each individual attack began with awareness of a particular bodily sensation or set of sensations (e.g., shortness of breath). These sensations were misinterpreted as signals of impending danger, which in turn triggered the anxiety (or fight or flight) response. Increased respiration, a normal part of the anxiety response, led to hyperventilation in the absence of either flight or fighting, which in turn produced more sensations. Together, these sensations would be misinterpreted as signals for suffocation, and so on in a vicious circle of panic (see Figure 5.5). The spiral would be ultimately broken by flight, which would involve action (thereby reducing the effects of hyperventilation).

What is important to note is that the formulation of the panic attack is not original to the present authors. Rather it draws on the literature about panic attacks and the seminal work of David Clark (1986) conceptualizing the panic in terms of a cognitive model. Substantial research laid an empirical foundation for the proposal of the model and subsequently much research has supported the model (see Pilecki, Arentoft, & McKay, 2011; Taylor, 2000). Given this, it is not surprising that the model serves as a useful clinical heuristic. It allows the clinician to organize the information provided by the client. It permits the clinician to take

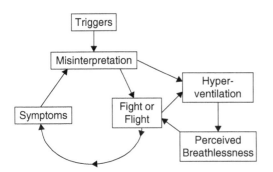

Figure 5.5 Clark's (1986) cognitive model of panic attacks (adapted from Andrews et al., 2003).

shortcuts by building upon the theoretical and empirical work of others. It was Isaac Newton who said, 'If I have seen further it is by standing on the shoulders of giants' (in a letter to Robert Hooke, 5 February 1675) and professional psychologists can likewise 'see further' in their clinical practice by standing on the 'shoulders' of those in psychology who have synthesized clinical experience, as well as the empirical and theoretical literatures, into a clear and useful model of a clinical condition.

Not every client will present in a way that so neatly fits into the 'textbook case'. Some will include elements that are not found in models published in the literature, others will present with a blending of two or more models, and still others will present with symptoms or patterns of symptoms that appear unique. The strength of a case formulation approach is that it is applicable in every instance. What varies is the degree to which the psychologist can draw upon existing theoretical and empirical literature and clinical experiences to conceptualize the case (see Turkat & Maisto, 1985 for examples of applying case formulations to novel symptom patterns).

When the case formulation is novel, the link to treatment will need to be clearly articulated and the greater the burden of proof will be upon the psychologist to test and demonstrate the validity of the model. Even when applying an existing model to a client, it is important to test the validity of the formulation. This can be done by presenting the formulation to the client in a formal manner and asking for feedback as to its ability to consolidate the client's problems. A further way is to test aspects of the formulation with psychometric tests (see Turkat & Maisto, 1985 for some examples). With the client in question a personality inventory (the NEO-PI-R; Costa & McCrae, 1992) was administered to determine if the trait anxiety was elevated. The SCL-90-R was also administered to provide a standardized broad pre-treatment assessment that could be used to evaluate changes during and post-treatment. The results of testing are displayed in Figure 5.6. The scores for the personality dimension of Neuroticism (N) are very high, consistent with the expectations; however, interestingly, conscientiousness (C) is very low. The low conscientiousness was not a theme that had emerged during the interview and suggested an area that required further investigation, particularly as it might indicate a problem for compliance with treatment. Extraversion (E), Openness (O), and Agreeableness were average. The SCL-90-R showed elevations on somatization, anxiety, and phobia which were all consistent with the reports of panic attacks. In addition, the elevation on the obsessive-compulsive, interpersonal sensitivity, and depression dimensions all suggested the existence of symptoms that have not been discussed in the sections reproduced. This highlights one advantage of using broad symptom measures at the outset

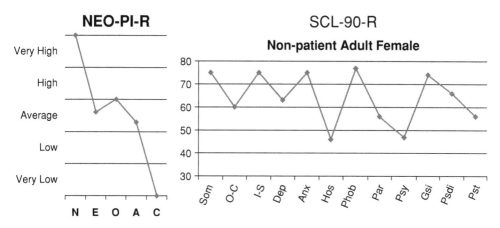

Figure 5.6 Results on the NEO-PI-R and the SCL-90-R of a female client with panic disorder and agoraphobia.

of treatment, in that they can identify areas of symptomatology that may have been ignored in the initial assessment interview(s).

A verbal interpretation of these test results was presented to the client along with the formulation and the client's response indicated that both seemed to summarize how she perceived herself. If anything, she expressed impatience and wanted to know what to do about these sensations.

Prescribed interventions

The evidence-based interventions for panic disorder and agoraphobia have been clearly documented in many difference sources (Andrews et al., 2003; Barlow, 2002; Clark & Salkovskis, 1996; Craske & Barlow, 2008; Sánchez-Meca, Rosa-Alcázar, Marín-Martínez, & Gómez-Conesa, 2010; Taylor, 2000). What is involved in these treatments will be discussed in later chapters, but for present purposes, the aim is to demonstrate the link between the formulation and treatment. This is displayed in Figure 5.7. The fear elicited by the trigger

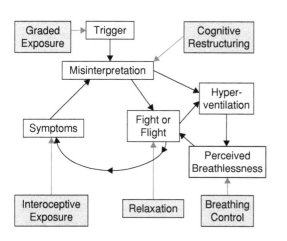

Figure 5.7 Adaptation of cognitive formulation to include treatments targeted at each component.

stimuli will be addressed using 'graded exposure', the misinterpretation of these triggers as potential threats will be addressed using 'cognitive restructuring', hyperventilation and its effects will be targeted using 'breathing control', anxiety about the bodily sensations will be treated with 'interoceptive exposure' (Forsyth, Fusé, & Acheson, 2009), and excessive reactivity of the fight or flight response will be dampened down with 'relaxation'. Thus, each important component of the model will be addressed with a particular treatment, and the rationale for each component can be demonstrated to the client with reference to the formulation. Importantly, the cognitive behavioural package that involves these components has been empirically validated in a variety of studies, lending further support to the use of these techniques (see Clum, Clum, & Surls, 1993; Cox, Endler, Lee, & Swinson, 1992; Gould, Otto, & Pollack, 1995; Mattick, Andrews, Hadzi-Pavlovic, & Christinesen, 1990; Taylor, 2000). In addition, there are studies demonstrating the individual efficacy of each component (Ito et al., 2001; Meuret, Wolitzky-Taylor, Twohig, & Craske, 2012; Rapee, Mattick, & Murrell, 1986; Michelson, Marchione, Greenwald, Testa, & Marchione, 1996; Öst & Westling, 1995; Salkovskis, Clark, & Hackman, 1991; Teachman, Marker, & Smith-Janik, 2008; Williams & Falbo, 1996).

Potential problems

The final component of a cognitive behavioural formulation (Figure 5.8) involves the identification of potential problems to treatment. The low conscientiousness identified by the NEO-PI-R (Costa & McCrae, 1992) represents a possible problem in treatment, suggesting that the compliance with treatment and homework exercises will need to be monitored carefully. The second problem, which flows more directly from the formulation, is the presence of worry and anxiety combined with the need for exposure to bodily sensations and situations associated with anxiety. It is likely that the client's motivation and their impatience to begin treatment will wane as the threat of elevated anxiety and panic looms; therefore these will need to be monitored and addressed if treatment is going to be successful.

This particular cognitive behavioural case formulation would represent a component of the entire clinical process outlined in Figure 5.1. As depicted in Figure 5.9, the case formulation (in the left hand callout box) represents the link between the client data and the treatment (in the right hand callout box).

Case formulations in interpersonal psychotherapy

Up to this point the discussion of case formulation began by describing behavioural (or functional) analyses and then developed this foundation into a broader cognitive behavioural formulation. However, it would be misleading to convey the impression that case formulations are unique to CBT. The diversity of case formulations is evident in Eells (2007b); however, not all of these therapies have strong empirical validation (Lipsitz & Markowitz, 2013). Therefore, we will review one more approach to case formulation to illustrate its application in evidence-based Interpersonal Psychotherapy (IPT) and in so doing contrast the approach with a cognitive behavioural formulation for the same case.

A case example

The transcript is designed to faithfully illustrate IPT as described in the treatment manual by Klerman, Weissman, Rounsaville, and Chevron (1984). To facilitate a synthesis with their work, many of the therapist's responses draw heavily from examples provided in their book.

Cognitive Behavioural Case Formulation Worksheet

Presenting problems

1. *Distressing bodily sensations* (*heart pounding, dizziness, choking, shortness of breath, and tingling in the extremities*)

2. *Fear of suffocation*_____   3. _____

4. _____   5. _____

Predisposing factors

1. *Parental anxiety*_____   2. _____

3. _____   4. _____

Precipitating variables

1. *Anticipatory worry*_____   2. *Situations where escape difficult*_____

3. _____   4. _____

Perpetuating cognitions and consequences

Cognitions   Behavioural Consequences

*I've just got to get out*_____   *Flee situation and panicky feelings decrease*

Sensations of shortness of breath mean I will   _____

*suffocate and die*_____   _____

Problem conceptualization

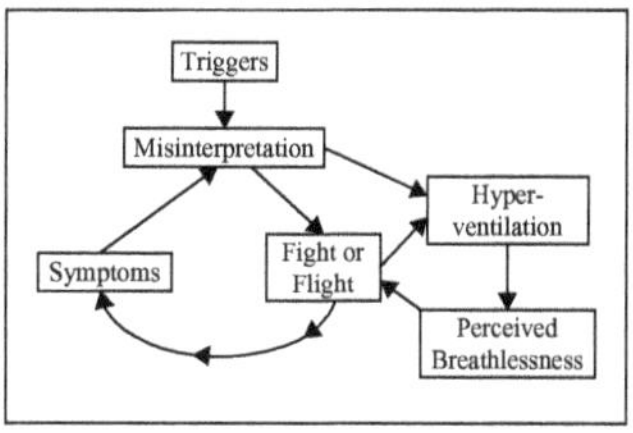

Prescribed interventions

1. *Graded exposure*_____   2. *Cognitive restructuring*_____

3. *Interoceptive exposure*_____   4. *Breathing control & relaxation*_____

Potential problems

1. *Low conscientiousness*_____   2. *Worry and anxiety about exposure*_____

3. _____   4. _____

Figure 5.8 Example of a completed Cognitive Behavioural Case Formulation Worksheet.

The client is an amalgam of individuals and draws upon a reference by Meighan, Davis, Thomas, and Droppleman (1999).

IPT is structured with three phases in mind. During the *early phase* an assessment is conducted to develop an interpersonal case formulation and a therapeutic contract is negotiated with the patient.[1] During the *middle phase* the psychotherapeutic work on one or two nominated problem areas is conducted, before the *termination phase* occurs. There are three tasks

---

[1] Note that the term 'patient' will be used in place of our term 'client'. IPT explicitly adopts a 'medical model' in which the therapeutic relationship is conceptualized in terms of a 'doctor and patient'.

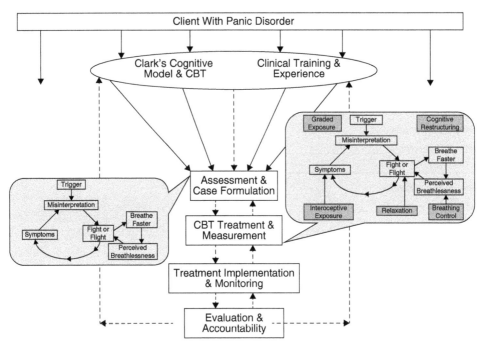

Figure 5.9 Inclusion of a particular case formulation for a client with panic disorder into a model of clinical practice.

to the early phase. These are to deal with the depression, conduct an interpersonal inventory, and negotiate the therapeutic contract.

Deal with the depression

IPT begins with the patient's problem. *Symptoms are systematically reviewed* with reference to diagnostic criteria, such as those outlined in the ICD or DSM systems. However, the process is not one of simply reading out a checklist and ticking off each item that is endorsed. It involves asking the person about the symptoms so that you gain a 'feel' for them. Once this is done the *diagnosis is confirmed* or communicated to the patient. This communication is an explicit statement that aims to make it clear that the cluster of symptoms is a whole. After this, is it possible to *explain the nature of depression* and identify ways that it can be *treated*. The patient is then encouraged to *adopt a sick role*. The psychologist is asked to legitimize the patient in the sick role without fostering dependency. Following Parsons (1951), the sick role means that the person is exempt from certain normal social obligations and certain types of responsibilities, and considered to be in a state that is socially defined as undesirable, to be gotten out of as quickly as possible. The person is in 'need of help' and should take on the role of patient, which means affirming that one is ill and cooperating with the doctor. The possible *value of medication* should be assessed, which for the psychologist would involve referral; but our experience is that most people who attend our clinic with depression have already consulted a general practitioner and been offered antidepressant medication. They have consulted a psychologist because they were reluctant to take medication, or stopped taking it due to side-effects, or the antidepressant has only been partially successful.

These steps are illustrated sequentially in the following excerpts. The interview opens with an examination of the problem and a systematic review of the symptoms. The client is a male in his late 20s who has presented with concerns about his mood.

THERAPIST: I was wondering if you could tell me what brought you here today?

PATIENT: Sure. Well, it began about two years ago now, after the birth of our son, Aubrey. Things seemed to be going very well and then the wheels fell off everything. My wife became really depressed. The depression was so bad that she had to see a psychiatrist, and then spent a few weeks in hospital. Things have really gone from bad to worse for me since then and I really don't know if I can cope any more. I think I'm catching her depression. That's why I came to see you, but I really don't want to be here because I should be able to cope, I should be able to keep things together. It's my wife who is sick and if I have a breakdown, then there will be no one left to look after Aubrey. I've got to be the stable one. I've got to keep the family together.

T: Life's been terribly difficult for you lately, with your wife's depression, your need to cope with everything that her being depressed entails, and starting to feel depressed yourself. We'll talk about each of these topics, but first of all, I wonder if we could talk about you and how you are feeling. I wonder if you could tell me something about these feelings of depression.

P: Well, I just feel empty all the time. I'm just like a hollow shell just doing the same things each day that I have to do, but there's no life left in me. I can't get out of bed in the morning, not only because I'm so tired due to not being able to go to sleep, but because I just haven't got any energy. I try to get myself motivated, but nothing appeals any more. I used to play golf, but I've given that up; and sex, well there's nothing in that department. I know they say that having a child is the most effective form of contraception known to man, but she's not up for it and quite frankly I could take it or leave it; and this is not like me at all. Eating too – I've lost 7kg in the past month because I can't seem to bring myself to eat. Food tastes bland and I just don't feel hungry.

T: These feelings seem to impact everything you do. Has this depression had an impact on your life; say looking after Aubrey or at work?

P: I've just received my second warning from my boss at work. I'm just not able to concentrate at work, so I keep making mistakes. Also, every couple of weeks I get a call from Suzanne, that's my wife, saying that she can't cope with Aubrey and I need to come home to rescue her before she does someone an injury. I'm just in a bind, I can't afford another mistake at work, but at the same time I worry that something bad will happen at home.

T: Often when people feel as depressed as you have been telling me you feel, they think about ending it all. Have you thought about killing yourself?

P: Every day. Usually as the day goes on I think about it more often, but I'd never do it. I'm all that there is holding the family together right now.

The therapist then moves on to confirm the diagnosis to the patient. The name of the disorder (in this case 'depression') is used. The use of the name is intended to organize what otherwise might be a group of seemingly unrelated symptoms into a condition that the psychologist knows about.

T: The feelings of depression, the lethargy, the lack of interest in previously pleasurable activities, the difficulties sleeping are all symptoms of depression. Although they don't seem to have a physical basis, this isn't to say that they aren't real. What you have told me are pieces to a puzzle, that when put together suggests to me these are all part of being depressed. Your eating and sleep are changed. You've lost interest in activities that you used to enjoy. Your thoughts about death, your tiredness, … are all part of the constellation of depression. Your symptoms are common ones for depressed persons.

P: So you really think I have depression? What am I going to do? When it was just Suzanne, that was bad enough, how are we going to manage?

The psychologist can respond to this question by leading in to a presentation of details about depression and its treatment.

> T: Depression has been called the common cold of mental disorders because it is so common. It affects about four out of every hundred adults at any one time. Although you may feel a lot of hopelessness right now, this is part of depression and the good news is that depression can respond to treatment. The outlook for your recovery is good. We know there are quite a few treatments that can reduce depression so many people with depression recover quite quickly with treatment. I expect that you will soon start to feel better and you will be able to resume your normal life and activities as the symptoms of depression decrease in response to treatment. One effective treatment for depression is Interpersonal Psychotherapy. It has been shown to be effective in a number of research trials. IPT helps you to understand the issues and difficulties that have produced this depression.
>
> P: Well I'm glad that you're hopeful, because quite frankly I've lost all hope. Life's just all too much for me right now. In fact, I can't even face up to having the parents-in-law over for dinner.

The next task for the therapist in IPT is to outline the 'sick role' to the patient.

> T: It's fine if you don't feel like being quite as sociable now. You are feeling depressed and so it's quite reasonable that since you are feeling so bad you won't be able to do many things you might feel you should. Perhaps you could speak to Suzanne and suggest that for the next month you'd like to keep social obligations to a minimum. The reason is that during the active phase of treatment for your depression we are going to be working towards your recovery. I expect you to be able to take up your normal life gradually. You will be able to become more active again, but for the time being the focus needs to be on getting you better.
>
> P: Can I tell Suzanne that you said this? I wouldn't want her to get the impression that I'm not handling everything. I've got to hold this family together. The way things are right now, I can't be the weak link.
>
> T: Yes you can, it's important that you talk with her and make sure that she is clear that you are going to need some time right now to work on yourself so that you are in a stronger position to help her.

For many psychologists, casting the patient in the sick role elicits a negative reaction. As a profession we are more likely to consider that clients need to take an active role in their recovery. In particular, psychologists who are expert at CBT will be familiar with the need to recruit and sustain motivation during treatment (Miller & Rollnick, 2012) and the importance of a collaborative relationship that includes homework activities. The notion that the 'patient' is 'sick' may feel like the psychologist is fostering dependency. These points are well taken, but take a moment to reflect on the experience of being depressed. The sufferer may have been struggling with their daily tasks and to the extent that they have not completed these, they may have felt a failure in meeting the real or projected expectations of others or themselves and the consequential guilt. Being instructed that treatment not only permits, but actually requires them and others to take things a bit easier could well make the person feel some relief from guilt and unattainable expectations. This is not to say that the psychologist should not consider the risks of fostering dependency, but that these risks need to be weighed up in light of the potential benefits.

Assess the interpersonal problems

Once the presenting problem has been addressed the interview moves to assess the interpersonal problems, and this begins with an Interpersonal Inventory. The psychologist asks questions to elicit information about what has been going on in the patient's present (or past) social and interpersonal life that is associated with the onset of the symptoms. Thus, the interview will focus upon important interactions, expectations of everyone in these important relationships, and the degree to which they are met. The satisfactory and unsatisfactory aspects of relationships are reviewed and the patient could be asked to identify ways they would like to change their relationships. The ultimate aim is to identify the main problem area or areas. Within an IPT framework there are four problem areas, which we prefer to summarize under the two headings of *Loss and Growth* and *Interpersonal Communication*. Under the heading of Loss and Growth, IPT identifies grief reactions (associated with the loss of a loved one) and role transitions. In a role transition the person loses past relationships and must grow into a new role and new relationships or ways of relating as they move from one stage of life to another (e.g., work to retirement, partner to parent, employee to manager, etc). Under the heading of Interpersonal Communication IPT identifies interpersonal role disputes (in which people in a relationship have unshared or unmet expectations) or interpersonal deficits.

T: Now, let's try to review what has been going on in your life. What else has been happening in your life about the time you started feeling bad?

P: As I said earlier, it seems that everything has happened since the birth of my son. Before Aubrey was born Suzanne seemed normal, and we had a great relationship. She seems to think that she was depressed, but I wasn't aware of anything.

T: Things seem to have changed after the birth.

P: I was so looking forward to our future together as a family. I had just got the promotion at work I'd been striving for, we now had the money to have a child and really give him the life that we wanted. But all that has changed. Before the birth, Suzanne was all clucky and maternal, but now she's so different. I've not seen that side of her before.

The patient is describing a role transition (from being a partner to being a parent), but what is also apparent, is that the patient is describing a loss. The patient is lamenting the loss of the previous relationship as well as the loss of the relationship that could have been. Both of these themes emerge during grief work, and for these reasons we tend to group the categories of grief and role transition under the same heading.

T: What is this side that you haven't seen before?

P: I'd get home and there she is holding the screaming baby. She hands me the baby and starts crying and screaming at me, blaming me for doing this to her. Then she collapses in tears saying she didn't mean it and she feels so guilty. All I know is that at one moment there was a crying baby to care for, then there was a crying wife to care for, and all I felt like doing was crying myself. The problem is there is no one to pass the baby to – the buck stops with me.

T: This seems like an incredible burden for you to carry.

P: I just wished I knew what to do. If she was a car I would have lifted up the bonnet, found the problem, fixed it and that would be the end to it, but nothing I did made any difference. This was the hardest thing to cope with – knowing that I couldn't fix it.

T: You felt hopeless even though you wanted to help your wife.

P: All I could do was hunker down for the duration. It was up to me to hold things together so I had to take care of them, no matter what the cost. I hate the way things are at work, but if that's what I've got to do, then that's what I'll do.

T: Do you take that 'hunker down' attitude home with you too?

P: I guess I'll do whatever it takes to get through this. I've tried to keep the peace at home. I had to sacrifice my own feelings. I didn't want Aubrey to be damaged by all this so I just put my feelings on hold.

T: This must have taken its toll on you.

P: I just feel so exhausted. I would get so tired doing my job at work and then coming home to another one when I got home. I'm on duty 24 hours a day, 7 days a week and all the time dreading the call from home when she'd say, 'you've got to come home, I can't take it another minute'.

T: It sounds like it took a toll on your relationship too.

P: There's no relationship between us anymore. We are just living day by day. It's like I've lost her and she's not even gone away. I'm learning that things have changed. There's nothing I can do to make her happy and I can't make myself happy now either.

T: What sort of things used to make you happy?

P: Work used to be my best source of happiness, but things have changed there.

T: How have they changed?

P: The promotion has changed everything. I used to just be able to do my job, but now I'm in charge of the whole purchasing department. I used to have heaps of friends at work, but now I don't know who my friends are. Sometimes I need to reprimand people who used to be my mates, and other people who never used to speak to me, seem to crawl to me all the time. I just hate it and wish I could have my old job back. The problem is I'm trapped, because we need the extra money now we've got the baby.

It appears that the patient is describing some ways of relating that might suggest interpersonal skill deficits. That is, the person's way of relating in past relationships appeared effective, but in the new relationship there could well be behaviours that are not in the patient's repertoire (e.g., reprimanding colleagues, assigning tasks, conducting performance reviews, etc.). A more detailed analysis of these situations could reveal the interpersonal skill deficits that need to be redressed.

T: Has work changed anything apart from your friendships?

P: I used to be really comfortable with my work. I knew my job and I knew that I could do it. Now everything's changed. I don't know what my job is anymore and I don't know if I can do it. My self-esteem has gone through the floor because I'm no longer confident that I'm succeeding.

The psychologist then moves to summarize this part of the interview and starts to draw out some interpersonal patterns. Although the two role transitions are different, there are common elements that suggest some recurring patterns that could well benefit from being addressed within the course of subsequent IPT sessions.

T: It seems from what you have been telling me that you have been having trouble in your marriage since the birth of your son and at work following your promotion. The problems can certainly lead to depression. I'd like to meet with you over the next few weeks, for about an hour each time, to see if we can figure out how you can cope better with the situation.

Negotiate a therapeutic contract

Finally, the psychologist and patient negotiate a mutually agreeable therapeutic contract. This involves explaining the role that interpersonal factors may play in depression. Patients are informed that they will be responsible for deciding on the focus of treatment, bringing new material, and choosing the topics to discuss. Following this, two or three treatment goals are set. These goals need to be potentially achievable within the time frame of therapy and may be symptom-related or interpersonal.

P: But what is causing this depression?

T: We live in a social world and we are social beings. People play a significant part in our lives. When depressed we are inclined to think we are alone, but we remain social beings. It is not surprising then that relationships play an important role in depression. So far we don't know all the causes of depression, but what is clear is that when you are feeling depressed you tend also to be having problems with personal relationships. These problems in relationships could include issues with your partner, children, family, or work colleagues. Sometimes relationship problems or bereavement may bring on depression. At other times or with other people, being depressed may stop them from dealing with other people as well as they would like (and used to). We will try to find out what you want and need from others and help you learn how to get it. We will try to understand how your relationships are related to your depression.

P: How long are we going to do this for?

T: My preference would be for us to meet once a week for about 16 more sessions. During this time we will work to understand how your relationships are related to your depression.

P: Okay, but what will we do?

T: From what you tell me, your depression began with recent transitions. One of the transitions was the birth of your son and your wife's depression, the other was your promotion at work. I'd like to discuss with you the critical areas you seem to describe as related to your depression. One is the kind of transition you've had to make from being a worker to a manager. The second issue centres on how you are relating to your wife, the impact of her depression on you and how you are acting in this relationship. Do these sound like the issues we should work on?

P: Sure.

Summary and contrast with CBT

In the preceding discussion and case example, the key aspects of an IPT formulation have been clarified. In the early phase of IPT the psychologist will deal with the depression, assess the interpersonal problems, and negotiate a therapeutic contract. To date there is little additional documentation in the IPT literature of the details of case formulation or psychometric assessments to identify which of the four interpersonal areas (i.e., role disputes, grief, interpersonal deficits, or role transitions) are present and warrant treatment (although see Markowitz and Swartz, 1997).

A case formulation from a CBT perspective will share many similarities with an IPT approach. However, the emphasis and treatment plan would be different. Therefore, let us consider how the preceding case might be conceptualized from a CBT perspective.

Under the heading of Presenting Problems would come the list of symptoms of depression that the client described. At this point there would be no difference between CBT and IPT case formulations. In terms of Predisposing factors, little attention was paid to predisposing factors and therefore minimal information is available in the IPT formulation. This highlights an important point, which is that the framework within which the case formulation is conducted has the capacity to influence the information elicited from the client. Considering the Precipitating variables, there appear to be a variety of factors. These precipitants include the birth of his son, the promotion at work, and his wife's onset of depression (and the impact and stress that this is having upon the relationship, his work, and so on). Once again, these are factors that would be drawn out within an IPT framework. One important difference arises when the Perpetuating cognitions and consequences are considered. The client describes quite a number of themes that would be relevant within CBT. For example, he comments, 'I *should* be able to keep things together. It's my wife who is sick and if I have a breakdown, then there will be no one left to look after Aubrey. I've *got* to be the stable one. I've *got* to keep the family together.' It is evident from these sentences that the client is identifying expectations that he has about himself that will be counterproductive and likely to enhance feelings of hopelessness, a lack of coping, and stress. In addition to these and other cognitions a CBT therapist would consider the consequences of his behaviours. Two patterns are evident. First, it is apparent that positive reinforcement is lacking and punishment occurs regardless of his responses, both at home and at work. That is, unpleasant consequences seem to arise whatever he does. The lack of sufficient positive reinforcement has been identified as an associate of depression (Lewinsohn & Graf, 1973; Soucy Chartier & Provencher, 2013) and so too has the occurrence of aversive stimulation that is not contingent upon any responses a person might give (Seligman, 1975). Putting this together, a provisional conceptualization might be that the client had certain beliefs about his role as a father (e.g., being the one to hold things together) and his wife's role as a future mother (e.g., she could be maternal and clucky), as well as expectations about his promotion. In each of these scenarios, the expectations he had of himself and others were not met. He did not modify these expectations and thus became depressed as he felt increasingly unable to control his negative emotional reactions and his inability to control his home and work life so that it met his expected ideal. Thus, a Prescribed intervention might involve behavioural activation to reinstate previously pleasurable activities, moving to identify the links between actions and moods and cognitions and mood. Cognitive therapy might then be used to modify the unhelpful cognitive patterns and behaviour management strategies implemented. Finally, some potential problems in treatment might be his wife's depression as well as his 'hunker down' attitude, which might lead to a reluctance to become involved in treatment and wait for it all to 'blow over'.

In summary, case formulation is a process of obtaining and organizing data about a client's problem into a format that guides treatment. Case formulation has been illustrated in the context of cognitive, behavioural, and interpersonal interventions for various psychological problems. However, case formulation is not unique to these approaches to psychological problems and Eells's (2007b) book is a good source to develop an appreciation of the diversity of approaches to case formulation. In routine clinical practice, case formulation will be relevant with every client; however, it will be most straightforward when a client's problems conform to the mythical 'textbook' case, in which the disorder is well documented and the treatment well validated. For instance, in Fairburn's (1995) treatment manual for bulimia, case formulation is used to help the psychologist decide in which order to present the empirically validated treatment modules (see Wilson, 1996a and 1996b for a discussion). Therefore, the topics for consideration in the next chapter are some of the available psychological treatments.

Chapter 6

Treating clients

Much effort has been expended trying to partition the variance attributable to the specifics and non-specifics of therapy; however, for a practitioner the specifics of a therapy are invariably delivered in the context of a therapeutic relationship. Clinical psychologists generally consult with clients in person, be this individually or in groups. In Chapter 2 we considered some of the important aspects of the therapeutic relationship but in the present chapter we will turn to some of the specific psychotherapeutic techniques that have empirical support.

As evident from the model in Figure 6.1, treatment planning follows from a careful assessment and formulation of the client's problems. The selection of treatment involves a considered and critical evaluation of the empirical literature. Although this consideration also draws upon clinical training and experience, published literature has passed through a peer review process and hence deserves greater weighting in the selection process.

One recent review of the psychotherapy literature has been provided in *A Guide to Treatments that Work* edited by Nathan and Gorman (2002, 2007; see also Roth & Fonagy, 2004). The process adopted in this review was that criteria for standards of proof were established and then the available literature was summarized in a way that the quality of the empirical support for the treatment of each disorder could be coded. The strongest support came from Type One Studies which used a randomized, prospective clinical trial. To qualify at this high level, the study needed to involve random assignment to conditions, blind assessments, clear exclusion and inclusion criteria, sound diagnosis, adequate sample sizes, and clear and appropriate statistical methods. Type Two Studies were similar to Type One Studies, except that some aspects were absent (e.g., non-random assignment). Weaker empirical support again was taken from Type Three Studies, which were open treatment studies and case-control studies collecting retrospective information. Type Four Studies were those that involved secondary data analysis (e.g., meta-analysis). Type Five Studies were reviews without secondary data analysis and Type Six Studies included case studies, essays, and opinion papers.

Clearly any interpretations based on reviews such as the one reported by Nathan and Gorman (2007; see also Weisz & Kazdin, 2010 for a review of children and adolescents) are open to allegations of being incomplete and potentially biased. For example, conclusions can only refer to treatments that have a broad research base and the review will omit newer treatments (e.g., Emotion-Focused Therapy; Elliott, Watson, Goldman, & Greenberg, 2004) or those that may be effective but have not been well-researched to date. The conclusions may be biased because some psychotherapies might not lend themselves as readily to empirical evaluation according to the specified criteria; the treatments included may be ones that emphasize efficacy over effectiveness, focus on ICD and DSM diagnoses, and some procedures (e.g., *in vivo* exposure for specific phobias) may suffer from the bulk of the research being

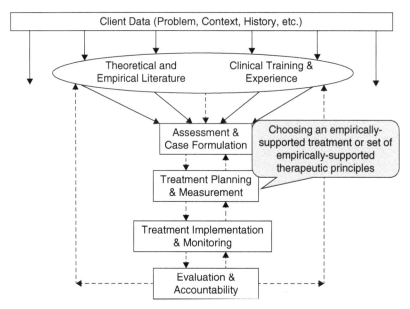

Figure 6.1 A science-informed model of treatment selection.

conducted during times when the criteria for conducting and reporting outcome research were less stringent. However, while a scientist-practitioner must always recognize the limitations of any data set upon which interpretations are based, critical evaluation must acknowledge that the products of a systematic review place individual practitioners in a strong position to lay empirical foundations for the practice of clinical psychology. In comparison to the state of the empirical foundation of clinical psychology when Hans Eysenck (1952) claimed that psychotherapy was no more effective than spontaneous remission, it is now possible to identify some broad areas where psychotherapy is efficacious. This is the nature of science. Our conclusions will always be tentative, more and better data available tomorrow will alter the inferences we would draw today, but scientist-practitioners must allow their treatment decisions to be influenced by a careful appraisal of the best data currently available.

When examining the conclusions of Nathan and Gorman (2007), it is clear that psychological and pharmacological treatments can alleviate a wide array of psychological problems. Focusing on the psychotherapies, Behavioural (including variants such as Dialectical Behaviour Therapy; DBT) and Cognitive Behavioural Therapies (CBT) have fair to strong empirical support in the treatment of Attention Deficit Hyperactivity Disorder, Alcohol Use Disorders, Avoidant Personality Disorder, Body Dysmorphic Disorder, Borderline Personality Disorder, Bulimia Nervosa, Conduct Disorders, Depression, Generalized Anxiety Disorder, Hypochondriasis, Obsessive-Compulsive Disorder, Paraphilias, Panic Disorder (with and without Agoraphobia), Post-Traumatic Stress Disorder, Schizophrenia, Sexual Dysfunctions (e.g., erectile dysfunction), Sleep Disorders, Social Phobia, Somatoform Pain Disorder, and Specific Phobias. Interpersonal Psychotherapy (IPT) has a demonstrated efficacy only for depression, and Dynamic/Psychoanalytic Psychotherapy has some support in the treatment of Borderline Personality Disorder and other Personality Disorders. Thus, when making decisions about the direction of treatment, a clinical psychologist will need to be cognizant of the relevant empirical literature to best inform these decisions. One way to keep abreast of current developments is to search the internet sites that list the evidence for particular treatments. For instance, there is the Cochrane Collaboration (cochrane.org) which publishes systematic reviews of health care (including psychological and psychosocial) interventions. Another listing, which focuses on broader social welfare interventions, is the Campbell Collaboration (campbellcollaboration.org). The remainder of this chapter will introduce some elementary components of these evidence-based treatments, but more detailed presentations can be found in the books listed in the Bibliography. Further, since many techniques are modified for application in many different clinical problems and psychological disorders, we will concentrate on providing a description of particular procedures that are broadly applicable.

Behaviour therapy

In contemporary clinical practice, behaviour therapy is often delivered alongside cognitive interventions, but for didactic purposes it is useful to consider them separately. The theoretical underpinnings of behaviour therapy have a long tradition (Pavlov, 1927; Watson, 1924) but recent learning theory emphasizes contingency over contiguity (Rescorla, 1988; Rapee, 1991). That is, the important relationships are those in which there is a contingency between two events, rather than a temporal contiguity between a stimulus and a response. Thus, in contrast to its early roots, behaviour therapy is much more 'cognitive' and learning theory emphasizes the learning of relations between events (if X then Y learning). Consequently, the aim of behavioural interventions is to modify learning by changing the parameters that control the acquisition of the 'if X then Y' rules. Broadly speaking, there are two approaches to modify behaviours. First, we can attempt to modify behaviours by managing the contingencies that control the behaviour. Second, we can attempt to modify behaviours by training the client in self-control strategies. Let us consider contingency management first.

Contingency management

Contingency management refers to the presentation of reinforcers and punishers in a contingent manner where the goal is to manage or modify behaviour. Learning theory assumes that there are general laws that govern the effects of different contingencies but it also acknowledges that due to the variability in learning histories, clinical practice must take into consideration the unique aspects of each individual. It is necessary to measure every intervention and monitor throughout the treatment process to ensure that the laws are in operation. Treatment begins, therefore, with a baseline measurement against which changes can be measured and monitored. Reminiscent of the methods of case formulation, these ratings will be direct measures of the behaviour in question, its antecedents, and its consequences.

In considering what to measure and how to intervene, one of the first questions is, 'What is a reinforcer?' This is an important theoretical issue with clear clinical implications. The Skinnerian definition states that a reinforcer is anything that changes the frequency of a behaviour if it is applied contingent upon emission of that behaviour. This suggests that identifying a reinforcer is an empirical question; you just have to try them out until you find what works. In clinical practice this would lead you to consult lists of possible reinforcements or speak with clients (or a person speaking on the client's behalf) and ask them to rate the reinforcing value of the alternatives. A second definition comes from the work of

Premack (1959) and avoids the apparent circularity in the Skinnerian definition. Premack's principle is that given two responses, the more probable will reinforce the less probable and not vice versa. Premack's principle implies that to isolate a reinforcer, you just have to identify a behaviour with greater probability than the behaviour in question, and then make the target behaviour contingent upon the high probability behaviour. For instance, Flavell (1977) sought to increase studying, so looked for a behaviour with a higher frequency than studying (in this case, showering), and made showering contingent upon studying. The effect was that studying increased. In this example, you could argue that showering was more pleasant than studying, but according to Premack's principle, the key is not the pleasantness but the natural frequency of a behaviour. Independent of definition, reinforcers are generally divided into primary (i.e., those which satisfy an innate, biological need; e.g., food) or secondary (i.e., conditioned; e.g., money) reinforcers.

Increasing desired behaviours

Positive reinforcement (sometimes called reward) seeks to increase the likelihood of a desired response by applying a reinforcer contingent upon the desired behaviour. When doing so, it is recommended that once a target behaviour has been selected as needing to be increased in frequency or intensity, you deliver the reinforcement immediately after a target behaviour and that you do so contingently and consistently. You may need to vary reinforcers to avoid loss of potency, and while you reinforce often to begin with, it is important to fade out and allow the natural reinforcement to take over. For this reason it is also desirable to use social reinforcement whenever possible as you fade out primary reinforcers to ensure that they are replaced with social reinforcement. For example, to increase peer interaction, you might use a star chart with primary reinforcers to reinforce social contact with peers, but then ensure that the inherent reinforcement from social interactions is brought to bear as the primary reinforcers are faded out. Another method of fading out is to use a 'pyramid chart' in which the number of behaviours (i.e., stars on a chart) required to obtain a primary reinforcer increase in a linear manner so that as time goes on, the reinforcers become more sparse.

Another way to increase desired behaviours is to use *negative reinforcement*. Negative reinforcement is not punishment (which *decreases* undesirable behaviours), but negative reinforcement involves removing a reinforcer contingent upon some behaviour, which in turn increases the likelihood of that behaviour being emitted in the future (e.g., a client with tension headaches who finds that using a newly learned relaxation technique successfully alleviates the headaches, will be more likely to use relaxation exercises in the future). Similar to positive reinforcement, the termination of the reinforcer should follow immediately, contingently, and consistently after the behaviour. The time between trials must not be too brief otherwise the offset of the reinforcer (e.g., the 'relief') is not of sufficient intensity or duration. If there is no progress, you might need to check that the 'aversive' experience that is being terminated is aversive to the person in question or you may move to avoidance conditioning (i.e., emission of a behaviour avoids the presentation of a stimulus).

Decreasing problem behaviours

Contingent *punishment* describes any procedure that decreases the future probability of a response being emitted. It is important to note that just because something is aversive, it does not mean that it is a punisher. For instance, yelling at a child may be aversive, but it may be positively reinforcing because of the attention that the child is receiving. There are two problems with using punishment. One is that in the past it has often involved physical punishments, which often are not socially acceptable or legally permitted. The other problem is that while punishment decreases behaviours it does not facilitate desirable behaviours. Thus, if punishment is used, then it needs to be used in conjunction with positive reinforcement of desirable behaviour. As with all behaviour management processes, but particularly in the case of punishment, it is useful to inform the client of the contingency. The punisher should be immediate, contingent, and on a continuous schedule with a duration and intensity that is minimal enough to be effective and a plan to promote generalization of any learning. For example, the bell and pad (Lovibond, 1964; Mowrer & Mowrer, 1938) is an arrangement to treat nocturnal enuresis in which the bed-wetting is reduced by an alarm triggered by the presence of a liquid-sensitive alarm placed beneath the sheet. The alarm needs to be sufficiently loud to wake the child during urination from sleep and therefore, the intensity of the alarm is not to 'punish' in the conventional sense of the word and there is no need for it to be aversive. Rather, the aim is to rouse the child from sleep and permit learning of the cues that signal nocturnal urination. However, it meets the technical definition of a punisher, in that the onset of the alarm is associated with a decline in the frequency of an undesired behaviour.

Another method of reducing undesired behaviours is to use *time-out from reinforcement*. Time out from reinforcement (and response cost) are sometimes distinguished from response-contingent punishment by calling them 'negative punishment' and the contingent punishment 'positive punishment'. Time-out from reinforcement describes a period in which previously available positive reinforcement is unavailable. It is useful to use the full title, rather than the abbreviated 'time out' because it will help you remember what the necessary conditions are. Namely, there needs to be an ongoing schedule of positive reinforcement and the person needs to be removed from the environment where the positive reinforcement is ongoing at least for long enough to have missed out on one reinforcer. Many discussions arise because people forget that it is time out *from reinforcement*. For instance, parents may send children to their rooms but find this is ineffective because they like being there. Another signal that you have forgotten the nature of the procedure is if you start to identify the optimal duration of time out with respect to a clock rather than with reference to the schedule of reinforcement that the person is being removed from. It also indicates that if a person is a reinforcer, removal of the person (rather than the client) for a specified period of time (e.g., a mother ignoring a child and going off to read a magazine) may also be effective. As with punishment, time out from reinforcement needs to be used in conjunction with reward of desired behaviours. It is useful to identify a time-out area that is safe and free of reinforcement. Shorter durations are preferred because while the person is in time out from reinforcement they are often removed from learning opportunities.

Undesirable behaviours can also be reduced with *response cost and extinction*. Response cost involves a previously acquired reinforcer being forfeited contingent upon the emission of an undesired response (e.g., removing marks for a late assignment). Response cost needs to be used in conjunction with positive reinforcers (to increase desirable behaviours). It requires the clinician to identify an effective reinforcer to be lost, the magnitude of which is commensurate with the undesirable behaviour. It needs to be instituted immediately after behaviour which can later be brought under verbal control. Extinction involves the cessation of reinforcement of a previously reinforced behaviour. It is important to note that extinction is not unlearning, but is the learning of a new contingency. Once extinction has occurred, the person has two 'If X then Y' rules, but one is given more weight. Remembering this aspect of learning theory helps you to expect four phenomena that regularly occur in clinical practice. First, there is reinstatement of the response. As the Rescorla–Wagner (1972) model predicts, learning can be reinstated by the presentation of the Conditioner Stimulus or the Unconditioned Stimulus. Therefore, experience of the US may reinstate old learning. For instance, once a phobia has been extinguished, the occurrence of fear may be sufficient to reinstate fears (Jacobs & Nadel, 1985; Menzies & Clarke, 1994, 1995). Second, changing the context can lead to renewal of responding (Rosas, Todd, & Bouton, 2013). Bouton (1991) has outlined this in detail; extinction is context-specific and therefore, once you change contexts, the learning that you have achieved may be lost. Contexts can be locations, but they can also be interoceptive (e.g., a drug-induced state), temporal (passage of time), and so on. A third factor is re-acquisition, such that previously extinguished behaviours are much more rapidly learned. For instance, tolerance is more rapidly acquired following each period of detoxification. Finally, there is rebound (extinction burst). That is, when you put a behaviour onto an extinction schedule, there is an increase in the behaviour (e.g., tantrums).

Satiation is another way to reduce the undesirable behaviours. Reinforcers lose their reinforcing qualities over time. This may be a danger when trying to increase one response, but it is useful when trying to decrease another. The essence is to use continual exposure to a reinforcer, so that it loses its reinforcing qualities. In practice, there are a number of potential problems. First, the reinforcer must be identified and able to be provided in sufficient quantity (e.g., Allyon [1963] took 635 towels to satiate a client's hoarding of towels!). Second, reinforcers may be harmful in high doses or frequencies. Third, some reinforcers may not be accessible to satiation (e.g., social reinforcement).

Two other ways to reduce undesirable behaviours are positive practice and overcorrection. *Positive practice* involves reducing unwanted behaviours by encouraging the repeated practice of adaptive or desired behaviours. *Overcorrection* involves two components: restitution and positive practice. Restitution requires that the environmental disruption of the undesirable behaviour is restored and the positive practice component involves restoring the environment to a better state than before. An example might be being asked to clean up the entire playground after dropping a single piece of paper.

Differential reinforcement

Sometimes, the goal of a behaviour modification strategy is the increase or decrease in rate or frequency, rather than just the absence or presence of a behaviour (e.g., eye contact). Therefore, rates of behaviour can be differentially reinforced in a variety of ways. Differential reinforcement of low rates (DRL) of behaviour encourages slow responding. Behaviours are reinforced only when they occur after a certain amount of time after the last response. Differential reinforcement of high rates (DRH) of behaviour encourages rapid responding. Behaviours are reinforced only when they occur after a short amount of time after the last response.

As discussed earlier, one problem with punishment, response cost, and time out is that they do not encourage new and more productive behaviours. To overcome this weakness, differential reinforcement of other (DRO) behaviour can be used. Rather than punishing one response, or in addition to punishing a response, some other response is reinforced. For instance, you may choose to ignore rudeness in a child (e.g., putting the behaviour on an extinction schedule if attention was maintaining it) and attend to constructive play. A related schedule is the differential reinforcement of incompatible (DRI) behaviours. That is, another behaviour is chosen to reinforce and the selection is based upon the fact that it is incompatible with the undesired behaviour. For example, hand or finger waving in a child with autism may be 'punished' (with contingent delivery of smelling salts) and then followed by rewarding constructive manual play.

Contingency contracting

The presentation so far may have given the impression that behaviour therapy is a technology that is applied to a client, rather than involving a collaborative relationship. While it is true that contingencies can be effectively applied to unwilling clients (e.g., random breath testing), behaviour therapy can be delivered in a collaborative relationship. Contingency contracting is one way to achieve this end. Contingency contracting involves clearly specifying in advance the nature of the contingencies now in operation. Research indicates that the most effective contracts are those that specify the treatment strategies and the expected outcomes. Further, efficacy is increased if the contract elicits from the client an agreement to participate fully in the programme. One common form of contingency contracting is an interpersonal one. Two individuals agree to reciprocal rules such as, 'if you do this, then I'll do that'. Another common form of contract is the deposit contingency, in which a deposit is forfeited if a behaviour is not emitted (e.g., lose deposit if therapy is prematurely discontinued).

Habit reversal

Behaviour therapy techniques can be combined as required. An example of such a combination is a procedure called habit reversal. Developed by Azrin and Nunn (1973) it involves the practice of behaviours that are incompatible with or opposite to the habit in question. For instance, nail biting may be treated by practising hand clenching. The components of treatment are (i) self-monitoring in which the behaviours are identified, (ii) habit control motivation in which the clinician reviews the inconveniences of the undesirable behaviour, (iii) awareness training in which the normally 'automatic' and habitual sequence of behaviour is brought into conscious awareness, (iv) competing response training, where the client practises a behaviour incompatible with the habitual behaviour, (v) relaxation training, and (vi) generalization training in which high-risk situations are identified and contingency plans are organized and practised (see Stanley & Mouton,1996).

Variables that influence performance

Although operant procedures do not require the use of language, providing information and negotiating contracts will facilitate the process. It is also important to consider the variables that can affect performance. Subject variables that can affect performance include motivation and learning to learn. One example of subject variables can be seen in Azrin & Foxx's (1974) dry bed training. The treatment begins by encouraging the child to drink as much fluid as possible in order to create the environment for learning. Another example is learning to learn. This describes the observation that learning is faster the second time around. Harlow (1949) discovered the phenomenon, when he observed that monkeys were faster solving a novel problem after they had experience with a previous (but different) problem. In the words of Harlow, people acquire a learning set, a way of acquiring knowledge. Thus, a clinical implication of this is to identify not only a person's past learning, but try to identify their learning set (i.e., what sorts of ways have they learned in the past). You can then teach the new behaviour in the way that previous learning was acquired.

Another class of variables that influence performance are response variables. First, there is belongingness. Deriving from the work of Garcia and Koelling (1966), we know that certain stimuli are conditioned more readily to certain responses. This can be applied by framing the intervention in terms of the natural tendencies.

The third class of variables that influence performance are schedules of reinforcement. One of the simplest parameters is delay of reinforcement. The shorter the delay between the response and the reinforcer, the greater the probability of learning. Another parameter is the reliability with which the reinforcer follows the behaviour. Continuous reinforcement produces rapid learning, but extinction is more rapid than with partial reinforcement. Therefore, training usually begins with continuous reinforcement and moves to partial reinforcement. Note also that partial reinforcement produces the partial reinforcement extinction effect (that is, responding continues for a long time after extinction when responding has been partially reinforced). The number of responses required for a response is also important to consider. Ratios may be fixed or variable. Ratios produce a scallop (with a post-reinforcement pause and a ratio run), except that if the number of responses required is too great (i.e., the ratio strain is too high), responding will stop altogether. Instead of reinforcing the number of responses, you can reinforce responses that are emitted after a certain period of time. Once again, the interval schedules may be fixed or variable. In clinical practice, two points to bear in mind are, first, variable schedules of reinforcement produce more steady rates of responding than fixed rates, and second, ratio schedules are extremely motivating because the person is encouraged to respond at higher rates.

Introducing new behaviours

Sometimes the aim is not to increase a desirable behaviour but to introduce a new behaviour or set of behaviours to an individual's repertoire. For instance, desired behaviour may not appear in its complete form during the early stages of a programme. One strategy to introduce new behaviours is to use *shaping* and reward successive approximations. That is, the clinical psychologist reinforces behaviour that approximates the desired behaviour, but as time goes on, the rules for reinforcement become more stringent and the requirements move towards reinforcing behaviour that more closely approximates the desired behaviour. When using shaping, it is recommended to identify a high frequency behaviour similar to the target behaviour and then establish a criterion for first approximation (low). After this, the clinician will arrange the context to maximize the probability of a response occurring and then differentially reinforce variants of the desired behaviour and withdraw reinforcement from behaviours incompatible with the desired behaviour. Over time the clinician will shift the criterion for reinforcement as there are shifts in topography of the behaviour towards the desired behaviour. Sometimes verbal or gestural prompts may be used to guide and encourage approximations of the target behaviour. Prompting is useful in the initial stages of a training programme. A cue is delivered that initiates the response, so that the response can be reinforced.

Another strategy to introduce new behaviours is *chaining*. If complex behaviours (e.g., tying shoe laces) are to be trained, often shaping will not work because the behaviour will not occur even with prompting. Therefore, chaining can be used, when the behaviour can be broken down into a series of elements that need to be performed sequentially. The behaviour is broken down and each element is reinforced either beginning with the first or last behaviour in the sequence. Forward chaining is when the reinforcement begins with the first behaviour in the sequence (e.g., brushing teeth). Backward chaining is when the reinforcement begins with the last behaviour in the sequence (e.g., tying shoe laces).

Maintenance of behaviours

The main problem with contingency management is that of stopping the contingency but maintaining the desired behaviour. One way of solving this is to ensure that the behaviour soon comes under the reinforcement of natural contingencies. For instance, reinforcing peer play may soon be unnecessary if peer interactions become inherently rewarding. However, thought needs to be given to fading out the contingency. Generally, this involves moving from continuous to partial reinforcement, fading from some situations and not others, and providing self-control.

Among the issues involved in behavioural maintenance is generalization; both the acquisition of new and inhibition of old responding. The general rule is that generalization should be programmed rather than assumed to be a natural consequence of therapy. Thus, work done in the clinic or with the clinician needs to be conducted in or translated into the natural environment. This will also involve identifying the important cues that control behaviours and ensuring that the behaviour is acquired or extinguished in the presence of these. You will need to train the client to identify the discriminative stimuli that operate in the environment and fade out prompts and reinforcement.

In terms of the context, it is useful to identify a class of stimuli that learning theorists have called occasion setters (see Bouton & Todd, 2014; Pearce & Bouton, 2001). These variables do not cause a response in and of themselves, but they set the stage for the occurrence of a response. For instance, a context may act to indicate that a particular set of contingencies are in operation (e.g., police warning that on a public holiday weekend they are going to punish speeding with higher fines). Related are conditioned excitors and conditioned inhibitors. For example, a conditioned inhibitor is a stimulus that acts to suppress responding (e.g., a person with agoraphobia may learn about safety signals, in that panic may be less likely to occur in the presence of some stimuli, so these acquire the ability to suppress fear).

Self-management

Contingency management involves procedures to increase desirable and reduce undesirable behaviours. The client tends to be viewed as a passive recipient of treatment in that behaviour is controlled by the environment and modifying the environment will modify the client's behaviour. In contrast, self-management therapy is based upon a participant model of treatment (e.g., Kanfer & Gaelick-Buys, 1991; Page, 1991b). The responsibility for change is viewed as lying within the client and therapy is part of a transition to self-control. The therapist continues to play an important part in providing the context for change, but the burden of engaging the change process is left with the client. The main reasons for a self-management role are that (i) many behaviours are not easily accessible for observation by anyone but the client, (ii) change is often difficult, unpleasant, and conducted with ambivalence, and therefore collaboration and negotiation are needed, and (iii) the aim of psychotherapy is to teach generalizable coping strategies, not only management of specific problems. That being said, self-management is best considered as a way of delivering contingency management rather than as a distinct technology.

Self-regulation develops out of social learning theory in which behaviour is seen to arise from learning, and complex chains of behaviours become more automatic through repetition. The greater the automaticity of a behaviour, the harder it will be to control. Self-management procedures are then required when new behaviours must be learned, choices need to be made, goals are to be achieved or blocked, or when habitual response sequences are interrupted or ineffective. Self-management brings into play controlled cognitive processing.

Finally, there is a self-reinforcement phase in which the person reacts cognitively and emotionally to the self-evaluation which motivates change. During the final stage two attributional processes come into play. The person must correctly *attribute both the cause and the control* of a behaviour to something under their influence/control.

Since self-management will require a degree of motivation, the strategies of *Motivational Interviewing* (Miller & Rollnick, 2012) will be useful in recruiting and building motivation for change. Motivational interviewing will be described later but for now some of the key interventions and techniques involved are summarized in the following:

Express empathy: Warm reflective listening during which you work to understand the clients, accept them as who they are, and acknowledge their feelings without judging, criticizing, or blaming. Acceptance is not identical to approval, but will facilitate change, while confrontation will inhibit change.

Develop discrepancies: The discrepancy in life goals between where a client is and where they would like to be can be used to motivate change.

Avoid argumentation: Arguments encourage resistance and are frequently counterproductive and for this reason they are best avoided in psychotherapy.

Roll with resistance: Respond to force by sidestepping and then using the force for your own end.

Support self-efficacy: Although the non-contingent encouragement of self-esteem has been questioned (Baumeister, Campbell, Krueger, & Vohs, 2003), self-efficacy is an important predictor of behaviour and its enhancement (discussed later) increases the probability that a desired behaviour will be engaged in.

Use behavioural contracting

One particular motivational strategy is behavioural contracting. Contracts can help to assist clients to initiate specific actions, identify criteria for success, and to clarify the consequences of particular behaviours. When negotiating contracts with clients it is useful to (i) describe the behaviour in detail, (ii) identify criteria (e.g., duration or frequency) for completion of a goal, (iii) specify the nature and timing of contingent positive and negative consequences upon fulfilment and non-fulfilment of the contract along with a 'bonus' indicating additional positive rewards if a minimal criterion is exceeded, and (iv) clarify how the behaviour will be observed, measured, recorded, and conveyed back to the client (if a third party is involved). If possible, a public commitment to the contract can be useful as a means to enhance compliance, but caution needs to be exercised if the consequences of a 'public failure' would be detrimental.

Once a sufficient motivational foundation has been laid, self-regulation begins with the self-monitoring stage, in which clients monitor and evaluate their behaviour. Self-evaluation involves a comparison between the person's actual behaviour and his or her standards for that behaviour. Even though self-monitoring may lack validity for experimental purposes, many of the reasons that make it problematic for research, become assets for clinical work. In particular, we know that performance is reactive, and therefore monitoring may have a therapeutic effect. Baseline data can be used to provide an incentive to change and as encouragement when change occurs. You can also select to measure a response that is incompatible with the problem behaviour. For example, spouses may be asked to record the interactions that lead up to a fight. This makes them conscious of those interactions that are leading to a fight and by inducing the awareness, increases the chances that alternative responses will be engaged.

Once monitoring has begun it is possible to start to modify the environment and the contingencies. Stimulus control is a useful self-management procedure since the client can construct conditions which reduce the possibility of an undesired behaviour. For example, a person with a gambling problem may put restrictions on a bank account and a person with a drinking problem may choose who they are going to drink with. Alternatively, stimulus narrowing may be used to decrease the range of stimuli or environments under which the behaviour occurs. That is, the behaviour is gradually put under the control of certain discriminative stimuli. For instance, sleep hygiene rules (Van Brunt, Riedel, & Lichstein, 1996) encourage the use of a bed for sleeping, and stipulate that other behaviours (e.g., watching TV, reading, etc.) are to be carried out in other locations. The aim of these procedures is to narrow the stimuli that are associated with sleep.

When introducing self-management procedures, it is helpful to consider how difficult they are for the client to execute. Task assignment is managed so that assignments are graded in difficulty and begin with the easier ones. These 'homework' (sometimes more fruitfully called 'active practice') assignments need to be presented to clients as essential to the process of therapy. To learn self-management, clients need to practise self-management. This will involve (i) information, in which the requirements of task are made explicit, (ii) anticipatory practice, in which the client imagines and practises the assigned task within the safety of the therapeutic context (e.g., role-plays), (iii) active practice (or response execution) in everyday settings, followed by (iv) a review. The review aims to translate the episodic memory that the person will have of an event into a semantic memory so that clients will form general rules and create knowledge about themselves and appreciate the meaning of events. The data routinely collected as part of measurement and monitoring activities can be useful in demonstrating the effectiveness of the behaviours to the client.

In summary, when using self-management models, the client controls the contingencies of reinforcement. Behaviour is then rewarded or punished according to specified rules, as in contingency management, but their implementation is under the control or management of the client. However, learning can occur without the use of external reinforcement and one important method is through procedures associated with social learning theory.

Modelling

Modelling and its use in behaviour therapy (and CBT) draws on an extensive empirical literature in psychology more generally (Bandura, 1977; Frith & Frith, 2012; Rosenthal & Steffek, 1991). Modelling describes the learning that occurs from the observation of others and any imitative change in behaviour that may follow. Therefore, it refers to changes in the behaviour of the individual who observes another (i.e., the model). Two subsets are observational learning and imitation. Observational learning is learning that occurs from observing others (e.g., children observing adult behaviour) and imitation refers to the behaviour of a person who observes and then copies the actions of others. There is some evidence (Litrownik, Franzini, & Turner, 1976) that observational learning is relatively more important than imitation for the transfer of learning because seeing repeated instances of a behaviour in different contexts allows an observer to formulate the rules that are important for generalization. In contrast, the imitative component facilitates acquisition because the observer engages in repeated practice.

For modelling to be most effective (Bandura 1977) the observer must attend to the modelled events. Optimal models are distinctive. By being unusual, the model gains attention but, if too distinctive, the model will be perceived as dissimilar from the observer and modelling will be reduced. Other factors to consider in modelling are the affective valence of the behaviour (pleasant behaviours are more likely to be modelled than ones which are anxiety-provoking or unpleasant to perform), complexity (complex behaviours may be broken down into simpler and shorter components to facilitate attention to the relevant components), the functional value to the client (behaviours that are valued by the client are more likely to be attended to), and the prevalence of models (the greater the number of and the greater the consistency within the models, the greater the likelihood that the observer's attention will be gained).

When using modelling it is important to take into consideration the characteristics of the observer to ensure that they have the appropriate sensory capabilities and that their perceptual set will allow them to perceive the important features (priming an observer about what to look for is useful). A therapist will need to ensure retention of relevant information and describe the behaviours in terms the client can understand. Consequences that flow from engaging in the behaviour can strengthen recall and encourage imitation. Motor reproduction of the model's behaviour with therapist feedback will facilitate greater acquisition of the desired behaviour. Finally, it is important to ensure that, when the client exhibits the desired behaviours, there is external reinforcement, such as praise by the therapist, self-reinforcement, or the natural rewards that occur from performing the responses in the natural context, and that the client identifies the positive consequences that follow the desired behaviour.

Modelling can be divided into a variety of types. First, graduated modelling is used when clients are capable of performing some components of the desired behaviour. Graduated modelling often involves assistance in the patterning of behaviours so that the appropriate elements are performed in their correct sequence. Guided modelling is also graduated but adds guided practice. For instance, you may guide the observer to correctly emit an appropriate behaviour that has been modelled and then reinforce appropriate responding. Participant modelling involves modelling by the therapist, who then remains with the client and participates during the task. The presence of the therapist provides social support as well as enabling the therapist to solve problems that arise during the process. Covert modelling allows the client to imagine a model performing the appropriate behaviour. This requires careful description by the therapist and the outcome is maximized when similarity of the model to the observer is greatest. In all of these different forms, an important dimension to consider is the difference between coping and mastery. Mastery models show perfect performance and depict the ideal behaviour that the observer is to imitate and acquire. Coping models, on the other hand, exhibit flawed performance that gradually becomes more competent and the model demonstrates coping with errors and setbacks. Coping models are often preferred to mastery models. For example, in our training clinic we have found that trainee therapists initially prefer to observe more senior trainees engaged in clinical work than experts, since while they can see the skill of master therapists, these skills seem too far beyond them at the present.

Modelling has many applications, but we will illustrate one usage in the training of social skills. In this context a clinical psychologist will begin with an assessment of social skill deficits, including the expressive features of language, speech content, the paralinguistic elements (e.g., volume, pace, pitch, tone, etc.), non-verbal behaviours (e.g., proxemics, kinesics, eye contact, facial expression), response timing, receptive features of social interactions (e.g., attention, decoding, etc.), contextual and cultural mores, and specific deficits (e.g., assertiveness). Once the deficits have been specified, appropriate behaviours are taught using direct behaviour training. Role-plays, in which the client makes an attempt to produce the desired behaviour, are used along with a demonstration by the therapist of the target behaviour in the form of a modelling display. Thus, there is role-reversal. This role-reversal will provide extra information about the client's perceptions and abilities. The role-reversal also provides an opportunity to allow the client to experience thoughts and feelings associated with being the other person in the interaction. The role-play is repeated, but the client now tries to incorporate the new behaviours into their repertoire. The clinical psychologist will provide response-specific feedback, giving praise for successive approximations and concrete instructions for change in future rehearsals. When giving feedback it is useful to begin with positive feedback, then negative, and finally some more positive feedback so that the client does not feel overwhelmed with criticism. The role-reversal continues with repetition of the cycle that may include response escalation and variation, to enhance the flexibility of the client's skills and to overtrain responses, so that they appear more 'naturally'. Initially role-plays should be brief, highly structured, and deal with relatively benign topics, until the client becomes comfortable with the procedure and has begun to acquire the principles. Finally, the client practises outside the therapy sessions to consolidate skills to and generalize the behaviours.

Dialectical behaviour therapy (DBT)

Dialectical Behaviour Therapy (DBT; Linehan, 1993a, 1993b) is an adaptation of the behavioural techniques and is worth considering in some detail for two reasons. First, the treatment has empirical support for managing symptoms of Borderline Personality Disorder (e.g., Bedics, Atkins, Comtois, & Linehan, 2012; Kliem, Kröger, & Kosfelder, 2010; Panos, Jackson, Hasan, & Panos, 2013). Second, it is an illustration of how existing therapies can be modified to suit particular domains and the techniques of acceptance and validation are being incorporated into many newer variants of CBT with promising empirical bases (e.g., Acceptance and Commitment Therapy – ACT; Hayes, Strosahl, & Wilson, 2011; Hayes & Strosahl, 2004; Veehof, Oskam, Schreurs, & Bohlmeijer, 2011). Thus, rather than describing the particular techniques of DBT (see Linehan, 1993b), we will focus on the novel ways that Linehan presents psychotherapy. Linehan suggests Borderline Personality Disorder evolves within an emotionally vulnerable individual who develops in an 'Invalidating Environment'. Individuals who are emotionally vulnerable are more sensitive to stress and therefore stressors elicit excessive responses and it takes a long time to return to a baseline level of functioning when the stressor has finished. An invalidating environment occurs when a child's experience and behaviours are disqualified or discounted by people who are important to the child. The children's utterances are not accepted as valid descriptions of their feelings, or even if they are accepted, the person rejects the feelings as a valid response to the stress. When a high value is placed upon self-control then any perceived deficiencies in self-reliance are taken to indicate that the child lacks motivation or is disturbed.

DBT recognizes the difficulties faced by an emotionally vulnerable person living in an invalidating environment and identifies three dialectical dilemmas. Individuals may not learn to identify and comprehend feelings. When feelings are recognized, they will be judged to be invalid. Further, growing up in an invalidating environment may inhibit children learning appropriate coping strategies to manage intense emotions. The paradox of the invalidating environment will cause an alternation between excessive emotional inhibition (to elicit acceptance from significant others) and extreme emotional expression (to elicit acknowledgement of feelings by others). This seemingly erratic behaviour will bring about erratic schedules of reinforcement, which in turn will strengthen the erratic behavioural patterns.

To Linehan (1993a) this situation is the primary dialectical dilemma: both inhibition and expression of emotions become distressing.

A second dialectical dilemma arises because one emotional trigger is not resolved before another stressor occurs. This blurring of unresolved stressors and the associated emotional reactions produces a series of unrelenting crises. A third dialectical dilemma is the alternation between active passivity and seeming competence. This will convey a sense of competence in an effort not to be determined by a current mood state, while simultaneously seeking out people to solve the problems. Thus, Linehan's (1993a) therapy is dialectical because it presumes that for any issue (i.e., the thesis), there is an alternative position (i.e., the antithesis), and that one arrives at a synthesis through the clash of these two positions. The synthesis is not a compromise, but is a third way that takes the assets of each position, leaves their deficiencies, and resolves any contradictions.

The key dialectic in DBT is the balance between acceptance on the one hand and the change on the other. Any attempt by the patient at self-invalidation is balanced with training in adaptive problem-solving techniques. In addition, given the emotional vulnerability of clients with Borderline Personality Disorder the therapeutic relationship is of central importance within DBT. Therapists are responsive to clients, and express warmth and genuineness. They use appropriate self-disclosure on the one hand and 'irreverent communication' on the other. The irreverence involves confrontational communications that aim to nudge the client when therapy appears stuck or moving in an unhelpful direction. Linehan (1993a) encourages therapists to adopt a perspective that, despite appearances, clients are doing their best. Therapists are reminded of the therapeutic model within which the behaviour can be understood as a reasonable reaction of an emotionally vulnerable person to an invalidating environment. This acceptance is balanced with the dialectic of change. That is, even though the reaction is understandable, clients need to work to change the situation. The client may not be the (sole) cause of their current circumstances, but they can choose to be responsible for change.

One valuable contribution of DBT is that it identifies a therapeutic hierarchy. Decreasing suicidal behaviours is the first priority in therapy and therapy interfering behaviours is the second. Therefore, if either of these behaviours is signalled, these become the focus of therapy until they are dealt with. Other goals moving down the hierarchy are to decrease behaviours that interfere with the quality of life, to increase behavioural skills, to decreasing behaviours related to post-traumatic stress, and to improve self-esteem and specific behavioural targets. However, a drawback of a rigid, therapist-supplied hierarchy is that it could be at odds with both a science-informed approach to clinical practice and with a key ingredient in the therapeutic relationship shown to be related to positive treatment outcome. That is, the order of treatment goals should be informed by a case formulation incorporating practice-based evidence and should be negotiated in a collaborative manner with the client.

In summary, behaviour therapies extend from relatively straightforward contingency management to more complex treatment regimes found in DBT. In addition, they are typically delivered alongside cognitive interventions, even though they evolved separately.

Cognitive therapy

One of the central techniques in cognitive therapy is Cognitive Restructuring. Cognitive therapy has a strong evidence base (Beck & Dozois, 2011; Hofmann, Asnaani, Vonk, Sawyer, & Fang, 2012; Tolin, 2010). Within Ellis's (1962) Rational Emotive Therapy (RET) it is argued that *A*ctivating events (called A's) do not cause emotional and behavioural *C*onsequences (called C's), but that thoughts or *B*eliefs (called B's) intervene as mediators (J. S. Beck, 2011). For example, an activating event, such as preparing to consult with one's first client, does not cause the emotional consequences of anxiety, but the emotion is mediated via beliefs such as, 'I must be a perfectly competent therapist or I am a professional failure.' Psychological disorders arise when the beliefs are irrational. By 'irrational' Ellis means that they are unlikely to find empirical support in the person's immediate environment and do not promote survival and enjoyment. Although there are many irrational beliefs, Ellis argues that they can be distilled into a relatively small set of basic irrational thoughts (see Ellis & Harper, 1975). Therefore, Ellis would argue that the preceding example is an illustration of a basic irrational belief such as, 'you must prove thoroughly competent, adequate and achieving' (Ellis & Harper, 1975, p. 102).

Treatment adds D and E to the 'ABC' model, where D refers to *D*isputing the irrational thoughts and replacing them with more rational thoughts. This is achieved through a Socratic dialogue and a logic-empirical method of scientific questioning, challenging, and debating. The consequence of replacing the old beliefs with the new more rational ones is more positive *E*motions (i.e., E's). Rational thoughts are based on objective facts and if acted on will lead to a preservation of life, a more rapid achievement of one's goals, and prevent undesirable conflict (Ellis & Harper, 1975). Thus, the procedural steps of RET are to (i) *persuade* the client that an RET analysis of the problem is useful, such that the client is convinced of the mediating role of cognitions, (ii) *identify* the most important irrational beliefs underlying the present complaint, which can be achieved using a case formulation approach described in Chapter 5, (iii) show the client how to *dispute* the irrational thoughts, and (iv) to *generalize* learning so the client can apply the newly acquired knowledge and skills without the assistance of therapy.

Once the core irrational beliefs have been identified the aim is to challenge them. The clinician achieves this goal by asking questions such as, 'What thinking errors are you making?', 'What is the evidence for what you thought?' and 'What is the effect of thinking the way you do?' In so doing Ellis would argue that one looks for thinking errors such as 'Awfulizing' (e.g., 'It's awful when I'm stood up'), 'I can't' thoughts (e.g., 'I can't bear it when you ignore me') and 'Damning' (e.g., 'You deserve to burn in hell for what you did to me').

Similar to Ellis's RET is Beck's cognitive (behaviour) therapy. Beck's approach clearly focuses on cognitions, but there is an added behavioural emphasis, especially with behavioural experiments (Bennett-Levy et al., 2004) that is less apparent in RET. Beck (1967) assumes that emotional difficulties such as depression and anxiety arise from negative automatic thoughts. They are negative in emotional content and automatic in the sense that they appear to occur involuntarily, and consequently are not easily dismissed. Depressed thinking is characterized by a cognitive triad: negative thoughts about the self, the world, and the future. Overlaid on this content are cognitive processes (attention, abstraction, and encoding) that transform environmental stimuli. Beck argues that these cognitive processes are biased (cf. Williams, Watts, MacLeod, & Mathews, 1997) which has the consequence that anxious and depressed individuals tend to make judgements in a systematic and consistent manner. The biases identified are: (i) *selective abstraction*, which describes forming conclusions based on isolated details of a single event (e.g., 'I had a bad therapy session because I forgot one question'), (ii) *overgeneralization*, which involves holding extreme views based on particular events and then generalizing the conclusion (e.g., 'I had trouble with my first client, therefore I must be a failure as a clinical psychologist'), (iii) *dichotomous thinking*, which includes thinking in all-or-nothing terms (e.g., 'My first client was a success, but I just know my second will be a failure'), and (iv) *personalization*, which describes incorrectly making an inference about one's self, based on an external event (e.g., 'My client has cancelled, therefore I must be a bad therapist'). These cognitive processes harden into stable characteristic cognitive beliefs (called schemata) that Beck argues render people vulnerable to anxiety or depression.

To identify and modify these dysfunctional beliefs, the first step is to identify automatic thoughts. This is achieved by getting the client to monitor *automatic thoughts*, which are verbal thoughts or images that seem to arise without effort and are associated with negative emotion. Clinicians can elicit these thoughts by asking clients to introspect (e.g., 'What's going through your mind right now?'). For instance, you might ask a client to try to identify the automatic thoughts that occur when you notice an abrupt shift in mood in a session; you could use evocative, personally relevant role-plays; you might model the process by 'thinking aloud' your own automatic thoughts.

Burns (1980, 1999) has described a *downward arrow* technique that can be very helpful. The clinical psychologist identifies an important automatic thought that could arise from an underlying dysfunctional belief. By repeatedly asking the client the meaning of the thought (e.g., 'What's the worst thing that could happen?' or 'What would be upsetting about that?' or 'What would that mean?') the clinician aims to spiral down towards the dysfunctional belief. Other methods to help clients focus on the content of cognitions are to help them to attend to global words (e.g., always, never) and imperatives (e.g., must, should, and ought), exploring a client's explanations of negative or positive moods, and attending to self-referent thinking. The clinical psychologist might also want to focus on the form of the cognitions, by drawing the client's attention to typical cognitive biases and asking about the degree to which these are used in other areas, especially those where emotional problems are observed. Therefore, during the session with a client, the observation of intense emotion may suggest the activation of more central automatic thoughts.

Outside the cognitive therapy session, clients are encouraged to maintain a record of the automatic thoughts and their effects. In a series of columns, clients record activating events, the accompanying emotion (rated from 0–100 in terms of intensity), a written verbatim record of the automatic thought, and finally the degree of belief in the thought (0–100). Clients are then encouraged, first within the therapy session and then more often on their own outside of therapy, to challenge the automatic thoughts. Similar to RET clients will (i) assess the evidence for a thought by asking 'What is the evidence?' or 'How could it be tested?'; (ii) evaluate alternative ways of thinking, by posing the questions 'Is there another way to look at it?' or 'What can I do about it?'; (iii) consider the implications of a way of thinking by asking 'What is the effect of thinking?' or 'What is the worst that could happen?'; and finally (iv) identify any thinking errors. The aim in each of these activities is to identify a new, more helpful and believable thought that leads to a more positive emotional reaction.

One issue of relevance to cognitive therapy is the role of unconscious thoughts. For example, it has been long argued that we only have access to cognitive products, not cognitive processes (Nisbett & Wilson, 1977). We might know that we decided to choose clinical psychology as a profession, but we do not have direct access to the reasons why we made this choice (even though we believe we do). That is, much thought is unconscious and inaccessible but we continue to answer 'why?' questions, even though we arguably do not have access to the data. This could be a problem for cognitive therapies if one believes that clients truly cannot get access to their automatic and irrational thoughts. However, it is also possible to assume that in therapy we are evaluating the evidence for and against different thoughts and we decide on which are best accounted for by the data. This latter position is agnostic as to whether we have direct access to automatic thoughts, by only assuming that we can evaluate and change our belief structures.

Presenting a rationale for cognitive therapy

When conducting any psychological treatment, presentation of a rationale is critical. Giving a rationale is part of the broader goal of orienting a client to treatment, which has been identified as a clinical activity that is predictive of positive therapeutic outcomes (Orlinsky et al., 2004). The challenge when giving a rationale for cognitive therapy is no different to any other therapy, since it is important to present the treatment in a manner such that the client understands it sufficiently well to be *able to comply* and so that sufficient hope and motivation are recruited to encourage the client to *want to comply*. Therefore, the principles of treatment need to be outlined and any potential objections must be addressed.

For example, in outlining a rationale for cognitive therapy in which cognitions are postulated to mediate the emotional responses to antecedent events, a few points are worth bearing in mind. First, the language must be clear, simple, and appropriate to the client. By way of example, if you consider the first sentence in this paragraph, you could well find that phrases such as 'cognitions are postulated to mediate emotional responses to antecedents' could be better expressed for clients as, 'You've been telling me that your husband makes you angry, but although it might feel as if he causes you to feel angry, it is what you think about in your head that causes you to feel bad. Now, I understand that the idea that he doesn't cause you to be angry may sound pretty strange so let me give you an example...' The jargon has been avoided and also a common client reaction to a cognitive rationale has been anticipated by using the phrase '... I understand that the idea ... sounds pretty strange'. Our rule of thumb is that if any word of phrase needs an explanation, then you do better to deliver the explanation than to use the word. That is, if you need to tell the client what 'cognitive' means, why use the word in the first place? Sometimes it will be useful to teach clients names and phrases to facilitate communication, but the main goal is therapy not education about therapy and so we suggest keeping jargon to a minimum. A second point is to try to make the rationale memorable. Since the rationale is a key point in therapy, you want to do everything you can to help the client focus on it and remember it. One way to do this is to use a memorable metaphor/illustration. Sometimes the client will have already given you an illustration (e.g., a client with panic disorder and agoraphobia might have said, 'as I stood in the queue at the supermarket I started to worry that I might not be able to get out in case of a panic and then whoosh, there was the panic') or you might choose a metaphor based around a client's interest. One example might be as follows:

'Let me try to show you what I mean about thoughts causing feelings. The other day I was driving along like normal and feeling fine. All of a sudden I caught sight of a police speed camera by the side of the road and I thought "did I just see it flash?" I quickly braked; I felt panicky; my heart started to beat fast and my hands got sweaty; I began to worry that I'd have to pay a fine and I didn't have the money. Then I realized that the camera hadn't flashed and so I hadn't been caught. A wave of relief swept over me and I drove on comfortably.'

You can then discuss with the client what caused your emotional reactions, by asking if the speed camera had caused your emotional response (e.g., 'how did the speed camera sitting by the side of the road cause my heart rate to increase?') and what caused the changes in emotions (e.g., 'how did the unchanging speed camera cause both anxiety and relief'?). Sometimes starting with these illustrations can be difficult, if the client responds by indicating that their emotional problems are different to the example given. Usually, however, they can help clients to see clearly relationships that can be obscured when they try to reflect upon event–emotion sequences that have been occurring for a long time or when the emotions are very intense. Thus, beginning to develop a suite of rationales is a good therapeutic skill.

In the process of presenting a cognitive rationale, clients will often object to the ideas and it is wise to tackle this head on. For example, clients may say that a cognitive approach is cold and cerebral. One way to respond to this is to ask them to imagine a distressing situation and see if it elicits an emotional response. If so, then you can respond that it is this kind of emotional response that can be triggered even by memories and thoughts that therapy is trying to tackle and the aim is to bring runaway emotions under control. Another objection clients may raise is that you are asking them to deny reality. One response is to reject this assertion and to indicate that the goal is not to deny reality, but to avoid making false assumptions, for example that the actions of others or events in the world can cause my feelings. Sometimes clients will respond that they must express their feelings and that cognitive therapy is about denying these feelings and their expression. A possible response to this concern is to highlight that once you have a feeling it may be useful to express it, but suggest that cognitive therapy involves asking if you needed to have the feeling (or one of that intensity) in the first place. Clients might also claim that thoughts happen too quickly or automatically/unconsciously. One response to this client concern is to try an experiment. Write on a piece of paper, 'a pen without ink is no use' and ask the client to read the sentence aloud. Then write, 'I prefer to use a pen that works' and ask the client to do the same. When the client has said these two sentences, ask them why they pronounced the word 'use' differently. Some clients will recall enough grammar to explain why, but most will respond that they 'just knew it from the context' but we have not found a client who will attest to having consciously articulated the grammatical rules to decide between possible pronunciations. This allows you to illustrate that there are rules/beliefs that we have learned and we can infer their current operation from our behaviour, but they may be so practised that they no longer need to be articulated. Having made this point, the question needs to be turned back on the client by posing the question; just because it has been that way does it always have to be that way? At this juncture, examples of learning to drive and then travelling to a country where the practice is to drive on the opposite side of the road may be useful. Although driving on one side of the road was learned and became automatic, nonetheless it is reversible with effort and concentration. Sometimes clients might respond that cognitive therapy sounds too idealistic, to which one could respond that therapy is about giving choice. Emotions are a cue to initiate a self-inventory and change associated thoughts if you wish. There is no imperative to changing your unhelpful thoughts. Finally, clients later on in cognitive therapy may indicate that they believe the rationale intellectually, but not emotionally. One way to address this concern is to reframe 'believing intellectually' as an initial sceptical belief. It reflects an openness to be convinced by the evidence and therefore the client can be encouraged to take the cognitive rationale and 'try it on for size' or to 'borrow the belief for a while and see what happens'. Thus, the issue becomes an empirical question that client and therapist work on together.

In summary, cognitive therapies focus attention on modifying psychological problems by identifying and then working with the client to modify thoughts and beliefs that are postulated to intervene between the activating event and the problem emotion or behaviour.

More recently, cognitive therapies have started to move away from a focus on the content of cognitions and towards the underlying cognitive processes. For example, some research has emphasized the role that metacognitions play in selecting cognitive processes which in turn can influence cognitive content. In a similar vein, Hayes and colleagues (Hayes et al., 2011; Hayes & Strosahl, 2004) in their Acceptance and Commitment Therapy focus on the cognitive processes clients use when responding to unwanted thoughts and emotions, and suggest replacing avoidance with an attitude of acceptance. These treatment developments are promising, but to date there has not been sufficient time for them to enter the listings of evidence-based treatments.

Basics of interpersonal psychotherapy

In contrast to the focus of behavioural and cognitive therapies, interpersonal psychotherapies emphasize different factors in treatment. Interpersonal psychotherapies have been found to be efficacious for depression, eating disorders, and some personality disorders (e.g., Cuijpers et al., 2011; Gunlicks-Stoessel & Weissman, 2010; Rieger et al., 2010).

As you may recall, an IPT (Klerman et al., 1984; Klerman & Weissman, 1993) approach conceptualizes treatment as falling into three phases with treatment mechanisms specific to each phase (Lipsitz & Markowitz, 2013). The first phase of assessment and orientation to therapy has been covered earlier. Therefore, the present discussion will focus on the middle phase, in which problem areas are selected and treatment is engaged in, and the termination phase.

During the middle phase the clinical psychologist using IPT will (i) facilitate a discussion of topics that are relevant to the problem area, (ii) maximize self-disclosure by fostering a strong therapeutic relationship and identifying topics which heighten the client's affective state during therapy, and (iii) ensure the smooth passage of the client through therapy by identifying therapy-interfering behaviours. A session of IPT will often begin by asking the client, 'Where should we focus today?' This contrasts with CBT, where the direction of treatment is more often managed by the therapist. Thus, the client chooses the topic for discussion and can change focus from a previous session. One particularly good point about this opening is that it gives a client licence to bring up previously unmentioned problems; however, the novice clinical psychologist needs to be cautious at this point because you run the risk of having therapy 'hijacked' by clients who skip between topics without resolving any issue.

Notwithstanding, once the focus of the session has been decided upon, the therapist will move through four developmental stages in therapy: the clinical psychologist will (i) explore the problem area, (ii) focus on the client's expectations and perceptions, (iii) analyse alternative ways to handle the problem area, and (iv) work with the client to initiate new behaviours.

For example, if the problem area is one of an abnormal grief reaction, then the first stage of problem exploration could involve an analysis of points at which a client fails to move through the grieving process or in which the mourning process has become distorted (e.g., depression in the absence of sadness), delayed (e.g., when grief is experienced long after a loss), or prolonged. The perceptions and expectations could be explored by a discussion of the client's life with their loved one and their life in the present. This discussion will move into treatment, which will aim to facilitate the mourning process and help the client re-establish interests and develop new relationships. The particular strategies that could be used include a non-judgemental elicitation and exploration of feelings by encouraging the client to consider the loss, to discuss events surrounding the loss and the consequences of those events, with a view to bringing out any associated feelings. Often clients need reassurance that grief is not a sign of abnormality and therefore a discussion of both the typical grief process (and the variability therein) can be beneficial to facilitate the client discussing, experiencing, and 'owning' the distressing feelings. During IPT a clinical psychologist might try to shift a client from the death per se, because a fixation on the death can lead to avoidance of some of the complexities within the relationships with the deceased. By discussing both the factual details of the dead person and the client's affective experiences with the dead person (both when alive and in the present context) it may be possible to move through some of the negative feelings feared and avoided by the client. In so doing, the client will be able to identify a new formulation of the relationship and understand the memories of the dead person that incorporates both the strengths and the weaknesses of the relationship. As treatment moves into behavioural change, the clinical psychologist will seek to help the client to become more open to developing new relationships and in this way, the therapist can lead the client to consider new and different ways of re-engaging with people.

A second area of focus in IPT is interpersonal role disputes, where the client and another person significant to them have non-reciprocal expectations about the conduct of a relationship or the roles therein. For instance, a married couple may have a dispute about the work–family balance of each partner. The clinical psychologist begins by trying to identify the chief issues and clarify the nature of any dispute by highlighting differences in expectations and values between the client and their significant others. This will also entail considering both the client's wishes about the relationship and the options and resources available to them. In addition, it is worthwhile spending time searching for patterns in behaviours (e.g., has the same issue appeared in previous relationships or does the same conflict manifest in a variety of presentations?) and if they exist, exploring the possible reasons. Moving to consider new ways to handle the issues, it can be useful to focus on avoidance of confrontation and an unwillingness to express negative feelings. If these unassertive behaviours are occurring, then treatment can involve assisting clients to devise strategies for managing the disputes and to resolve differences.

A third target of IPT is role transitions, in which a person has moved from one social role to another (e.g., promotion, marriage, childbirth, etc.). Since people who do not cope adequately with transitions are at risk of developing depression, treatment will try to enable a client to view their new role in a more positive manner. By exploring both the (usually forgotten) negative as well as the positive aspects of a previous role, it may be possible to develop a more balanced view of the present circumstances while simultaneously working to restore the client's self-esteem. In terms of new behaviours, IPT will encourage the client to initiate new relationships in their new role. This will require an assessment of the client's social skills to determine the degree to which previously successful social skills may generalize to the new context and whether new skills are required. Since some of the difficulties with role transitions arise because there is a loss of familiar social supports and attachments (often accompanied by a reduction in self-esteem to the extent that it was bound up in the previous role), and because there are demands for new social skills, the therapist should address these deficits. Once identified, the clinical psychologist will try to put the lost role in perspective by evaluating the activities and attachments that were given up, and by using the processes in IPT, such as encouragement of the expression of affect and training of required social skills, to help the client establish a new system of social support.

Finally, IPT will focus on interpersonal deficits. These are targeted when it is apparent that a client lacks the skills for initiating or sustaining relationships. These deficits may be observable in the therapeutic sessions or from a review of the client's life. Since interpersonal skill deficits remove a person from a major source of enjoyment, a major goal of the treatment is to reduce any social isolation. Maladaptive patterns in previous relationships will be sought and, if identified, the clinical psychologist will discuss with the client negative and positive feelings associated with these relationships. At this point the clinician may explore with the client the feelings about the therapist and the therapeutic relationship, with the aim of using this relationship as a model for other relationships. That is, the therapeutic relationship can be used to help clients learn interpersonal skills which they can then apply outside therapy.

In summary, IPT focuses treatment upon the interpersonal difficulties that may cause the presenting problem or may arise from it. In so doing, the treatment seeks to reduce the presenting problem by addressing issues that may cause or exacerbate the client's difficulties.

Delivering evidence-based treatments

Having described some of the basics of behaviour therapy, cognitive therapy, and interpersonal psychotherapy, it is worth bearing in mind that no psychotherapy can be completely captured in a description of its components. This is not to say that components cannot be isolated, manualized, and even automated using computerized technologies (Tate & Zabinski, 2003), but the ability to deliver the treatment in a manner that connects with the client is a critical skill. Therefore, we will conclude the chapter with two detailed examples of particular treatments, illustrating how they might be presented to a client. We present these not as scripts to follow, but as illustrations of how a treatment may be delivered to a particular client. Putting this another way, the manualization of psychological treatments has facilitated the dissemination and reproduction of treatments in the same way that musical annotation facilitated the dissemination of music. However, in the same way that a skilled musician interprets the notes or arranges a piece for different instrumentation, a skilled clinical psychologist will modify and adapt treatments so that they meet a client's needs. The first example is graded exposure for a phobic anxiety and the second is relaxation.

Example 1: exposure to feared stimuli

Exposure to feared stimuli is another broadly applicable treatment (Andrews et al., 2003) that has a strong empirical foundation. However, while the efficacy of exposure is not in question, the mechanism whereby the beneficial effects are brought about is not as clear as once thought. Procedurally, confronting a feared stimulus in the absence of aversive consequences parallels extinction as it involves the repeated presentation of a conditioned stimulus (CS) in the absence of the unconditioned stimulus (US), with the end result that a new contingency is learned. However, the procedure also parallels that of habituation and counterconditioning. For example, in systematic desensitization counterconditioning occurs as a client is first taught relaxation training so that they are able to elicit the relaxation response rapidly and effectively. Once this skill has been taught, the client is taught to construct anxiety hierarchies so that feared stimuli are organized into a 'stepladder' of fear. For example, a 100-point 'fear thermometer' is used to help clients rank feared situations and stimuli in terms of the amount of fear elicited. Exposure (often in imagination) is then conducted, beginning with the least fear-provoking, and during stimulus presentation the client is encouraged to relax, with the goal being that relaxation functions as a competing response inhibiting anxiety. If anxiety begins to escalate, exposure is terminated or reduced until relaxation dominates over anxiety. At this point exposure is recommenced. However, in contrast to counterconditioning, exposure is also effective when conducted *in vivo* without the buffering of anxiety and when high levels of anxiety are elicited (i.e., flooding). Further, a client needs to confront a feared stimulus, yet in some circumstances distraction from the stimulus appears to enhance the anxiety reduction both within (Johnstone & Page, 2004; Penfold & Page, 1999) and between (Oliver & Page, 2003) sessions. The variety of procedures (e.g., imagination versus *in vivo*; distracters present versus absent) and differences in the intensity of anxiety (e.g., systematic desensitization versus flooding) present difficulties for many different theories of anxiety (see Barlow, 1988; Craske, 1999, 2003). However, for a scientist-practitioner these differences are non-trivial, because a good conceptual understanding of the mechanisms whereby an intervention brings about its clinical effects is essential to good clinical practice. Without a strong theoretical foundation it is unclear how to apply a treatment under conditions that differ from a 'textbook' situation, what factors to consider when a client does not respond as expected, and when clients present with a complex mix of different problems.

One theory that can accommodate the variety of circumstances in which exposure reduces anxiety is self-efficacy theory. Bandura (1977) argued that all anxiety-reducing treatments share the common property that they increase the sense of competence in mastery regarding a fearful situation. Thus, successful mastery enhances self-efficacy that in turn reduces avoidance. Self-efficacy predicts therapeutic outcome more accurately than arousal during treatment, anticipated danger, or perceived danger. Further, it guides treatment by suggesting that effective therapy will maximize the elements that enhance a sense of mastery.

Another approach that can also accommodate the variety of situations within which exposure is effective is the more pragmatic approach typified by Barlow's (1988) essential targets for change. Barlow first suggests that exposure should address *action tendencies.* Anxiety primarily involves action tendencies that are typified by vigilance, or a chronic state of readiness to respond. Consequently, exposure treatment should aim to modify these action tendencies by encouraging approach rather than avoidance. All varieties of exposure share this as both a process and a goal. Second, Barlow claims that a key belief structure/ meaning proposition in anxiety appears to be the *perception of a lack of control.* Exposure exerts its effect in part by enhancing perceived control. Thus, during successful exposure and in combination with anxiety management strategies clients learn that they have increased control over the feared objects and situations themselves as well as the anxiety response. Finally, Barlow identifies *self-focused attention* as a critical variable. Anxiety is associated with self-focused attention in general and a self-evaluation in particular. Barlow cites evidence that clients fail to exhibit reductions in anxiety when they are in a self-evaluative mode, but that reduction of anxiety is greatest when attention is focused on the external and non-emotional aspects of the environment.

Both Bandura's and Barlow's approaches mesh with an interesting review by Clum and Knowles (1991) about the factors that predicted which people with panic attacks would go on to develop agoraphobic avoidance. They claimed that it was not severity or frequency of panics, the age of onset, and probably not the duration of panic or location of first panic. Rather agoraphobic avoidance was predicted by negative outcome expectancies, the perception of a link between situation and panic occurrence, and self-efficacy. To the extent that these factors are generalizable, exposure should aim to do more than simply confront a person with the feared stimulus. The treatment should also aim to change outcome expectancies, which it could do through psychoeducation and successful experiences of confronting feared stimuli and situation. Secondly, the treatment would aim to modify a perception of a link between situations and panic and anxiety, by changing causal assumptions through cognitive therapy and by using exposure to test false beliefs about the danger inherent in situations and establish new learning that promotes less anxiety. Thirdly, exposure treatments should aim to enhance self-efficacy. It appears that exposure to feared stimuli is associated with enhanced self-efficacy per se (e.g., Oliver & Page, 2003) but these changes could be enhanced by teaching emotion and problem-focused control strategies in addition to successful experiences of confronting feared stimuli.

With these principles in mind, it is possible to examine some questions about the conduct of exposure to feared stimuli. A first question is, how much anxiety should be permitted? Given the aims are to extinguish anxiety, it is important to have as much as possible, but since the aim is also to change cognitions and enhance self-efficacy, this goal can be balanced with the aim of eliciting as much anxiety as the client can manage (most often achieved by grading the exposure tasks). Although grading exposure does not appear to be essential, graded exposure is preferable because it tends to have lower dropout rates than flooding. A second question is, how similar to the feared situation or original trauma does exposure need to be? In general the closer the exposure situation resembles the actual situation, the greater the anxiety-reducing effects will be (Andrews et al., 2003). This is important to remember when using imaginal exposure, but it also needs to be borne in mind that although *in vivo* is generally superior to imaginal exposure, better imaginers improved more with imaginal exposure (Dyckman & Cowan, 1978). Further, imaginal exposure is excellent for 'filling in steps' that aren't possible in real life (e.g., having a plane take off for one metre and land again) or undesirable or impractical to replicate (e.g., a trauma), but transfer from imagination to real life is only around 50%. A third issue concerns the temporal parameters of exposure. Broadly speaking, the more frequent and the closer the sessions, the stronger the treatment effect, and longer sessions (i.e., until anxiety reduced to around 10–20%) appear better than shorter ones (due to the risk of sensitization). These factors allow anxiety to reduce and the person's expectations and beliefs to change as they come to feel in greater control of their anxiety.

Having discussed these general principles, we will illustrate how a therapist may present a rationale for exposure to a client and then proceed to introduce exposure hierarchies.

THERAPIST: A universal truth about anxiety is that avoidance makes fears worse. This is the case because first, anxiety is unpleasant, second, avoiding fear-provoking situations or activities stops anxiety, and third, escaping when anxiety is rising brings enormous relief.

CLIENT: It sure does. Getting away from spiders is the best thing I can do.

T: In the short term, avoiding is the most sensible thing to do, but what have been the longer-term effects?

C: I've just got more fearful and had to avoid not only spiders, but places where they might be.

T: And what happens when you escape or avoid these places?

C: I feel relief.

T: That relief is a problem because in the short term, avoidance and escape give you a sense of control over your anxiety but in the long term you spend more and more time organizing your life to avoid what your fear. In this way fear spreads throughout your life. Phobic avoidance develops a little like a child's tantrum to get something to eat when out shopping. Supermarkets are designed so that the aisle containing the candies is far enough from the entrance that children have had time to get tired and hungry. When the candies finally come into view, the child throws a tantrum. To a frustrated parent, the candies provide a simple solution to stop the noise and embarrassment. The problem is that the next time the parent ventures into the supermarket, a tantrum is even more likely. Avoiding or escaping from what you fear is like giving a kid a candy to stop a tantrum. Every time that you flee before your anxiety subsides, you make it more likely that you will be anxious the next time.

C: But I've tried to face my fears, but it hasn't worked.

T: A common mistake made by people trying to manage fears is to progress too quickly. Their anxiety reaches very high levels and never goes down until the person runs away from the frightening situation. Is this what happened to you?

C: It almost sounds like you were there! But I've tried so hard and it hasn't worked.

T: Putting in so much effort and not seeing any benefit can be very demoralizing. For that reason we are going to carefully monitor your anxiety to make sure that we can tell what we are doing is working and if it isn't, we can rethink our strategy. What I am going to suggest is that we try a different way and face your fears gradually. To face your fears step-by-step, you first must clearly identify what you want to achieve. Your goal may be to go somewhere or do something that you presently find frightening. Remember, a goal is something to strive towards; don't worry if you can't achieve it yet. Later you'll be able to break it down into easier steps. Let's try to write down a goal.

C: Well, I'd like to be able to walk into my house like a normal person and not have to check each room for spiders before I can feel comfortable.

T: OK, let's try to break this goal into smaller, easier steps. Each step must be specific and we'll try to build a 'stepladder' so that we begin with steps that cause little fear and anxiety and work up to something that is quite scary.

C: Well I could begin by standing outside a room, but not going in.

T: How much anxiety on our fear thermometer would that cause?

C: About 10 out of 100.

T: OK, that sounds like a good place to be. What might be a little more fear-provoking for the next step. Say around 20?

The client and therapist then continue to work out the hierarchy.

T: Now we've got the anxiety stepladder, let's get some guidelines in place for when we start to face these fears. First, I want you to agree that you are going to do everything you can not to leave because of fear. Only leave once your anxiety has begun to decline. You will become panicky and fearful, but you can use the anxiety management techniques we've covered to control it.

C: Is this absolutely necessary?

T: What do you think?

C: I guess so, because otherwise I'll keep reinforcing the anxiety through relief.

T: Well done. I know it's going to be difficult, but this is the way to break the cycle. The next guideline will be that you will repeat each step until anxiety has decreased and your confidence has increased enough for you to attempt the next step. I'll work with you to make sure that you don't go too quickly or too slowly, but by facing your fears regularly and systematically, they will decrease.

C: If that's the only way.

T: I know it will be hard, so don't forget that after each attempt you reward yourself. No one else understands how frightening your steps are for you, so praise yourself or give yourself a treat whenever you face your fear and your anxiety decreases.

C: OK, I think I'm ready.

T: Before we start, there is one last thing to mention and this is an important point to remember. When people start to face their fears, they feel as though they are getting worse. Their anxiety feels stronger and their ability to control it weaker. This experience is not only normal; it is a signal that you are beating your anxiety. Your anxiety is behaving like the child in the supermarket who screams to get a candy. The more you say 'No', the louder your anxiety will scream to make you give in. Expect a tantrum – and we'll work together to manage it without avoiding or escaping.

Example 2: relaxation

One treatment technique that has a broad application is relaxation. Borkovec, Grayson, and Cooper (1978) reported that progressive muscle relaxation was superior to a control condition in alleviating tension and the effects were maintained over five-month follow-up. Although the effects of relaxation do not appear to be mediated by therapeutic suggestions (Borgeat, Stravynski, & Chalou, 1983), Agras, Horne, and Taylor (1982) found that client expectations do affect outcomes. Clients were told to expect an immediate improvement or no immediate improvement and the results (for systolic blood pressure) were more favourable for participants in the former group. Perhaps related to the enhanced expectations, Brauer et al. (1979) found that therapist-directed progressive muscle relaxation was more effective than audiotaped relaxation. Thus, the live training appears superior, perhaps because it enhances therapeutic expectations, or perhaps because the relaxation can be paced appropriately and the therapist can use visual cues to correct errors. However, relaxation requires sufficient practice and training to be effective. With the downward pressure on the duration of therapeutic contact, it is important to note that, on average, studies that find that relaxation is effective use *over five sessions* of training (Borkovec & Sides, 1979; Hillenberg & Colins, 1982). Studies finding no effect average only 2.3 sessions of training. Thus, relaxation is an effective method of anxiety management, but how is it to be delivered? In the following example, we illustrate how one might deliver a rationale and treatment with a client (see also Bernstein & Borkovec, 1973) who has already been explained many elementary aspects of anxiety and fear (e.g., the fight–flight response).

CLIENT: But I keep getting these headaches from all the tension I've got. What can I do about that?

THERAPIST: Do you remember we talked about the flight or fight response and how it involves increased muscle tension?

C: Yes, so, is that why I've got this muscle tightening when I'm worried or panicky?

T: Yes, and have you noticed what happens if the physical tension remains too high for too long?

C: I get exhausted and have headaches.

T: That's right. So to overcome problem tension you will need to do three things. First, you'll need to learn to recognize when you've got excess tension. Second, you'll need to learn to relax it away and third to learn how to keep the excess tension away. The first step in all this is to separate good tension from bad tension.

C: But all tension's bad. I want to be relaxed don't I?

T: Think for a moment about playing tennis. Just before you receive a serve, what do you do?

C: I crouch and get ready to whack it back as hard as I can.

T: You tense up?

C: I guess so, but that's so my muscles are ready for when the ball is served.

T: And when the point is over, what happens to your muscles?

C: They relax until I get ready to receive the next service.

T: So you see how throughout the game you alternate between being tense and relaxed? If you remained too tense between points you'd tire out, but if you relaxed before a serve you wouldn't be ready. This tension is *good* tension because it is not too high for the task and it lasts as long it needs to. In the same way, you need to be more and less tense throughout the day. It is necessary to be more tense when driving a car than, for example, when watching television.

Table 6.1 Tension identification chart

Body area	Where am I tense right now?	Where am I usually tense?
Neck and Head		
• Neck		
• Scalp		
• Forehead		
• Eyes		
• Temples		
• Jaw		
Upper Body		
• Shoulders		
• Top of back		
• Chest		
Hands and arms		
• Hands		
• Lower arms		
• Upper arms		
Lower body		
• Stomach		
• Base of back		
• Buttocks		
• Groin		
Legs		
• Thighs		
• Knees		
• Calves		
• Feet		

C: I see that the tension increases my alertness when I'm driving, but I don't need it when I crash in front of the TV.

T: Absolutely. Now ask yourself, where you feel tense *right now* and then where you *usually feel tense*. On this sheet [Table 6.1], put a tick against every area which is relaxed. Put a cross against every area that is tense. Leave blank any area which is neither tense nor relaxed.

T: See how the areas of tension seem to group together, especially around your neck, head, and face.

C: No wonder I get these damned headaches. What can I do about them?

T: What we need to do is to learn how to relax every muscle in your body by learning the art of muscle relaxation. I'll give you a bit of the theory first and then go on to the practice, so we can start to learn it here and now.

C: Let's get on with it.

T: OK. Well, you can defeat tension with relaxation because they work *against* one another. The more tense you become, the less relaxed you are. The more relaxed you become, the less tense you are. Both the flight or fight response and the relaxation response are controlled by part of your brain called the involuntary nervous system. One half of the involuntary nervous system triggers flight or fight, while the other half controls the relaxation response. These two halves work like a pair of scales. If you load one side of the scales with panic, fear, and worry, you will have more tension than relaxation (because you feed the flight or fight response). If you load the other side with relaxation, you will have more relaxation than tension (because you feed the relaxation response).

C: So this tension is why I feel keyed up and headachy?

T: Tension can lead to all those things as well as backaches, sore muscles, nausea, stomach upsets and 'butterflies', and even trouble sleeping. What we've got to do now is to see how to control this tension with something called progressive muscle relaxation. Let me show you what I mean. Try to tense the muscles around your eyes.

C: Erm … I don't know what you mean. How do I do that?

T: Yes, when we try to get tense it's difficult. Now try another way. Close your eyes tightly. You are now taking control of your muscles, making them do what you want. Once this tension is under control, relax the muscles by opening your eyes.

C: I can see that. They were tense and then relaxed.

T: Switching between tensing and relaxing in this way shows the two principles of physical relaxation. First, the muscles are deliberately tensed to take control of tension. The idea is not to *increase* physical tension, but simply to tighten the muscles sufficiently for you to *recognize* physical tension. Second, the muscles are then relaxed. You can progressively work through your body, gently tensing and relaxing all your muscles in turn. In this way you can totally relax your whole body. Let's start by learning how to identify and relax each muscle area, then you can begin a whole body relaxation session. Make yourself comfortable by sitting back in the chair with your legs uncrossed, feet firmly on the floor, and hand resting on your thighs.

T: Try to relax your hands by first tensing them by curling them into fists. Then relax them by stopping making a fist and letting it fall. What did you notice?

C: I could feel the tension grow and then fall away when I let it go.

T: Excellent, that's the funny thing about progressive muscle relaxation. Putting the tension in is the way to get control of it and let the tension go. Now let's move up to your lower arms. Tense your lower arm muscles by lowering your hand. Bend it down at the wrist as though trying to touch the underside of your arm. You should feel the tension in your forearm. Relax the muscles by straightening the wrist again.

T: Moving up now to your upper arms. Can I ask you to tense your biceps by bending your arm at the elbow, curling your hand towards your shoulder? This is the same movement that bodybuilders use to show off their biceps. Relax the arm by straightening it.

T: Now let's try the shoulders. Tense the muscles by lifting your shoulders. Hunch them up as if trying to cover your ears with them. Now relax by letting your shoulders drop again … To work on the neck, lean your head to the left until you feel the muscles tighten in the right side of your neck. Slowly and carefully roll your head forward, around to the right and then all the way back to where you started. One side of the neck will tense while the other is relaxing. If you feel any pain, you are stretching too vigorously. How does this feel?

C: This is hard because it all feels pretty tense to begin with and the relaxing doesn't seem as effective.

T: It's really good that you notice these things because remember that one of the goals was that you learned to recognize the tension. With practice you will get better at relieving the tension, but the first step is to become aware of the tension. Now have a go at the forehead and scalp. Tense these muscles by raising your eyebrows. Release the tension by letting your face resume its normal expression once more. How was that area?

C: Not as much tension as the neck.

T: OK, let's try the eyes. Tense the muscles around the eyes, hold, and then relax … We can do the jaw now. Tense the jaw by clenching your teeth (enough to tighten the muscles and no more). Relax by unclenching them … OK, moving to the chest, inflate your lungs to expand and tense your chest muscles. Hold the tension, then release by breathing out … Tense and relax the stomach. To do this, push your tummy out to tense your stomach muscles. Release by letting your stomach return to its normal position … Next we can do the upper back. Tighten the muscles by pulling your shoulders forward while leaving your arms by your sides. To relax, let your shoulders swing back to their usual position. Can you notice the difference between the tension and relaxation?

C: Yes. The tension makes it easier to relax because all you've got to do is let the tension go. It is as if the relaxation happens automatically.

T: That's right. The relaxation response isn't something that you force to happen, but something that you just let happen. Let's see if you can do the same with the remainder of your body. To focus on the lower back, try to arch your lower back by dropping your head forward. Your back should roll into a smooth arc, tensing the lower back as you lean forward. Now relax the muscles by sitting up straight again. When you've done this you can move to your buttocks. Tighten your buttocks by pulling them together. You'll feel yourself rising in your chair. Release the tension by sinking back into the chair … Then we'll move down our legs, beginning with your thighs. While sitting, push your feet firmly into the floor to tighten your thigh muscles. Relax by stopping pushing … Now try to relax your calves. Lift your toes towards your shins to tighten your calf muscles. Now release the tension by dropping your toes again … Finally, with your feet, curl your toes down so that they are pressing against the floor. Now release by letting the feet straighten back to their normal position.

C: I feel quite relaxed now.

T: Are some places more relaxed than others?

C: Yes, my neck and head still feels pretty tense, but my back and lower body feels better.

T: That's probably because the muscle groups where you notice the most tension need more work, so now that we've practised each exercise, we'll do them all in turn to relax your whole body. When you do this on your own at home you'll probably find it is best to do these exercises while sitting in a comfortable but straight-backed chair, with your feet flat on the floor, and hands resting in your lap. Sitting is preferable to lying down, otherwise you may find the urge to sleep may become overwhelming. Allow yourself around 15–20 minutes in which you will not be disturbed. You may like to play soothing music, dim the lights, and draw the curtains. However, what we'll do now is repeat the actions we've practised, but in the way I'd like you to try at home.

C: So you want me to do this for like homework?

T: Yes, I want you to repeat this so that with practice you can get better at the progressive muscle relaxation and that you learn better to notice when you're getting tense. Then you'll be able to use some faster and more targeted relaxation exercises.

C: That would be good, because I'm not sure I'll always have 15–20 minutes to relax.

T: Although you won't always have time, with more practice, you will get more benefits. We'll talk about the practice a bit later, but for now let's do a run through. I'd like you to sit back comfortably in the chair and close your eyes. Are you comfortable?

C: Yes, I'm ready.

T: OK. Well your body has a natural rhythm to it. You may have noticed that as you breathe in, you tend to tense. As you breathe out, you tend to relax. That's why it is easiest to breathe in as your tense your muscles and breathe out as you release the tension. We'll work through the same muscle groups as before but as we do each one I'd like you to do the following routine. First, as you're breathing in, apply enough pressure to feel tension to the muscles so that they are about 75% tight. Hold the tension for 7–10 seconds and while you're holding the tension try to breathe as easily as you can. After about 10 seconds, on the next breath out, let the tension go. Sometimes people find it good to mentally say the word 'relax' as they breathe out. Once the tension has gone from the muscles, wait 10 seconds and then apply tension again or move on to the next area. I'll talk you through this first time …

C: That was good. I feel very heavy now.

T: When you've finished relaxing, you will probably want to remain seated for a few minutes to enjoy the pleasant feeling. Try not to jump up too quickly as you may tense up again; you may even feel dizzy, as your blood pressure drops when you relax. But while we're sitting here, what did you notice happened to your mind during the exercises?

C: I found that my mind started to wander. That was a bit distressing and I forgot what I was supposed to be doing.

T: That is perfectly normal. As you relax, your mind becomes less focused and it will wander. Recognize this sign of relaxation, because it is the opposite of being tense and stressed, when your mind is very stuck on one or two things. However, as you notice your mind has wandered off, gently bring your mind back to the exercises. Was there anything else you noticed?

C: I'm not sure what you mean.

T: Sometimes people find the bodily sensations of relaxation unusual and possibly worrying but whatever sensations you feel, it is important that you label them as part of the relaxation process. With practice, you'll find that the sensations aren't frightening and they become less noticeable over time. Bear in mind that physical relaxation is an art that takes persistence to master. Only a few people enjoy their first attempt; it is only with patient practice over a two-month period that relaxation becomes a useful strategy in managing excess tension.

C: I'm willing to give it a go, but does it always take so long?

T: One of the main benefits of whole body relaxation is that you learn to recognize excess tension and replace it with relaxation. This means that taking time regularly to do the whole body relaxation is a good use of time even though it is time-consuming. However, when time is short, you can modify the normal progressive relaxation to a quick relaxation programme. Quick relaxation can be adapted to any situation. Although it may not bring the same degree of relaxation as the full 20 minutes of progressive muscle relaxation, it can be targeted at particular muscles. To relax quickly you need to identify which muscles are too tense, tense those muscles (as you breathe in) for 7–10 seconds, and then allow the muscles to relax (as you breathe out) for 7–10 seconds.

Embedding evidence-based psychological treatment in a health care system

Although the focus of the present chapter has been on the provision of psychological care within individualized treatment, it is useful to note that this is not the only manner in which psychological treatments can or should be delivered. This point is well-made by Kazdin (2011) who notes that within the United States, one quarter of people meet criteria for a psychological disorder in any one year while more than two thirds of these do not receive treatment. More telling, is the observation that in most countries mental health services tend to be concentrated in affluent, urban areas which results in those in rural and remote locations being underserviced. Thus, the problem of unmet need is greatest among those from minority and disadvantaged groups because the barriers to access services are more significant.

While in the past these challenges were insurmountable, current developments in the delivery of psychological services are providing effective and efficient solutions. Video-conferencing as well as telephone and video calls allow for psychological therapy to be delivered at a distance. For instance, telephone quit lines allow smokers to be provided with evidence-based treatment services. These can be mailed to them and supplemented with a combination of pre-recorded messages and access to a counsellor (Lichtenstein, Zhu, & Tedeschi, 2010). Similarly, cognitive behavioural interventions have been adapted with great success to delivery over the internet for a variety of psychological problems, such as pain and headaches (Cuijpers, van Straten, & Andersson, 2008), anxiety and mood disorders (Andersson, Cuijpers, Carlbring, & Lindefors, 2007; Andrews et al., 2010; Richards & Richardson, 2012), and many other health issues (Lustria et al., 2013). Yet despite the great potential of these technologies to address many challenges, clinical psychologists have sometimes viewed these developments with caution.

One concern that clinical psychologists may have about the internet and other self-help strategies is that they may be less effective than face-to-face treatments. While it is self-evidently true that self-help cannot be adapted in the face of a complex clinical presentation, there is little evidence that it is unhelpful. In fact, in a meta-analysis, guided self-help was more (albeit by a small margin) effective than face-to-face psychotherapy (Cuijpers, Donker, Van Straten, Li, & Andersson, 2010). Thus, guided self-help is effective with an apparent saving in resources. This point can be made more forcefully from a study of social phobia treatment (Andrews, Davies, & Titov, 2011). Not only were treatment effects comparable between internet-delivered and face-to-face treatment, the total therapist time was 18 minutes per patient for the internet group and 240 minutes per patient for the face-to-face group. Thus, the significant saving in terms of staff time makes the internet treatment a worthwhile consideration. But should psychologists worry about the future of the profession if internet-delivered treatments are effective?

Returning to an earlier point; there are more people with psychological problems than a society can treat and this has implications for how clinical psychologists should respond to new treatments and delivery modes. Many people who deserve treatment cannot access the services they require and therefore a stepped care model appears a viable solution. Clients may access services in a hierarchy of intensity. Clients could begin with internet-delivered therapies or guided self-help. Clinical psychologists may provide oversight to assist in the assessment of people who require different or additional, more intensive treatment. Problems (such as elevated suicide risk) may occur and when these events are monitored, decisions will need to be made about how to manage these risky situations. Furthermore, there is no reason to believe that the internet-delivered treatments will be immune from the iatrogenic effects that occur in psychotherapy more generally (Barlow, 2010), but unlike psychotherapy, there is not always a psychologist monitoring the situation. Therefore, clinical psychologists have nothing to fear as a profession. There will always be an abundance of cases to treat.

By way of explanation, we can consider Kazdin's (2011) claim that over two thirds of clients deserving treatment do not receive therapy. Even if we assumed that everyone in the entire population who needed treatment received an internet-based therapy (rather than came to see a clinical psychologist in the first instance), would there be a lack of work? Not at all. Internet-delivered treatment will probably have rates comparable to psychotherapy generally of clients who deteriorate or show no reliable change (i.e., over 50%; Lambert, 2010; Newnham, Harwood, & Page, 2007, 2009). Consequently, the number of 'treatment failures' would still exceed the number of people that clinical psychologists could provide services to. Thus, there is no need for the profession to shy away from other modes of delivering psychological treatment. We should embrace it.

This is why, in the first chapter, we argued that clinical psychologists are at a crossroads. Clinical psychology is faced with a demand for mental health services that far exceeds our ability to meet it. However, that challenge will be met as other professional groups become involved. Clinical psychologists can take what is best practice and adapt it to novel delivery methods. We can research the programmes to guide the refinement of existing treatments; we can train other professionals and para-professionals to assist in providing treatment; and we can continue to invent new treatments. By taking an active role in the research process we can demonstrate leadership and continue to show how science-informed practice remains the foundation of good clinical care in the twenty-first century.

Internet-delivered psychological treatments are not an alternative to psychotherapy delivered by clinical psychologists; they are a supplement to it. By supplementing the array of treatment options, we improve the overall effectiveness of the service provided. To give one example, in Germany at the University of Trier, Wolfgang Lutz has implemented a regime at their public clinic, in which clients on the waiting list are first offered internet-based treatment. This addresses a practical problem (i.e., how do you care for the welfare of clients on a waiting list?) while ensuring that the clinic only deals with clients whose problems were resistant to the front-line treatments. To date it is not clear what the best models of treatment delivery are. Does stepped care improve the overall outcomes of a service? Which psychological treatments do not transfer well to the internet? (For example, Carlbring et al., 2012 found that attentional bias modification did not appear to translate well to the less-controlled environment of the internet.) What happens when psychologists incorporate internet-delivery into standard psychotherapy? Which clients are less well-suited to internet treatment (e.g., Lancee et al., 2014)? Clinical psychologists will continue to contribute to and deliver science-informed practice in the way they have for years. What will change is the focus and scope of the treatments.

Summary

In conclusion, clinical psychologists have an array of psychotherapies that have an evidence base for a variety of conditions. However, there are psychological problems for which empirical support is still lacking and there are no doubt psychotherapies that do not yet have 'empirical support' which will in time be so identified. Thus, as a scientist-practitioner it is important to be familiar with evidence-based treatments, and to continually evaluate the psychological literature to identify and become familiar with new treatments as they become supported (e.g., Emotion-Focused Therapy – Elliott et al., 2004; and Mindfulness-Based Cognitive-Behaviour Therapy – Khoury et al., 2013; Segal, Williams, & Teasdale, 2002). Behaviour Therapy (and variants such as Dialectical Behaviour Therapy – Linehan, 1993a, 1993b), Cognitive Therapies, and Interpersonal Psychotherapy (Klerman et al., 1984) represent some current treatments it is important to be familiar with. However, it is one thing to use an efficacious treatment, but another to be an effective clinician. Thus, even when using treatments with a known efficacy, it is necessary to evaluate the effectiveness in your setting by measuring and monitoring the progress of clients in therapy. Furthermore, with pressures to make treatment not only effective, but also efficient, there has been an increasing awareness of the occasions when brief interventions and group treatment are valuable treatment options. Therefore, we will now turn to consider the delivery of brief interventions and then group treatment.

Chapter 7

Brief interventions

It is likely that demand for health care will always outstrip supply. Stepped care approaches provide a partial solution by aiming to detect health problems at an early stage and offering efficient, less costly, low-intensity interventions before problems become more complex and less tractable. Known as the prevention paradox (Kreitman, 1986; Spurling & Vinson, 2005), more problems can be averted by intervening with a large number of people at low risk than with a small number of people who are already at high levels of risk. Brief interventions target people with health-compromising behaviours at the lower end of the risk spectrum who are not formally seeking help, but are offered the intervention opportunistically whenever they present to health professionals including psychologists.

Here we focus on brief interventions for alcohol use. The aim of these interventions is to raise awareness of alcohol-related risk and reduce hazardous and harmful drinking behaviour. There are at least two reasons why clinical psychology trainees need to develop competencies in brief interventions for alcohol. First, many patients when presenting to the clinician focus on their primary presenting symptoms (e.g., depression or anxiety) and may not mention alcohol use or any associated problems. The brief intervention protocol allows the clinician in just a few minutes to conduct a formal screening for potentially risky alcohol use and – if indicated – provide personalized advice to motivate the client to do something about it. Unidentified alcohol use problems can otherwise hinder therapy progress with the primary presenting problems. Second, the motivational interviewing principles and strategies that often complement the brief feedback and advice are universally applicable in all types of interventions (brief or intense) aimed at positive behaviour change.

Brief interventions for alcohol address four levels of alcohol risk as identified by the Alcohol Use Disorders Identification Test (AUDIT; Babor & Higgens-Biddle, 2001). Education and positive reinforcement are provided to individuals at low risk including abstainers. Simple advice including personalized feedback and information about strategies to reduce drinking and avoid hazardous drinking is provided to those identified as risky drinkers. This is often combined with brief counselling and motivational interviewing especially for those at higher levels of risk. Finally, those at the highest, possibly dependent, level of risk are strongly encouraged to seek specialist help.

The effectiveness of brief interventions at reducing alcohol-related problems is well established especially in primary health care (O'Donnell et al., 2014) and university settings (Carey, Scott-Sheldon, Elliot, Garey, & Carey, 2012). However, the evidence to date does not support the effectiveness of brief interventions for drinkers in the dependent range who will require specialist care and more intense monitoring and support (Saitz, 2010). Nonetheless, as it is inevitable that excessive drinkers at the dependence end of the spectrum will be

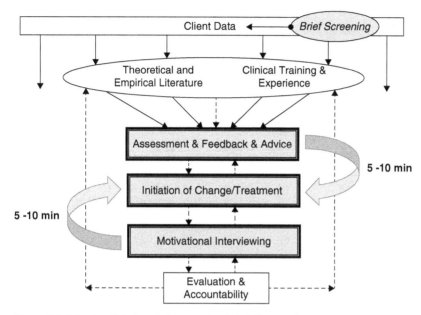

Figure 7.1 Adapting clinical psychology practice for brief interventions.

identified though routine screening, the brief intervention contact can be used to encourage the person to consider and accept a specialist referral.

Figure 7.1 shows that the client data to inform the brief intervention are gathered via a brief screening instrument. A copy of the AUDIT adapted for Australian standard drinks is shown in Figure 7.2 (a copy of a version used in the UK can be found in Kaner, Newbury-Birch, & Heather, 2009). In *brief* interventions, assessment information is limited and targeted. It is not used to inform a comprehensive case formulation, but the screening score is used to immediately provide feedback following guidelines for a giving risk category, and offer advice on how to act on that feedback. If a person is willing, this can flow on into a brief motivational interviewing segment to increase the likelihood that a person initiates behaviour change by following the strategies listed in a brochure handed out during the intervention, or if possible dependence is identified by accepting specialist referral information. These interventions typically last between 5 and 25 minutes (O'Donnell et al., 2014), and the key steps in the intervention are based on the '5 A's' model – Ask, Assess, Advise, Assist, and Arrange.

1. Persons are **asked** if they would be willing to fill out a short questionnaire and discuss their drinking.
2. Their drinking (and risk of alcohol-related harm) is **assessed** using the Alcohol Use Disorders Identification Test (AUDIT).
3. Persons are **advised** about the meaning of their AUDIT score, the likely consequences of their drinking pattern, and provided with simple strategies for modifying their drinking (if necessary). A structured information brochure is typically used to facilitate this feedback (for an example see Kaner et al., 2009).
4. Students who drink at levels considered to be risky or very risky are encouraged to discuss their motivation for change. The aim of this motivational interviewing segment is to **assist** students to increase their motivation to change.

Drink Check AUDIT

Number of standard drinks in common beverages

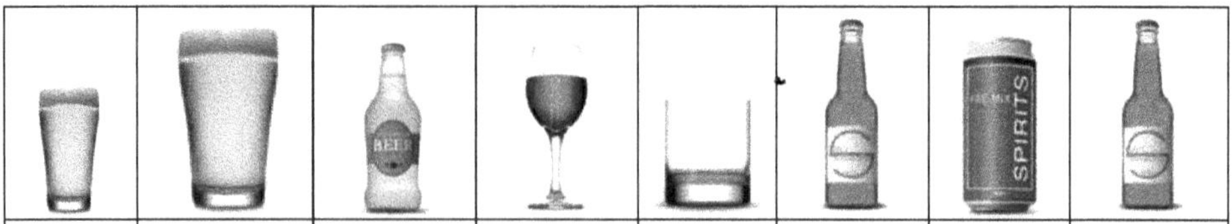

1 middy of full strength beer (285ml)	1 pint of full strength beer (568ml)	1 can or stubbie of full strength beer (375ml)	1 average restaurant serve of wine or Champagne (150ml)	1 shot of spirits (30ml)	Premix spirits Full strength (5%) 330 / 600ml	Premix spirit can Full strength 375 / 440ml	High strength (7%) spirits bottle or can 330 / 660ml
1	**2**	**1.4**	**1.5**	**1**	**1.3 / 2.6**	**1.5 / 1.7**	**1.8 / 3.6**

Please circle the response that best fits your drinking.

Questions	Scoring system					Your Score
	0	1	2	3	4	
1. How often do you have a drink containing alcohol?	Never	Monthly or less	2–4 times per month	2–3 times per week	4+ times per week	
2. How many standard drinks do you have on a typical day when you are drinking?	1 or 2	3 or 4	5 or 6	7–9	10 or more	
3. How often do you have 6 or more standard drinks on one occasion?	Never	Less than monthly	Monthly	Weekly	Daily or almost daily	
4. How often during the last year have you found that you were not able to stop drinking once you had started?	Never	Less than monthly	Monthly	Weekly	Daily or almost daily	
5. How often during the last year have you failed to do what was normally expected from you because of your drinking?	Never	Less than monthly	Monthly	Weekly	Daily or almost daily	
6. How often during the last year have you needed an alcoholic drink in the morning to get yourself going after a heavy drinking session?	Never	Less than monthly	Monthly	Weekly	Daily or almost daily	
7. How often during the last year have you had a feeling of guilt or remorse after drinking?	Never	Less than monthly	Monthly	Weekly	Daily or almost daily	
8. How often during the last year have you been unable to remember what happened the night before because you had been drinking?	Never	Less than monthly	Monthly	Weekly	Daily or almost daily	
9. Have you or somebody else been injured as a result of your drinking?	No		Yes, but not in the last year		Yes, during the last year	
10. Has a relative or friend, doctor or other health worker been concerned about your drinking or suggested that you cut down?	No		Yes, but not in the last year		Yes, during the last year	
					Total	

Figure 7.2 A drink check audit. Based on material provided by the National Health and Medical Research Council.

5. Students with AUDIT scores that suggest dependence on alcohol are helped to **arrange** a referral or follow-up with a specialist health professional.

The structure of the brief intervention using the 5 A's is shown in the flowchart in Figure 7.3. We next explain each step of the intervention in detail. This training protocol

Flow Chart for Brief Alcohol Intervention

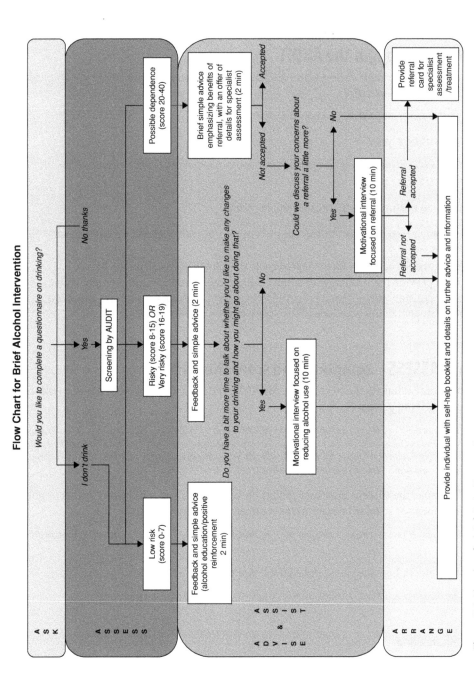

Figure 7.3 Flowchart for brief alcohol intervention.

was developed in collaboration between our clinical psychology training programme at the University of Western Australia and our university's health promotion unit and medical centre. Students undergo training in a half-day workshop, followed by supervised experience in the delivery of brief interventions to the campus community.

Step 1: ASK – begin the AUDIT

The first step in the intervention is to ASK the student if he/she is interested in completing an alcohol use questionnaire.

'Would you like some feedback about your current drinking levels?'

If the student says 'yes':

'Great. I'll get you to fill out this form. I'll then be able to provide you with some feedback on your drinking.'

Responding to students who say they do not drink

If the student responds that he/she does not drink, then ask question 1 from the AUDIT to clarify this.
- If the student never drinks, do not complete the full AUDIT (i.e., skip Step 2)
- Then provide the student with some feedback and positive reinforcement about their decision not to drink, referring to Step 3a (Feedback for low-risk drinkers).
- If the student drinks occasionally, then complete the AUDIT as usual.

Step 2: ASSESS – complete and score the AUDIT

Once the student has agreed to complete the AUDIT, you are ready to **ASSESS** how risky the student's drinking pattern is.

'Now I'll ask you to fill in this questionnaire called the AUDIT, which will only take a minute or two. It was developed by the World Health Organization and is extensively used worldwide. Some of the questions ask about standard drinks. There's some information at the top of the form that will help you work out how many standard drinks you normally have each time you drink. What do you drink most often?'

As an example, the student may answer that he or she usually drinks beer. Use this to point out the number of standard drinks in the student's usual alcoholic drink.

'Ok, well you can see here that there's 1 standard drink in a middy, 1.4 standard drinks in a can, and 2 standard drinks in a pint.'

Once the student has completed the AUDIT, you need to work out his/her total score.

'Thanks for filling this in. I'll add up your score now and give you some feedback about your results.'

Troubleshooting

If a student says he or she drinks a beverage that is not featured at the top of the AUDIT, you can refer to the **Standard Drink Chart**. This chart contains a wider range of drinks than listed on the AUDIT – use this to work out how many standard drinks the student typically consumes.

After calculating the AUDIT score, determine the category into which the student's score falls (low risk, risky, very risky, or possible dependence).

Scoring procedure for the AUDIT

- The response to each item is scored from 0–4, according to the number at the top of the response column.
- Write this number into the column titled 'Your Score'.
- Sum the scores for each response to give a total score and write this at the bottom of the page next to 'Total'.
- Determine which drinking category the total score falls into.
  - Scores from 0–7 are categorized as 'low risk'.
  - Scores from 8–15 are categorized as 'risky'.
  - Scores from 16–19 are categorized as 'very risky'.
  - Scores from 20–40 are categorized as 'possible alcohol dependence'.

Step 3: ADVISE and ASSIST – give feedback about the AUDIT score

After scoring the AUDIT, you need to **ADVISE** and **ASSIST** the student by:
- providing **feedback** about his/her AUDIT score
- where necessary, providing **simple advice** about how to reduce alcohol consumption.

During this step you should use the **Drink Check Brochure** to guide the discussion.
This step should take two minutes or less to complete.
The intervention will progress differently depending on the student's AUDIT score.

(a) If the student scores in the **low risk** range, provide feedback, simple advice and positive reinforcement.

(b) If the student scores in the **risky** or **very risky** range, provide feedback and simple advice and encourage the student to participate in a brief individualized discussion about their drinking, using motivational interviewing.

(c) If the student scores in the **possible dependence** range, provide feedback and simple advice that focuses on the importance of seeking a referral for further assistance and advice about drinking. If the student is resistant to this idea, encourage him/her to participate in a brief discussion about referral using motivational interviewing, with the intention of encouraging the student to take up the referral.

These steps are now described in detail, according to the AUDIT score.

STEP 3a: feedback for low risk drinkers (score 0–7)

The main goal of feedback with low risk drinkers is to provide positive reinforcement and encouragement for them to continue drinking at safe levels. You need to:
- Tell the student that their level of drinking falls in the low risk range.
- Point out that, like them, most UWA students are low risk drinkers.
- Reinforce the benefits of low risk drinking.
- Encourage the student to continue drinking at a low risk level.

Steps in detail

Important

As you work through the Drink Check Brochure with risky, very risky, and dependent drinkers, it is important to try and engage the student in conversation, rather than talking *at* them.

Showing respect for the student and their views may encourage them to participate in the Motivational Interviewing part of the intervention.

Write the student's score on the beer glass on the **How Risky is My Drinking?** section of the Drink Check Brochure.

'Your AUDIT score is X.'

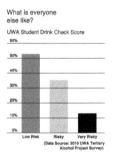

Point to the graph titled **What is everyone else like?**

'Congratulations, this means that you're drinking at a low risk level. About 53% of UWA students are also low risk drinkers.'

Point to the **What does your score mean?** section of the brochure.

'Compared with students who drink at risky levels, you're likely to feel better, study more effectively, and are unlikely to suffer from health problems. Basically, drinking is unlikely to have a negative impact on your life.'

Low Risk

Compared to risky drinkers, you have a greater chance of…

- ⬎ Feeling happy
- ⬎ Feeling relaxed
- ⬎ Feeling sociable
- ⬎ Studying effectively
- ⬎ Being physically healthy
- ⬎ Being mentally healthy
- ⬎ Staying safe
- ⬎ Having good relationships

Motion to the relevant parts of the brochure as necessary.

'This brochure also provides information for those students who are drinking at more risky levels, with suggestions on how to cut down and support services available on campus should you or someone you know ever need them.'

Provide encouragement.

'I'll leave the brochure with you. Keep up the low risk drinking! Enjoy the rest of your day.'

STEP 3b: Feedback for risky (score 8–15) and very risky (score 16–19) drinkers

For students with an AUDIT score in the *Risky* or *Very Risky* range:

- Tell the student that his/her score falls in the Risky or Very Risky range.
- Point out that most UWA students are low risk drinkers.
- Point out the negative consequences of risky/high risk drinking.

- Point out the potential benefits of reduced drinking.
- Show the student the list of drinking targets.
- Advise the student about where he/she can access further information and support.

Steps in detail

Write the student's score on the beer glass on the **How Risky is My Drinking?** section of the Drink Check Brochure.

'Your AUDIT score is X.'

How risky
is my drinking?

40

20
16

8

0

Point to the graph titled **What is everyone else like?**

'This is in the risky/very risky category. About 32%/13% of UWA students fall into this category. Most UWA students are low risk drinkers. Does that surprise you?'

What is everyone
else like?

UWA Student Drink Check Score

60%

50%

40%

30%

20%

10%

0%
Low Risk   Risky   Very Risky
(Data Source: 2010 UWA Tertiary
Alcohol Project Survey)

Point to the **What does your score mean?** section of the brochure.

'If you continue to drink at your current level, you may experience some negative effects, like poor judgement and decision-making, hangovers, and health problems. Have any of these things been a problem for you?'

Risky

Compared to low risk drinkers, you are more likely to be affected by these problems...

↘ Impaired judgement

↘ Slurred speech

↘ Sexual encounters
that you later regret

Point to the section titled **Drinking Targets**.

'This shows Australian drinking guidelines to help avoid alcohol related problems. It's recommended that people should have no more than 2 standard drinks a day on average, with no more than 4 drinks at a time, and should have at least 2 alcohol free days each week.'

Drinking targets

↘ Aim for 2 or fewer standard drinks per day
↘ Have no more than 4 standard drinks at any
one time, no more than 3 times a week
↘ Make at least 2 days each week alcohol free

Remember, if at first you don't succeed, try again!

Motion to the section titled **Benefits of Reducing Your Drinking.**

'If you reduce how much you drink you'll experience some of the benefits listed here, like having more money and energy, and you'll be less likely to experience health problems.'

Benefits of reducing your drinking

↘ Improve your
relationships with
friends and family

↘ More positive mood
↘ More likely to make
sensible decisions

Motion to the **Ways to Cut Down** section.

'If you want to reduce your drinking then there are some strategies listed here that other students have found helpful, such as drinking more slowly and having water in between drinks. Are there any things that you already do to try to slow down your drinking?'

Ways to cut down

↘ Eat before and during
drinking

↘ Count how many drinks
you have

Motion to the **Further Information** section of the brochure.

'You could visit or telephone these centres if you'd like more information.'

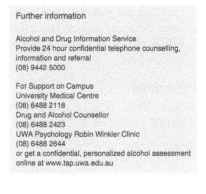

Further information

Alcohol and Drug Information Service
Provide 24 hour confidential telephone counselling, information and referral
(08) 9442 5000

For Support on Campus
University Medical Centre
(08) 6488 2118
Drug and Alcohol Counsellor
(08) 6488 2423
UWA Psychology Robin Winkler Clinic
(08) 6488 2644
or get a confidential, personalized alcohol assessment online at www.tap.uwa.edu.au

Give the student the brochure to keep, and **seek permission** to undertake the Motivational Interview.

'If you have a few more minutes I'd like to talk to you about whether you'd like to make any changes to your drinking and how you might do that. Is that OK?'

If the student declines, give them the **Self-Help Booklet** to take away.

'That's fine. I'll give you this to take away – you could use it to help you decide whether changing your drinking pattern is something you'd like to do. Enjoy the rest of your day.'

If the student consents, move on to the fourth A – Assist (i.e., conduct a Motivational Interview). This is discussed below; but first we show how to give feedback to someone in the possibly dependent range.

STEP 3c: Feedback for drinkers who are possibly dependent (score 20–40)

For students with an AUDIT score in the *Dependent* range

- Tell the student that his/her score falls in the Very Risky range, and that a score above 20 usually indicates alcohol dependence.
- Point out that most UWA students are low risk drinkers.
- Point out the negative consequences of high risk drinking.
- Point out the potential benefits of reduced drinking.
- Show the student the list of drinking targets.
- Show the student the contact details for further support.
- Encourage the student to make an appointment with a health professional.

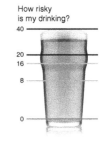

How risky is my drinking?

Steps in detail

Write the student's score on the beer glass on the **How Risky is My Drinking?** section of the Drink Check brochure.

'Your AUDIT score is X.'

Point to the graph titled **What is everyone else like?**

'This is in the very risky category. As you can see here, most UWA students are low risk drinkers. About 13% of UWA students are like you, which is a high risk drinker. However, not many students score over 20 – only around 6%. A score of 20 or more suggests you might be experiencing alcohol dependence. Do you know what that means?'

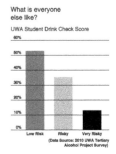

What is everyone else like?

UWA Student Drink Check Score

(Data Source: 2010 UWA Tertiary Alcohol Project Survey)

Encourage the student to talk to you. If necessary, give the following explanation of dependence:

'*Dependence means that your alcohol use can cause a lot of problems but you might feel like you can't, or don't know how to, reduce how much you drink.*'

Point to the **What does your score mean?** section of the brochure – discuss both the '*Risky*' and '*Very Risky*' sections.

'*If you continue to drink at your current level, you're likely to experience some negative effects, like poor judgement and decision-making, hangovers, conflicts with friends and family, and you'll be at risk of serious health problems. Do any of these things concern you?*'

Motion to the section titled **Benefits of Reducing Your Drinking**.

'*If you reduced how much you drink you might experience some of the benefits listed here, like having more money and energy, and you'll be less likely to experience health problems.*'

Point to the section titled **Drinking Targets**.

'*This shows Australian drinking guidelines to help avoid alcohol related problems. It's recommended that people should have no more than 2 standard drinks each day on average, with no more than 4 drinks at a time, and at least 2 alcohol free days each week.*'

Motion to **Ways to Cut Down** section.

'*There are some strategies listed here that other students have found helped them reduce their drinking. However, because your AUDIT score was in the dependent range, it might be helpful for you to speak with a health professional like a GP or alcohol counsellor about your drinking, rather than trying to follow these strategies on your own. What do you think about that idea?*'

Motion to the **Further Information** section of the brochure.

'*There is more information here about where you can get help on campus, as well as telephone lines and internet sites you might find helpful.*'

Very Risky

Any of the above, plus...

↘ Memory loss and blackouts

↘ Problems getting and keeping a job

Benefits of reducing your drinking

↘ Improves your relationships with friends and family

↘ More positive mood

↘ More likely to make sensible decisions

Drinking targets

↘ Aim for 2 or fewer standard drinks per day
↘ Have no more than 4 standard drinks at any one time, no more than 3 times a week
↘ Make at least 2 days each week alcohol free

Remember, if at first you don't succeed, try again!

Ways to cut down

↘ Eat before and during drinking

↘ Count how many drinks you have

Further information

Alcohol and Drug Information Service
Provide 24 hour confidential telephone counselling, information and referral
(08) 9442 5000

For Support on Campus
University Medical Centre
(08) 6488 2118
Drug and Alcohol Counsellor
(08) 6488 2423
UWA Psychology Robin Winkler Clinic
(08) 6488 2644
or get a confidential, personalized alcohol assessment online at www.tap.uwa.edu.au

Provide students who have expressed an interest in getting professional help with a copy of the **referral card**.

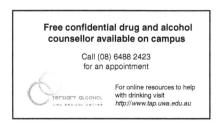

'The number on this card is for a person who regularly talks with students about their drinking. All you need to do is telephone and make an appointment. Do you have any other questions? ... Ok, well thanks for your time today and I hope things go well when you speak with (whoever is on the referral card).'

For students who indicate that they are unsure whether they want to make an appointment – ask if they are willing to discuss this further.

'I understand that you're not sure what you want to do from here – many people feel the same way. Can we talk a bit more about your concerns?'

Next, move onto the **Motivational Interview**.

Step 4: ASSIST and ARRANGE – motivational interviewing (and referral if indicated)

The broad aims of the final step in the intervention are to:

- **ASSIST** students by increasing their motivation to change their drinking pattern.
- **ARRANGE** for the student to seek professional help (if this appears necessary).

These aims are achieved by conducting a brief **motivational interview** with the student. Because our protocol was designed for trainee psychologists at the beginning of their practical training, and for health promotion volunteers to administer peer-delivered brief interventions, we also designed a **flip chart** to guide both the interviewer and interviewee through this more challenging part of the intervention. This step of the intervention is only conducted with students whose AUDIT scores are in the *risky, very risky,* or *dependent* drinking ranges (i.e., scores of 8 through 40). The focus of the intervention differs depending on whether the student's AUDIT score is in the risky/very risky range (8–19), or in the dependent range (20–40).

Step 4a For students with AUDIT scores between 8 and 19, the motivational interview should focus on increasing the student's motivation to reduce their alcohol consumption.

Step 4b For students with AUDIT scores between 20 and 40, the motivational interview should focus on increasing the student's motivation to seek help from a health professional.

The Motivational Interviewing Stance

When you are conducting a motivational interview, you should try to keep the following things in mind.

Be empathic

- Try to put yourself in the shoes of the student. Show a respect for and a genuine interest in the student's concerns and views.

Be non-judgemental

- Don't fall into the trap of negatively judging students who are drinking at risky levels, or who are ambivalent about change. Remember that change is difficult. Your job is to support the student by increasing their motivation to change. Ambivalence can be an important first step towards change.

Use summary and reflective statements

- Try to summarize and reflect back to the student the things they say to you. For example, if they tell you a list of negative things about drinking, repeat these back to them. For example, you might say, 'It sounds like some of the things you dislike about drinking are x, y, and z.'

Develop discrepancy

- Try to point out contradictions in the student's current behaviour (e.g., drinking excessively). For example, the student may say they enjoy drinking but it may be causing them lots of problems. For example, you could say, 'So, on the one hand there are things you like about drinking, but on the other hand there are things about drinking that you don't like, such as …'

Enhance self-efficacy

- Try to build the student's sense of confidence that they can reduce their drinking. This is achieved by equipping them with strategies they can use to reduce their drinking, as well as by providing encouragement.

STEP 4a: Assisting risky or very risky drinkers (AUDIT scores 8–19)

- The **interview** should focus on encouraging the student to reduce their alcohol consumption.
- Use the **flip chart** to guide the interview.
- The same information covered in the flip chart and interview is in the **Self-Help Booklet**, which the student will take away after the interview.

Steps in detail

Work through each page of the **flip chart**.

Start with the **Thinking about Drinking 1** exercise in the flip chart.

The aim of this exercise is for the student to consider and contrast the positive and negative consequences of their drinking, and to increase their motivation to change.

Thinking about Drinking ❶
↓

Continue present drinking pattern	Reducing my drinking
Positives (benefits)	
↘ e.g. "My social life won't change"	↘ e.g. "I won't get hangovers"
↘	↘
↘	↘
↘	↘
↘	↘
↘	↘
↘	↘
↘	↘
Negatives (costs)	
↘ e.g. "I will contine to spend too much money on booze"	↘ e.g. "My friends might make fun of me"
↘	↘
↘	↘
↘	↘
↘	↘
↘	↘
↘	↘

'People often feel unsure whether they want to make changes. This is understandable, since there are positive and negative aspects to every decision. Thinking about these positive and negative aspects might help you to clarify how you feel about drinking. First, we'll focus on your current drinking patterns.'

'Tell me some of the benefits that drinking has for you.'

'What are some things that aren't so good about your drinking at the moment?'

Some extra prompting questions about the negative aspects of drinking might be:

'What don't you like about xx?'

'How does xx affect you?'

Use a **double-sided reflection** to **summarize** what the student has said to you.

'So on the one hand you like drinking because … On the other hand, there are things about drinking that you don't like, such as …'

Turn to **Thinking about Drinking 2** and discuss the positives and negatives of reduced drinking.

'Now, imagine that you decide to reduce your drinking. What do you think would be some of the likely benefits of reducing your drinking?'

'OK, what would be some of the negatives of reducing your drinking?'

Use the examples in the Drink Check brochure to prompt discussion of the benefits of reducing drinking if need be.

Again, use a **double-sided reflection** to **summarize** what the student has said.

'It sounds as though it would be worthwhile for you to reduce your drinking because … but some barriers to you deciding to reduce your drinking would be that …'

Now move onto the page titled – **Are You Ready to Change? 1**. Ask the student to rate how important changing their drinking is, and how confident they are that they can change.
Write their answers on the back of the AUDIT.

'Now that we've talked about the pros and cons of reducing how much you drink or keeping things as they are now, how important to you is reducing your drinking, on this scale that goes from 0, for not at all important, to 10, for very important.'

Are you ready to change? ❶

How *important* is it to you that you reduce your drinking?

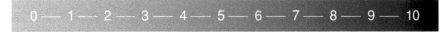

0 — 1 — 2 — 3 — 4 — 5 — 6 — 7 — 8 — 9 — 10

Not at all important   **Very important**

Are you ready to change? ❷

How *confident* are you that you can reduce your drinking?

0 — 1 — 2 — 3 — 4 — 5 — 6 — 7 — 8 — 9 — 10

Not at all confident   **Very confident**

Summarize the student's response. This may help him/her to elaborate upon it.

'Ok, you feel that it's not at all/somewhat/moderately/highly important to reduce your drinking.'

If the student picks a low number on the scale (e.g., 1 or 2), you could say:

'It seems that changing your drinking isn't something you think is very important at the moment.'

If the student picks a moderate number on the scale (e.g., 4, 5, 6), you might say:

'Changing your drinking is somewhat important to you, but you're not fully convinced it's something you want to do at the moment.'

If the student picks a high number on the scale (e.g., 8 or 9), you could say:

'So, reducing your drinking is very important to you.'

Then ask the student how confident they are that they can reduce their drinking, using the scale provided. Don't forget to write their response on the back of the AUDIT.

'How confident are you that you could reduce your drinking, if you decided to?'

Summarize the student's response, for example:

'Ok, you feel not at all/somewhat/moderately/very confident that you could reduce your drinking if you decided to.'

Then turn to **Are You Ready to Change? 2**. Discuss the similarity or difference between the student's perceived importance of change and their confidence in their ability to change.
    Example response to a student who feels that change is not important:

'So although you're confident that you could change if you wanted to, you don't feel that change is very important at the moment. On the other hand you were telling me before that drinking has ... (list negatives of current drinking). Can you tell me a bit more about how important, or unimportant, you feel it is to change your drinking?'

Example response to a student who does not feel confident that they can reduce their drinking:

'So although reducing your drinking is very important to you, you don't feel very confident that you'll be able to do it. What makes you feel like that?'

Move on to the **Plan to Reduce Your Drinking 1** section of the flip chart. The aim of this exercise is to encourage the student to verbalize the main reason(s) for and benefits of reducing their drinking.

'It sounds as though you'd like to make some changes to your drinking'

OR

'It sounds as though you're not wanting to make changes to your drinking at the moment, but perhaps you can just imagine that you're wanting to change your drinking.'

Plan to reduce my drinking ❶

↘ You may have decided that you would like to reduce your drinking.

↘ If you have not decided to reduce your drinking, then please just imagine that you are going to reduce your drinking.

What are your top 3 reasons for reducing your drinking?

Talk to the student about why they might want to reduce their drinking.

'What are your top 3 reasons for wanting to reduce your drinking?'

Reflect and validate the student's response.

'You're saying that you want to reduce your drinking because ... They sound like really important reasons.'

Ask the student to imagine what would change with reduced drinking.

'Can you tell me a bit about how your life might be different if you do reduce your drinking?'

Reflect the response.

'So if you reduce your drinking you expect that...'

Turn the flip chart to **Plan to Reduce My Drinking 2**. The aim of this exercise is to clarify the student's drinking goals and develop strategies for meeting the goals.

'A good way to make something happen is to make a plan. This increases the chances that you'll be successful. First, let's think about what sort of drinking pattern you'd like to have.

How many days each week do you want to drink?

How many drinks would you like to have each day?

What is the highest number of drinks you want to have at any one time?'

> ### Plan to reduce my drinking ❷
>
> ↘ How many days each week do you want to drink?
>
> ↘ How many drinks would you like to have each day?
>
> ↘ What is the highest number of drinks you want to have at any one time

Summarize and reflect the student's response, and compare them with the Australian guidelines for healthy drinking.

'So you think it would be realistic for you to have __ drinks on __ days each week.'

'This matches well with the Australian guidelines for healthy drinking.'

Or

'This is higher than the Australian guidelines, but seems like it would have a lot of benefits compared with how you're drinking at the moment.'

Turn to **Plan to Reduce My Drinking 3**. Discuss strategies for meeting the student's goals, dealing with lapses, and rewards.

'Do you have any ideas about some strategies you could use to help you meet your drinking goals?'

'Those are great suggestions that should help reduce how much you drink. It is common for students who are trying to drink less to sometimes slip up and drink more than they had planned. If that happens to you, what will you do to make sure you don't slip back into old habits?'

'Some people find giving themselves a reward for sticking to their goals helps motivate them to keep sticking to their goals. Would this be helpful for you? What rewards would you give yourself?'

> ### Plan to reduce my drinking ❸
>
> ↘ Can you think of some strategies you could use to reduce your drinking?
>
> ↘ What will you do when you have a lapse (drink more than you planned)?
>
> ↘ How will you reward yourself for drinking less?
>
> Reducing your drinking is challenging, but you can do it!

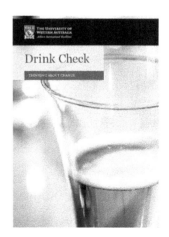

Finally, give the student a copy of the **Self-Help Booklet**, thank them for their participation and encourage them to reduce their drinking.

'Thanks for talking to me today. I'll give you this handout to keep, which covers everything we just talked about. It might be helpful if you filled it in, particularly the plan, and put it in a place where you'll see it regularly, like

on your fridge or next to your bed. Thanks again for talking to me today, and good luck in reducing your drinking. Enjoy the rest of your day.'

STEP 4b: Assisting possibly dependent drinkers (AUDIT scores 20–40)

- The **interview** should focus on encouraging the student to **seek professional help** to reduce their alcohol consumption.
- Use the **flip chart** to guide the interview.
- The same information covered in the flip chart and interview is in the **Self-Help Booklet,** which the student will take away after the interview.

Steps in detail

You will have just said something along the lines of:

'I understand that you're not sure what you want to do from here – many people feel the same way. Can we talk a bit more about your concerns about your drinking and about making a more formal appointment?'

If the student consents, work through the **flip chart**.

Start with the **Thinking about Drinking 1** page.

The goal is for the student to think about the negative consequences of their drinking, in order to increase their motivation to seek professional help.

'People often feel unsure whether they want to make changes. This is understandable, since there are positive and negative aspects to every decision. Thinking about these positive and negative aspects might help you to clarify how you feel about drinking. What are some things that you like about drinking? What are some things that you don't like about your drinking at the moment?'

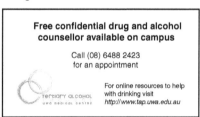

Free confidential drug and alcohol
counsellor available on campus

Call (08) 6488 2423
for an appointment

For online resources to help
with drinking visit
http://www.tap.uwa.edu.au

Use a **double-sided reflection** to **summarize** what the student has said to you.

'So on the one hand you like drinking because … On the other hand, there are things about drinking that you don't like, such as…'

Now turn to **Thinking About Drinking 2** and discuss the pros and cons of reduced drinking.

'Now, imagine that you decide to reduce your drinking. What do you think would be some of the likely benefits of reducing your drinking?'

'OK, what would be some of the negatives of reducing your drinking?'

Use the examples in the **Drink Check Brochure** to prompt discussion of the benefits of reducing drinking if need be.

Again, use a **double-sided reflection** to **summarize** what the student has said.

'It sounds as though it would be worthwhile for you to reduce your drinking because … but some barriers to you deciding to reduce your drinking would be that …'

Move onto **Are You Ready to Change? 1** and **Are You Ready to Change? 2** and have the student answer the questions about the importance of reduced drinking.

Are you ready to change? ❶

How *important* is it to you that you reduce your drinking?

0 — 1 — 2 — 3 — 4 — 5 — 6 — 7 — 8 — 9 — 10

Not at all important   **Very important**

Are you ready to change? ❷

How *confident* are you that you can reduce your drinking?

0 — 1 — 2 — 3 — 4 — 5 — 6 — 7 — 8 — 9 — 10

Not at all confident   **Very confident**

'Now that we've talked about the pros and cons of reducing how much you drink or keeping things as they are now, how important to you is reducing your drinking, on this scale that goes from 0, for not at all important, to 10, for very important.'

Write the student's answers on the back of the AUDIT.

Summarize the student's response. This may help him/her to elaborate upon it.

'Ok, you feel that it's not at all/somewhat/moderately/highly important to reduce your drinking.'

If the student picks a low number on the scale, (e.g., 1 or 2), you could say:

'It seems that changing your drinking isn't something you think is very important at the moment.'

If the student picks a moderate number on the scale (e.g., 4, 5, 6), you might say:

'Changing your drinking is somewhat important to you, but you're not fully convinced it's something you want to do at the moment.'

If the student picks a high number on the scale (e.g., 8 or 9), you could say:

'So, reducing your drinking is very important to you.'

Then ask the student how confident they are that they can reduce their drinking, using the scale provided. Don't forget to write their response on the back of the AUDIT.

'How confident are you that you could reduce your drinking, if you decided to?'

Summarize the student's response, for example:

'Ok, you feel not at all/somewhat/moderately/very confident that you could reduce your drinking if you decided to.'

Now, discuss the similarity or difference between the student's perceived importance of change and their confidence in their ability to change.

Example response to a student who feels that change is not important:

'So although you're confident that you could change if you wanted to, you don't feel that change is very important at the moment. On the other hand you were telling me before that drinking has … (list negatives of current drinking). Will you tell me a bit more about how important, or unimportant, you feel it is to change your drinking?'

Example response to a student who does not feel confident that they can reduce their drinking:

'So although reducing your drinking is very important to you, you don't feel very confident that you'll be able to do it. What makes you feel like that?'

Turn to **Are You Ready to Change? 3** and discuss whether the student will talk to a health professional. You might say:

Are you ready to change? ❸

1. How *important* do you think it is that you talk to a health professional (like a doctor or counsellor) about your drinking?

0 — 1 — 2 — 3 — 4 — 5 — 6 — 7 — 8 — 9 — 10

Not at all important   **Very important**

2. How *ready* are you to talk·to a health professional?

0 — 1 — 2 — 3 — 4 — 5 — 6 — 7 — 8 — 9 — 10

Not at all ready   **Very ready**

'Earlier on you were saying you weren't keen on talking to a health professional about your drinking. Now that we've talked some more about the pros and cons of your current drinking pattern, and the benefits of reducing how much you drink, has anything changed? How important to you is it that you speak with a health professional about your drinking?'

'Ok, so you feel that it's not at all/somewhat/moderately/highly important that you speak with a health professional about your drinking.'

'How ready are you to speak with a health professional about your drinking?'

If the student is keen to reduce his/her alcohol consumption but not keen to talk to a professional, highlight this discrepancy.

'It sounds as though on the one hand it's important to you that you reduce your drinking, but on the other hand you're not keen to talk to a health professional about how to do that. Will you tell more about that?'

Some prompters for this question might be:

'What would make you more likely to talk to a health professional?'

'What would be some of the pros and cons of this?'

Then move on to **Plan to Reduce My Drinking 1.**

'What would be your top 3 reasons for wanting to reduce your drinking?'

'Ok, you're saying that you want to reduce your drinking because ...

They sound like really important reasons.'

'How might your life might be different if you do reduce your drinking?'

'So if you reduce your drinking you expect that ...'

Plan to reduce my drinking ❶

↘ You may have decided that you would like to reduce your drinking.

↘ If you have not decided to reduce your drinking, then please just imagine that you are going to reduce your drinking.

What are your top 3 reasons for reducing your drinking?

Turn to **Plan to Reduce My Drinking 2** and discuss the student's goals.

'A good way to make something happen is to make a plan. This increases the chances that you'll be successful. First, let's think about what sort of a drinking pattern you'd like to have.

How many days each week do you want to drink?

How many drinks would you like to have each day?

What is the highest number of drinks you want to have at any one time?

So you think it would be realistic for you to have __ drinks on __ days each week.

This matches well with the Australian guidelines for healthy drinking'

Or

'This is higher than the Australian guidelines, but seems like it would have a lot of benefits compared with how you're drinking at the moment.'

> ### Plan to reduce my drinking ❷
> ↘ How many days each week do you want to drink?
> ↘ How many drinks would you like to have each day?
> ↘ What is the most number of drinks you want to have at any one time?

Turn to **Speaking with a Health Professional.**

Reinforce the importance and likely benefits of speaking with a health professional. Point out that talking to a professional is a recommended strategy for reducing very risky drinking patterns.

'Given the things we've discussed today, what would you like to do next? Would you like to make an appointment to speak with someone further?'

Yes

- Give the student a referral card.

'The number on this card is for someone who regularly talks with students about their drinking. All you need to do is telephone and make an appointment. I hope things go well when you speak with ...'

No, appointment not wanted

'There is more information here on the brochure about where you can get help if you change your mind later. Remember that if you decide to reduce your drinking it might be hard, but you can do it, and there is lots of support on and off campus if you want to access it.'

> **Free confidential drug and alcohol counsellor available on campus**
>
> Call (08) 6488 2423
> for an appointment
>
> Tertiary alcohol
> uwa medical centre
>
> For online resources to help
> with drinking visit
> http://www.tap.uwa.edu.au

> Further information
>
> Alcohol and Drug Information Service
> Provide 24 hour confidential telephone counselling,
> information and referral
> (08) 9442 5000
>
> For Support on Campus
> University Medical Centre
> (08) 6488 2118
> Drug and Alcohol Counsellor
> (08) 6488 2423
> UWA Psychology Robin Winkler Clinic
> (08) 6488 2644
> or get a confidential, personalized alcohol assessment
> online at www.tap.uwa.edu.au

Finish by giving the student a copy of the **Self-Help Booklet,** irrespective of whether they've made an appointment to speak with someone further.

'I'll also give you this handout to keep. It would be a good idea if you filled it in at home, particularly the plan, and put it in a place where you will see it regularly, like on your fridge or next to your bed. Do you have any other questions? Ok, well, thanks for your time today and for talking with me. Enjoy the rest of your day.'

Brief interventions are available for a number of health compromising behaviours other than alcohol use such as for smoking cessation (Aveyard, Begh, Parsons, & West, 2011) or suicide attempters (Fleischmann et al., 2008). Online versions of brief interventions are also becoming increasingly utilized (McCambridge & Cunningham, 2013), as well as freely available, self-directed, online training programmes (e.g., http://ndri.curtin.edu.au/btitp/). Such efficient, low-intensity interventions respond to an important public health need, but there remains a vital need for more intense speciality care in the delivery of psychological interventions. An alternative to brief interventions to achieve efficiencies in care is the delivery of interventions in a group format. Group treatments can be delivered just as intensely as one-on-one treatments, but are efficient in that they benefit a larger number of people at the same time. In the next chapter, we turn to the competencies involved in delivering a group treatment programme.

Chapter

8

Group treatment

Group-based interventions are available for almost every conceivable problem a person might experience over the course of a lifetime. Myriad therapeutic groups facilitated by trained mental health professionals exist alongside an even greater number of self-help and mutual support groups (Dies, 1992). The mushrooming choices in the group-helping field over the last few decades, compounded by a 'chaotic proliferation of theoretical orientations' with often limited empirical support and sometimes harmful consequences, resulted in much controversy and uncertainty (Scheidlinger, 2004, p. 266). Such a bewildering state of affairs is precisely the situation where a scientist-practitioner approach is helpful in separating the wheat from the chaff. For example, the long-term group therapy models derived from traditional psychoanalysis (e.g., Kutash & Wolf, 1993; Rutan, 1993) are incongruous with current health care systems that emphasize efficient, time-limited service delivery. In contrast, short-term group interventions based on a more substantial empirical foundation and designed to achieve relatively rapid relief from specific symptoms are increasingly popular in this era of accountability and cost-effectiveness (Dies, 1992). The latter are highly goal-oriented and use interpersonal interaction in small, carefully planned groups to effect change in individuals specifically selected for the purpose of ameliorating a circumscribed set of problems.

The use of interpersonal interaction as a therapeutic tool in the here-and-now context of a group is an inherent advantage of group interventions. The presence of others provides opportunities for vicarious learning and the experience of universality – the relief felt from realizing that one's concerns are not unique and are shared by others (Dies, 1992; Yalom, 1995). Moreover, by engaging with and helping others, patients learn to help themselves more effectively (Rose, 1993; Yalom, 1995). Finally, a group functions as a social microcosm that approximates the individual's day-to-day reality more than a therapist–patient dyad does (Dies, 1992). Thus, patients can rehearse change strategies in the group and, after trying out those strategies in the real world, the group helps the patients evaluate the outcomes (Rose, 1993). This iterative rehearsal in group and community increases the probability that learning will generalize beyond the immediate context of treatment. Given the unique therapeutic advantages and cost-effectiveness of group interventions compared to dyadic sessions, how does a therapist go about selecting, modifying, or developing a group treatment programme that meets the standards of science-informed practice and accountability in patient care?

Selecting a treatment programme

The first step in selecting a group programme is to determine whether there is an empirically validated treatment manual for the particular problem that is targeted by the intervention (see Figure 8.1). For example, excellent treatment manuals with step-by-step clinician guides and ready-to-use patient materials are available for group treatments of social phobia (Andrews et al., 2003) and obesity (Cooper, Fairburn, & Hawker, 2003). But what if such detailed manuals are not yet available? Consider the example of smoking cessation. Until the publication of a comprehensive *Tobacco Dependence Treatment Handbook* in 2003 (Abrams et al.), which included a chapter describing an eight-session behavioural treatment programme for smoking cessation, practitioners had to develop their own programme based on their knowledge of the literature. In the case of smoking cessation, this process was greatly facilitated by clinical practice guidelines, which had been derived from systematic reviews of treatment approaches and were disseminated by the end of the last millennium (Fiore et al., 2000; Miller & Wood, 2002; Raw, McNeill, & West, 1998; West, McNeill, & Raw, 2000). Practice guidelines identify the treatment strategies, formats, and parameters for which there has been sufficient evidence of their effectiveness. This may include recommendations about what treatment strategies to include or what the optimal number of sessions is, but the clinician is still left with the nuts and bolts of translating that information into a coherent treatment programme. For smoking cessation treatment groups there is now a programme available that is based on such a translation of clinical practice recommendations into a step-by-step treatment manual with a detailed session-by-session guide for therapists and ready-to-use client materials, activity sheets, and routine sessional monitoring tools (Stritzke, Chong, & Ferguson, 2009).

In the absence of clinical practice guidelines, the individual clinician has the additional task of critically distilling from the literature what a smoking cessation programme should entail and how it should be structured. Alternatively, if an available treatment manual focuses primarily on behavioural strategies (e.g., Brown, 2003), but the literature suggests that a combination of behavioural, cognitive, and pharmacological approaches outperforms either treatment alone, the clinician may want to modify the existing programme by incorporating a pharmacotherapy component (e.g., Goldstein, 2003) and other relevant principles of treating addictive behaviours (e.g., Miller & Heather, 1998), as well as cognitive behavioural strategies relevant to group treatments more generally (e.g., Rose, 1993). In either case, the onus is on the clinician to evaluate if this newly designed or modified treatment programme produces outcomes that are comparable to those published in the literature (see 'Evaluation & Accountability' box in Figure 8.1).

For example, the literature on smoking cessation treatment recommends the use of biological markers such as carbon monoxide (CO) to infer strength of habit from nicotine levels in the patient's body (Niaura & Shadal, 2003), to provide feedback on initial CO levels to increase motivation for change, and to assess post-cessation CO levels to demonstrate the positive physical health consequences of quitting (Emmons, 2003). From these general recommendations, it is not clear how closely changes in CO levels would correspond to changes in smoking levels. If CO levels are measured weekly, but are not sensitive enough to reflect small reductions in average number of cigarettes smoked per day over the previous week, then lack of change in the 'true' biological index undermines the boost in self-efficacy patients typically experience when realizing that the effort of executing small, planned, behavioural changes in daily routines has resulted in immediate, tangible reductions in their cigarette intake. If, on the other hand, changes in CO levels closely parallel those gradual reductions in daily cigarette intake, they can serve as a powerful motivator to stay committed to the ultimate goal of becoming smoke-free. Given that earlier available treatment handbooks did not offer explicit guidance on how to resolve the above issue, a scientist-practitioner would act as a 'local clinical scientist' (Stricker & Trierweiler, 1995) and evaluate

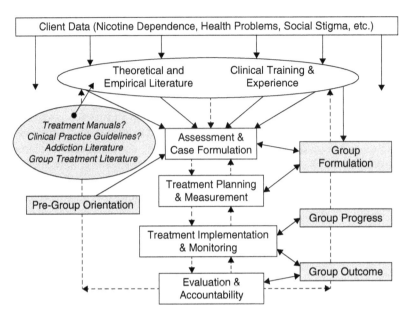

Figure 8.1 The process of integrating individual case formulation and treatment within science-informed, group-based interventions for the example of nicotine dependence.

the results of the decision to use weekly CO monitoring. We will return to this example in our Documenting Progress and Outcomes section below, but first, we will describe what factors need to be considered in selecting patients for a group, and how the process of individual case formulation and treatment is modified and enriched within a group-based intervention.

Selecting patients for a group

In goal-oriented groups where the emphasis is on support and reduction of a specific set of symptoms over a short period of time, the composition of the group by definition will be relatively homogeneous in terms of symptomatic complaints. One advantage of such homogeneous groups is that their concerns and goals for treatment are closely aligned, and therefore they can be quickly moved into a working mode by an active and facilitative therapist (Klein, 1993). The manageable size of groups ranges from 4 to 12 members, with 8 members usually regarded as the ideal number (Klein, 1993; Yalom, 1995). In order to approximate this ideal number, it is important to consider attrition rates. These can range from 17–57% (Yalom, 1995). It is therefore advisable to start with a group that is about 20% larger than the targeted size, so that the predictable dropouts of two or three members early in treatment do not affect the critical number needed for interactive group processes to occur.

The principal consideration in selecting individuals for a group is that they are able and willing to participate in the primary task of the group (Yalom, 1995). That is, they must be available regularly over a specified period of time, have a desire for change, and have the capacity to tolerate a group setting. Beyond these basic inclusion and exclusion criteria, the choice of patients is often determined by expedience, the availability of suitable candidates, and the need to respond flexibly to referral requests, especially when working in multidisciplinary settings.

Assessment and pre-group orientation

In group-based interventions, the process of linking assessment data and case formulation to treatment planning involves two components. One is the individual case formulation that follows from the synthesis and integration of the assessment information regarding each patient's history and circumstances with respect to the presenting problem. The other component is a group formulation (see Figure 8.1). That is, treatment planning is also informed by the unique constellation of individual group members' characteristics and circumstances. The aim is to anticipate and plan for likely patterns of group interactions and processes that can either facilitate or hinder individual patients' treatment goals. For example, some of the participants in a smoking cessation group may have been prompted by similar motives to join the group, such as worry about ongoing medical problems that are caused or exacerbated by smoking, or concern about exposing their children to the harmful effects of secondary smoke, or embarrassment towards work colleagues for engaging in a stigmatized behaviour. This information can be used at the start of the group to build cohesion and mutual support among group members. Likewise, some group members may report similar barriers to their aspirations of becoming smoke-free, such as high levels of stress, worry about weight gain following cessation, or significant others who are smoking in their presence. The group formulation determines which of these potential impediments to treatment success are particularly relevant in a given group, and thus influences the selection and timing of curricular elements during treatment planning (Rose, 1993).

In addition to adjusting aspects of the treatment delivery based on the group's pattern of factors specifically related to symptom presentation (for our example, this would include a detailed smoking history, level of dependence, craving, previous quit attempts, readiness to quit, etc.), group formulation and treatment planning are informed also by more general information about patient characteristics obtained during assessment. For example, patients may have other medical or psychiatric conditions that they may not wish to reveal in front of other group members, and that are not critical to address within the group's explicit purposes. Equipped with this knowledge, the group facilitators can plan their sessions accordingly and skilfully manoeuvre around such confidential issues to protect individual members from unintentional disclosure and embarrassment. Other general assessment information that is particularly relevant to the planning of groups includes pre-existing relationships between group members and interpersonal styles. It is not uncommon that problem-focused groups (e.g., smoking cessation, weight management, fear of flying) are attended by individuals jointly with a partner or a friend. The dynamic between such dyads within the group may require special attention and management. Similarly, considering which members are particularly talkative or timid during assessment can be helpful for facilitating group interactions while ensuring that all members receive equal attention. Finally, assessment yields a wealth of information on the particular personal meanings, circumstances, and events that individual patients associate with their struggles and tribulations with the presenting problem. The planned use of these patient-generated examples at the start of the group is an effective way to personalize explanations of the rationale, principles, and strategies underlying the treatment programme.

Besides the primary assessment function of informing individual case and group formulations as a basis for treatment planning, it is also essential that the therapist uses the assessment session to prepare the patient for the group and start the process of building a therapeutic alliance. Recently, this strategy of initiating pre-treatment processes has also been recommended for interventions with individuals to enhance informed patient choice in the treatment planning, especially when implementing new evidence-based treatments in a setting where patients might be unaccustomed to the new intervention mode and hence reluctant to engage with it (Karlin & Cross, 2014). Drawing on Yalom (1995) and others (Klein, 1993; Salvendy, 1993), we recommend the following preparatory tasks to be covered with a patient prior to entrance into the group:

Enlist patients as informed allies

Explain the rationale underlying the treatment programme. For a smoking cessation group, this would involve an explanation that nicotine addiction is not only maintained by the reinforcing pharmacological effects of nicotine on the brain, but is also powerfully driven by the behavioural aspects of the addiction. Consequently, both the pharmacological and behavioural components of this addiction need to be addressed in treatment. This is why patients need to hit the deck running and start from the first session implementing the behavioural strategies taught in that session, which are later complemented by chemical treatments such as nicotine patches.

Offer guidelines about how to best participate in the group

This will of course vary according to the purpose of the group, although some aspects are common to most groups. Emphasize that group therapy is hard work and that patients are expected to take responsibility for their treatment progress. Stress the importance of punctual and regular attendance. Explain that they will benefit the most by actively engaging with the programme and the other members. Introduce the mantra of treatment success, that is, *change comes from doing things differently*, and that they need to be prepared to do lots of things differently every day once treatment has commenced. Encourage them to provide support to fellow group members.

Clarify format and duration of the programme

Provide information on what to expect in the first session and beyond. If appropriate, preview the timeframe of critical treatment components and follow-up sessions. For example, in a smoking cessation group, patients might be informed about the relative timing of behavioural strategies, quit day, and nicotine replacement therapy. Explain the nature of between-session work with the help of patient handouts, worksheets, and goal-attainment monitoring materials. Describe the session structure and any key staff (co-therapist, supervisor, nutritionist, social worker, etc.) that may be part of the treatment team. Clarity on organization, structure, and procedures of the group helps to allay anticipatory anxiety that stems from uncertainty and misconceptions about group therapy.

Set ground rules

When it comes to setting rules for groups, less is more! Too many rules constrain the very processes by which group interactions add value over the narrower bandwidth inherent in one-on-one communications. Yet, two simple ground rules are essential for groups to fulfil their therapeutic potential. First, *what occurs in the group remains confidential*. This is not to say that patients are not permitted to share any of their experiences and the benefits they derived from them with someone outside the group. After all, many clients join a group on the recommendation from a family member, friend, or colleague, who was satisfied with attending the same or a similar group in the past. What must remain strictly confidential is any identifying information that could be linked to a person, place, or event associated with the other members of the group. Second, *time and attention in the group are shared equally.* Patients are asked to be active participants while being mindful of the needs and different views of other members in the group.

Anticipate frustrations and disappointments along the way

Patients often develop feelings of frustration or annoyance with the therapist when realizing early during the group programme that quick fixes are not forthcoming and that the responsibility for 'doing things differently' ultimately rests with each patient. Similarly, seeing some group members progress at a much faster rate, or another group member relapse after considerable treatment gain, can be upsetting and undermine motivation. It is important to communicate to patients from the outset that there are different paths to achieving the treatment goals and that setbacks are normal. Challenge the patient's perception of setbacks as failures and reframe setbacks as important opportunities for learning to do better the next time.

Instil faith in the programme and optimism about the outcome

One of the great benefits of adhering to a science-informed approach to practice is that even the novice group therapist can, with utmost confidence, assure patients that the programme works and has helped many patients to get better. In particular, if the therapist can refer to recent outcome data collected from previous groups conducted in the same clinical setting (see Figure 8.1 for feedback loop from 'Evaluation & Accountability' to 'Clinical Training & Experience'), patients will react to this information with hope and optimism about their own chances for success. This will go a long way in getting patients 'on board' with the rationale for the treatment and the methods to implement it.

Consider adaptations of typical practice to the particular group

Not all groups are equivalent and the nature of the presenting problem can affect the nature of the interactions and the manner in which the group is conducted. For example, in our social phobia group programme we begin the initial session with clients arranged in a semi-circle facing the therapists in order to reduce the discomfort, but move to a circle with therapists at either end of the room. The anxiety-generating effects of these changes and the anxiety reduction within sessions are then discussed as part of therapy. Likewise, we do not begin by asking people with social phobia to discuss their problems, but we ask them to write comments on paper which are then put in a bowl. The comments are then read out and discussed, but because they are anonymous, the anxiety generated is less intense. In other group formats, such as working with patients with Borderline Personality Disorder (Linehan, 1993a), patients are informed how the group treatment is to complement the individual treatment and which topics are for group discussion.

Getting the group under way

Yalom (1995) observed that the first session is invariably a success, because both patients and novice therapists tend to 'anticipate it with such dread that they are always relieved by the actual event' (p. 294). Although this should be reassuring to the novice group therapist, it cannot be overemphasized how important it is to get a group off to a good start. Given the brevity of many contemporary evidence-based group programmes (i.e., typically not exceeding 10–12 sessions), the first session constitutes an important anchoring function, a point of departure where patients are coached to rapidly embrace the rationale and treatment principles that are at the very heart of what makes the programme *evidence*-based and hence successful. A directive and purposive approach is essential.

A first meeting typically begins with a brief restatement of the ground rules, some housekeeping issues (when are breaks, where is the restroom, etc.), and an opportunity for group members to introduce themselves and their reasons for joining the group. Because generally these reasons are already known to the therapist from the assessment interviews, the therapist can use this knowledge to strategically plan a tentative outline of who to draw in to the interaction during this introductory phase on what occasions, so as to initiate the process of sharing and bonding among members. Thus, while this interaction may appear quite conversational and free-flowing to the patients, the therapist is hard at work and can guide the process into fairly predictable patterns with the aim to accelerate the establishment of group behaviour that is instrumental to change and sets the stage for the 'working phase' of the session.

Following the introductions, therapists will review the rationale of the programme, the strategies that will help patients change, and the reasons why these strategies will work for *them*! In other words, here is where scientist-practitioners give all the 'secrets' of the profession away. They demystify the process of treatment and make it clear that it is the patients' responsibility to engage in the change strategies that they learn and practise in the group, if they want to experience change. Change does not happen from doing things the same, change happens from doing things differently. Therefore, while therapists need to communicate warm and empathetic understanding of the patients' concerns and frustrations stemming from the presenting problem, it is equally important to communicate in a firm and directive manner that patients need to begin acting on what they learn in group from day one. For example, in the context of a smoking cessation group, this involves the introduction of a menu of options of change strategies, from which each patient must select at least one or two strategies to be implemented between the first and second group sessions. In addition to immediately engaging in active change behaviours, patients need to be educated about the benefits they can expect from monitoring and evaluating the outcomes of their efforts.

Monitoring and evaluating progress and outcomes

Just as treatment planning in group-based interventions is informed by an integration of individual case data within the overall group pattern, so is treatment monitoring and outcome evaluation (see Figure 8.1). While group programmes allow for flexibility in how and at what pace individual members progress towards the treatment aims, there are often phases or milestones that provide a common threat and that serve to gauge individual members' progress towards goal attainment relative to the change trajectory of the group as a whole. For example, in the first phase of a smoking cessation group, most members will be successful in gradually reducing their daily intake of cigarettes by increasingly adopting a variety of behavioural change strategies. This is followed by a preparation phase for planning a 'quit day' and the start of nicotine replacement therapy to ease withdrawal distress after becoming smoke-free. The last phase and follow-up assist with reducing relapse risk and adjusting

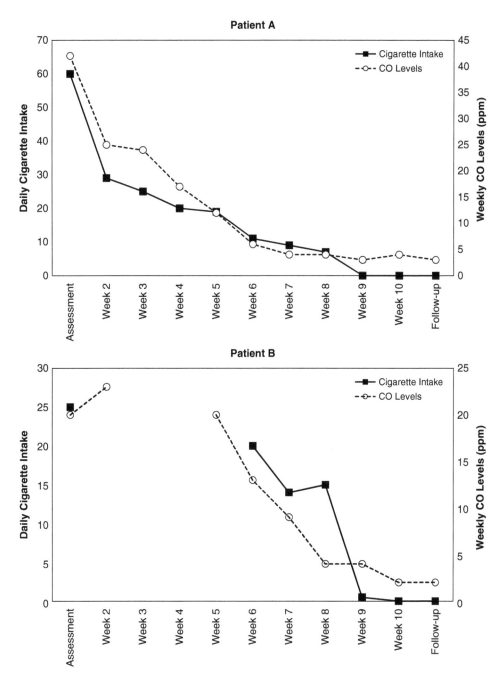

Figure 8.2 Change trajectories of two patients from a smoking cessation group.

to the significant lifestyle changes associated with becoming a non-smoker. As illustrated in Figure 8.2, two smokers from the same group can have different trajectories towards becoming smoke-free. Whereas Patient A showed a gradual progression towards goal attainment and was smoke-free by Week 9, Patient B experienced some significant health problems during the early weeks of the group which precluded her from attending for a couple of weeks. With the help of between-session materials supplied by the therapists, and by redoubling her motivation and effort upon rejoining the group, this patient was determined to 'catch up with the group' and hence showed a much steeper trajectory towards successful goal attainment than Patient A did.

As shown in Figure 8.1, treatment implementation is continually adjusted as a function of progress achieved by individual members within the parameters of the group's progress overall. In the case of Patient B in Figure 8.2, the lack of progress early on could be attributed to external factors associated with stressful medical procedures that interfered with her ability to fully adhere to the group's treatment plan. For other patients, lack of progress may be indicative of internal factors, such as ambivalent attitudes towards change or low motivation. In that case, the timing and intensity of programme components dealing with motivational interviewing techniques can be adjusted accordingly. At the same time, the group therapist can use the positive example set by Patient A, who started out with one of the highest levels of nicotine dependence and daily cigarette intake within the group (i.e. 60 per day), as tangible evidence that engaging with the treatment process leads to goal attainment. However, for therapists to fully exploit these opportunities for vicarious learning within groups, they need to wear a scientist-practitioner's hat. They need to be committed to regular, systematic evaluation and documentation of the group's progress.

Likewise, for patients to fully harness the benefits of making the link between implementation of the treatment strategies learned in group and the resulting gradual changes towards goal attainment, they first must be aware of these changes. Often these changes will be subtle at first and become obvious only when viewed as a trend over repeated measurements. It is therefore essential to provide group members with regular, easy-to-follow feedback on critical outcome measures such as those illustrated in Figure 8.2. Evaluation of individual and group progress with the help of clear graphs should be a routine component of any group treatment programme (Woody et al., 2003).

The value of systematic documentation of group progress and outcomes is threefold. First, routine examination of group progress data stimulates vicarious learning and mutual support among group members. Consider the pattern of treatment progress for five members of a smoking cessation group in Figure 8.3. Note that all patients show the predicted gradual decline in daily cigarette intake over the first six weeks, with Patient C showing the steepest decline (over 50% reduction) after initially starting out with the highest level of cigarette use. Because of her excellent progress, her determined and upbeat attitude, and her strong encouragement of others in the group, Patient C had become somewhat of a role model. After she experienced a severe relapse in Week 7, three things were particularly instrumental in getting her to re-commit to her treatment goal. One was a brief, caring phone call by the group therapist following her absence in Week 7 to encourage her to rejoin the group the following week. Another was the non-judgemental, warm, supportive reaction by her fellow group members following Patient C's return in Week 8. But particularly important to Patient C in overcoming this setback was the compelling evidence of her successful steady progress *prior* to her relapse, which reinforced her belief that she had the capacity to succeed at this difficult task. Equally important was the evidence *following* her decision to re-commit to treatment, which confirmed to her that she had overcome the setback and consolidated the treatment gains achieved prior to the relapse. Although Patient C was not smoke-free by the end of the last group session, she succeeded in becoming smoke-free prior to the follow-up session two months later.

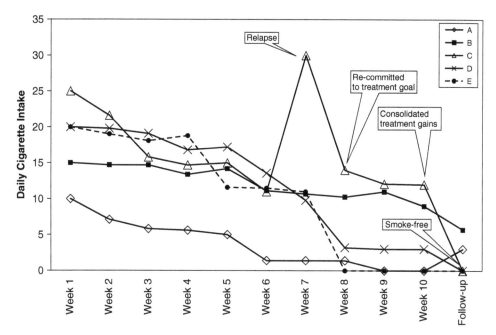

Figure 8.3 Pattern of treatment progress for five patients in a smoking cessation group.

Second, systematically accounting for group progress and outcomes is valuable because accurate feedback on partial improvements that fall short of the ideal outcome can still be therapeutically meaningful. For example, smokers who reduce their daily cigarette intake by at least 50% (see Patients A and B at follow-up in Figure 8.3), have an increased chance of becoming smoke-free in the future (Hughes, 2000) and have reduced their exposure to harmful levels of carbon monoxide in their body (see Figure 8.2).

Third, accurate documentation of successful group treatment outcomes adds value to any services offered in a competitive health care market. This is especially critical if the clinician had to newly design or modify a treatment programme. Recall the earlier example of incorporating the monitoring of CO readings as an outcome measure into a smoking cessation programme. If CO readings lacked sensitivity to accurately mirror small, gradual changes in smoking behaviour, then their addition to the treatment protocol could undermine motivation to continue with the behavioural strategies. The scientist-practitioner can use replication of positive outcomes across clients within a group (e.g., see the close correspondence between self-reported behavioural changes and CO reading for Patients A and B in Figure 8.2), followed by replication of this pattern across subsequent groups, to build confidence that the introduction or modification of a new treatment component was useful in improving treatment outcomes. If these treatment outcomes are comparable or exceed the average success rates of smoking cessation treatments published in the literature, the clinician can be confident that the newly refined treatment programme is providing value for money.

Treatment decisions and protocols can also be informed by evaluating these monitoring and outcome data over time across several groups. For example, in smoking cessation there is a certain dilemma when considering whether to encourage a 'cold turkey' or 'warm turkey' approach to setting a quit date for patients (Miller & Page, 1991). Patients have typically tried abrupt cessation many times before and failed each time; another failure at the start of treatment may prompt disengagement from treatment and hence should be avoided. In contrast, gradual reduction in cigarette intake before setting a quit date provides opportunities to become engaged in treatment, experience some success, and build confidence before attempting again to stop altogether. However, the latter approach can lead to procrastination and stalling of serious treatment engagement. So, the question becomes: when to gently nudge, and when to firmly push? An evaluation of our own monitoring and outcome data showed that abstinence at follow-up was associated with: (1) attending more treatment sessions, (2) completing treatment, and importantly, (3) achieving treatment milestones such as a 50% reduction in cigarette intake and a 48-hour smoke-free period *earlier* in treatment. This suggests that while patients can benefit from a gradual approach to quitting, this does not mean that effort can be at half throttle; patients must be encouraged to work towards critical change milestones from the outset and engage in vigorous early behavioural change.

Thus, using aggregate treatment process and outcome data to refine treatment protocols is central to the activity of a science-informed practice and this will be the focus of the following chapter on programme evaluation.

Chapter 9

Programme evaluation

The concept of *ongoing quality improvement* is inherent in the science-informed approach to clinical practice. The evaluation skills needed to ensure that treatment programmes and services are delivered in line with best practice standards and, as a whole, reliably achieve clinically meaningful improvements in patient health and satisfaction, are as important to acquire for clinical psychologists as the therapeutic skills involved in the actual treatment of individual patients (Health Service Psychology Education Collaborative, 2013). The role of psychologists as health care providers in a competitive health care market (see also Chapter 15) makes it imperative that empirically based outcome evaluation is not only conducted at the level of the individual patient, but is routinely extended to outcome evaluation at the aggregate level of the service provider or agency (see Figure 9.1).

Clearly, psychologists must be more than mere consumers of research, and detailed session-by-session outcome monitoring and ongoing evaluations of intervention programmes and services are integral to accountability, quality improvement, and innovation in clinical practice (Clark, 2011). Clinical psychologists by virtue of their combined training in research and clinical practice already have a solid grounding in research methodology and extensive experience in data management and analysis. This distinguishes them from many other health care providers and places them in a good position to make valuable contributions to addressing programme evaluation needs within their employment settings. However, programme evaluation involves more than competent data collection and analysis. In addition to data management skills, good evaluators need to develop good negotiation and communication skills (Owen & Rogers, 1999). Whereas research findings are instrumental in drawing conclusions that generalize to a broader context of a discipline or area of investigation, evaluation findings serve to inform decisions about specific aspects of a programme or policy within a local context. Hence, the conclusions that evaluators draw from quantitative and qualitative data will be influenced by the position held by various stakeholders. These may include consumers, policy-makers, funding bodies, and staff and management of the respective agency (see Figure 9.1). For example, evaluation data may be used to demonstrate that service provision achieves stated outcomes and is cost-effective, to account for the resources spent on developing and implementing a new service, to monitor quality of care, to articulate the value of particular services to management and funding bodies, to determine financial incentives to providers, or to market services to consumers. In order to achieve these goals, the views and values of relevant stakeholders need to be considered. Good negotiation skills in the planning stage of an evaluation are essential to clarify and endorse the purpose of the evaluation, and to maximize the quality and utility of the data to be collected. Good communication skills are needed because evaluation data need to be

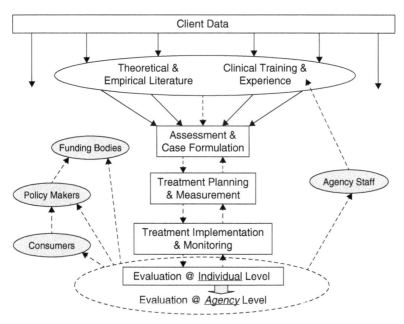

Figure 9.1 Programme evaluation extends routine evaluation of individual patient outcomes to evaluation of outcomes, procedures, and policies at the level of the service setting.

translated into effective recommendations. Effective recommendations are those that are specific, realistic in scope, easily translated into action, and mindful of any constraints within the organizational environment that might hinder their full implementation (Sonnichsen, 1994). Finally, the gathering of patient data for the purpose of quality improvement programmes must follow clear processes that protect the rights of patients (e.g., confidentiality, treatment preferences and choices), and respect the professional responsibilities and clinical judgement of treating staff (American Psychological Association, 2009).

Clinical psychology trainees typically experience two modes of skills training in programme evaluation: didactic teaching including practical experience in conducting small-scale evaluation projects, and modelling via exposure to and participation in ongoing programme evaluation activities within their training clinic and community placements. By embracing evaluation as a continuous learning process of asking questions, reflecting on the answers to these questions, and modifying actions and strategies in light of those answers, trainees learn to be committed to a process of continual improvement that forms the basis of accountability and good practice. As shown in Figure 7.1, members of the agency staff may be the direct beneficiaries of evaluation findings. To the extent that these findings are incorporated in continuing education and training of staff, programme evaluation adds to the wealth of clinical experience that practitioners bring to bear in treatment planning and implementation.

There is an enormous diversity in approaches to programme evaluation (Wholey, Hatry, & Newcomer, 1994), and the scope of many evaluation designs and purposes extends well beyond the local clinical context in which practitioners typically engage in programme evaluation. These more systemic evaluation projects are conducted by teams of professional evaluation contractors and are not the focus of this chapter. In this chapter, we introduce trainees to a few basic steps of programme evaluation that are common to the sort of evaluation projects that practitioners are likely to use in their respective local clinical setting on a routine basis. We will illustrate these steps with examples drawn from evaluation projects that clinical psychology trainees may encounter in their own clinical training setting.

Five basic steps of programme evaluation

1. Asking the right questions

The questions that form the impetus for a programme evaluation can be categorized according to their primary purpose. Owen and Rogers (1999) identify five conceptual categories. *Proactive* evaluation is conducted prior to the design and implementation of a treatment or programme. Questions addressed in proactive evaluation might include: Is there a need for a particular treatment or programme? (For example, should a women's health centre offer a smoking cessation programme aimed at pregnant women? Is there a need to offer clinical psychology trainees practicum experience in rural and remote settings?) What does the relevant literature or professional experience tell us about the problems and benefits of introducing a particular service? Have there been previous attempts to address this need or problem? Are there external sources or agencies that could contribute expertise and solutions to problems in implementing a programme?

Clarificative evaluation examines the internal structure of a programme or policy. It clarifies how the programme's elements and activities link to intended outcomes. Data will need to be collected that might address questions such as the following: What are the intended outcomes of the programme? What does the programme do to achieve those outcomes? Is the rationale for certain aspects of the programme plausible? One example of clarificative evaluation that clinical psychology students may experience with respect to their own training programme is accreditation. Accreditation aims to certify that the structure, components, and procedural guidelines of a programme are of a standard that instils confidence that the programme can deliver what it intends to deliver.

Unlike clarificative evaluation, which is concerned with the design and logic of a programme, *interactive* evaluation is concerned with implementation of a programme or its components. This form of evaluation is formative in nature and is particularly appropriate for the purpose of ongoing quality improvement. Questions asked in an interactive evaluation might include: Are there ways in which the delivery of services can be changed to make it more effective? Are therapists implementing agency practice guidelines? Do programme activities or innovative approaches make a difference? Are there changes in the type of patients and problems that present at the clinic? Are the skills taught in a training clinic up to scratch in meeting the demands of current and projected workplace requirements?

Monitoring evaluation aims to provide quantitative and qualitative information at regular intervals to gauge whether performance indicators are in line with specified programme targets and implementation is carried out as intended. Questions asked during monitoring evaluation might include: How do patient outcome and satisfaction indices compare with the previous year? Are the resources available to therapists sufficient to meet current and projected trends in service delivery and patient needs? What is the average length of treatment provided by therapists? What is the rate at which clinical psychology trainees accumulate supervised client-contact hours? This type of evaluation often uses *outcome monitoring* data. Unlike programme evaluation, outcome monitoring itself is not explanatory, but simply generates routine reports of programme results, which are then available for periodic evaluation and interpretation. Thus, results-oriented monitoring generates the 'proof' needed to satisfy the accountability mandate (Affholter, 1994). In addition, outcome monitoring facilitates the early detection and correction of problems as well as the timely identification of opportunities for innovation and performance improvement (Affholter, 1994).

Finally, *impact* evaluation assesses the attainment of intended outcomes against specified criteria or outcome indicators. This category of evaluation is often summative in nature and may assist in decisions to scale back, terminate, continue, or expand certain services or programmes. Impact evaluation may also include an analysis of unintended programme outcomes and of the integrity of implementation. Questions addressed in impact evaluation might include: Do patients receiving treatment in a training clinic achieve reliable and meaningful improvements in psychiatric symptoms and well-being? Are patients showing improvement in a timely and cost-effective manner? How long does it take graduates from a training programme in clinical psychology to find employment in their chosen field?

Once a set of critical evaluation questions has been determined that reflects the primary purpose and scope of the evaluation, the next step is to develop an evaluation plan.

2. Developing an evaluation plan

The second step of programme evaluation involves planning how to find answers to the critical questions agreed upon in the first step. Several issues need to be considered when negotiating an evaluation plan (Owen & Rogers, 1999). One consideration is who the recipients and users of the information are going to be. For example, if the question is how long it takes to find employment after graduation from a clinical psychology training programme, information will be primarily used by (a) current students from the programme for career planning, (b) future applicants to the programme for weighing the pros and cons of entering the programme, (c) potential employers for gauging the quality of graduates from the programme, and (d) programme directors for promoting the quality of programme graduates to employers and for advertising the strengths of the programme to prospective quality applicants.

A second consideration is what personnel and material resources are available to conduct the evaluation project. All evaluations are subject to resource and time constraints which determine the extent of information gathering, the complexity and sophistication of data management, and the range of dissemination strategies. If the people who deliver a programme are also part of the evaluation team, then time and resources need to be made available for the evaluation tasks. These tasks should not present an additional burden on normal workload and should therefore be integrated within the routine demands of day-to-day programme activities.

A third consideration in developing an evaluation plan is selecting the data collection and management strategies that are most appropriate for each evaluation question. It is important to bear in mind that the level of data analytic complexity should not exceed the sophistication of the intended audience. Clarity and utility are paramount. To answer the question of how long it takes for graduates to find employment, a brief survey could be designed that examines not only time taken to secure the first job, but also provides further informative details such as number of job interviews relative to job offers, success in obtaining most preferred positions, duration of first contracts, starting income level, and time taken to progress to more senior or permanent positions and/or higher income levels. If data on prompt employment of graduates are not only of interest as an index of recent training success, but are also viewed as a performance target to be maintained in the future, data gathering may also require the simultaneous elicitation of critical feedback. Thus, the plan for data collection may include some open-ended forms of information gathering where respondents can identify areas for improvement in training, so that future graduates are kept abreast of evolving trends in knowledge and skills expected of their profession. In addition, the evaluation plan would articulate sampling strategies and may identify potential external resources that could aid in data collection. For example, a survey of recent psychology graduates could be mailed with the help of existing mailing lists kept by the university alumni services and could be included in their regular mailings at no cost to the evaluators. Finally, the data management component of the evaluation plan must specify how data will be processed and analysed.

A fourth aspect in developing an evaluation plan concerns the strategies that will be used to disseminate the outcomes of the evaluation. This involves determining when and in what format reporting will take place, and what kind of results, conclusions, and recommendations will be included.

Finally, an evaluation plan must estimate the costs associated with carrying out the plan. The constraints imposed by the size of the budget and the amount of available resources have a direct impact on the timeline that can be set for achieving the various phases of the evaluation project. The timeline may also be constrained by any ethical issues that need to be addressed before and during the implementation of the evaluation. How these ethical issues will be handled needs to be made explicit in the evaluation plan. After completion of the evaluation plan, the data gathering phase commences.

3. Collecting and analysing data to produce findings

The third step of programme evaluation produces evaluation findings. These findings link the evaluation questions to answers that are then disseminated to relevant stakeholders (see Figure 9.2). The key tasks during the evidence gathering phase involve selecting and gaining access to the most appropriate sources of data, and then obtaining the data. Sources may include existing records and documents, as well as individuals who can either provide relevant information directly or are the gatekeepers of the information required. One of the most important tasks of data management is the maintenance of a reliable database. Clinical psychologists trained within a science-informed approach to clinical practice are usually very experienced in conducting and supervising the tasks involved in data reduction and analysis. Interpretation of the results of the analyses must, of course, be grounded in the evidence, but in programme evaluation it is also important to ensure that the interpretation of evaluation findings reflects the diversity of viewpoints by different stakeholders. Are the conclusions based on a valid and balanced reflection of the evidence? Are there any limitations of the evaluation findings? Could these limitations have different implications for different stakeholders? It is essential to remember that evaluation conclusions must win the support of relevant stakeholders if they are to be utilized and lead to action.

4. Translating findings into recommendations for action

The fourth step of programme evaluation produces recommendations based on the judgements and interpretations derived from the evaluation findings. All recommendations have the purpose of influencing organizational decision-making. They may be used to justify

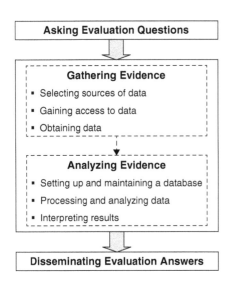

Figure 9.2 The collection, management, analysis, and interpretation of data link the evaluation questions to answers for the utilization by relevant stakeholders.

decisions already made or, more typically, they inform and shape decisions about courses of action intended to bring about organizational change (Owen & Rogers, 1999). Whereas the first three steps of evaluation look backward and examine the status quo, the recommendations developed in the fourth step as part of the written evaluation report are designed to think forward. They are prescriptive and present solutions to problems, which in turn provide the impetus for organizational debate and action (Sonnichsen, 1994). As such, writing good recommendations is the most pivotal component of the final evaluation report if the evaluation effort is to bring about desirable change.

Effective recommendations are characterized by several basic qualities (Sonnichsen, 1994). Foremost, recommendations must be delivered in a timely manner. Evaluation outcomes that are not available when they are needed are of little value to decision-makers. Recommendations must also be realistic. Unless factors that might constrain the implementation of a recommendation are carefully considered, the recommendation may be viewed as impractical and hence is likely to be ignored. For the same reason, it is wise to avoid recommending changes that are so fundamental that they threaten values perceived by staff to be core aspects of the programme under evaluation. Such radical proposals for change are bound to meet with strong resistance and hence have little chance of being implemented successfully. In addition, care must be taken to direct each recommendation to the appropriate persons who are in the position to act on and oversee its implementation. Otherwise, recommendations will collect dust and get bogged down in organizational inertia. Good recommendations are simple and specific. Each should focus on only one issue and make explicit what tasks are to be executed by whom to ensure its implementation. Finally, the link between each recommendation and the empirical findings that underlie it must be clear. This will enhance the credibility of the recommendations and thereby their potential for acceptance and implementation.

The written recommendations can be seen as the ultimate product delivered by the programme evaluators. Because they are embedded in the final evaluation report, it is important that evaluators present their final report in a way that makes it easy for readers to understand the evidence behind a recommendation, the benefits of implementing it, and how to get there. If recommendations are entombed in a thick, unwieldy report, they are likely to remain unread, and hence cannot have an impact on ongoing quality improvement of service delivery. Therefore, they need to be displayed prominently in the final report. Sometimes adding page references to the relevant sections of the report can make it easier for the readers to find sections of interest. Although the specific content, structure, and format of an evaluation report will depend on the target audiences and the guidelines imposed by funding bodies, most evaluation reports present upfront a brief section with an executive summary. This summary provides a brief overview of the evaluation aims, methods, and key findings, and highlights the recommendations that follow from these findings. The remainder of the report typically contains a more detailed introduction to the evaluation, a review of the literature, a description of the methodology, a succinct report of outcomes, and a discussion of the interpretations and judgements leading to the recommendations. Further details are usually relegated to appendices in the form of tables or figures.

Even if great care has been invested in writing effective recommendations and presenting them in a way that they are quick to absorb and easy to understand by the stakeholders, this is not a guarantee that they will be adopted and lead to change. It may be desirable and possible, especially within local clinical settings where interactive forms of evaluations are often useful, for evaluators to be also actively involved in facilitating the transition from recommendations for action to the actual initiation and follow-up of the recommended changes.

5. Advocating and promoting change

Evaluation findings produce recommendations, but recommendations do not always influence organizational decision-making. As Sonnichsen (1994) noted, 'some evaluators labor under the delusion that elegant methodologies, eloquent reports, and scientific neutrality are sufficient qualities to ensure that evaluation results will be used' (p. 535). Non-use of recommendations may in part be due to the judgemental nature of evaluation. If recommendations for change are perceived as criticism and elicit defensive reactions, they are not likely to be universally met with enthusiasm. For recommendations to lead to change, the evaluation process must include a plan and strategies for actively promoting that change. The onus is on the evaluators to market the benefits relative to the perceived risks of changing, while highlighting the risks of not changing. In clinical settings, failure to act on reliable and valid evaluation outcomes is costly and harmful, because it leads to overuse of unhelpful care and underuse of effective care (Berwick, 2003). Thus, the translation of evaluation recommendations into practice must be actively promoted as a value-adding organizational enterprise.

One important strategy of promoting recommended changes is to not wait for audiences to request information, but to actively seek opportunities for communicating key findings regularly and frequently in a variety of formats (Hendricks, 1994). The consequences of recommended changes may impact differently on individuals or groups within the provider organization. Thus, readiness for change can be enhanced if the recommendations are as compatible as possible with the values, beliefs, past experiences, and current needs of the various stakeholders (Berwick, 2003). When promoting change, simplify! Audiences tend to be busy and are not so much interested in general information than in the bottom line. They want guidance on what they are expected to do differently, and reassurance on how the benefits of doing things differently outweigh the costs of doing things the same. This means that delivering a recommendation only as part of a lengthy evaluation report may be insufficient to initiate and sustain change. Personal, concise briefings tailored to select individuals or small audiences, accompanied by the use of effective visual aids and handouts, and delivered with ample opportunities for questions, comments, and discussion, provide additional momentum for translating recommendations into action (Hendricks, 1994).

Another important strategy for promoting recommended changes is to form a team of individuals and invest them with sufficient power to lead the change effort (Owen & Rogers, 1999). These local change coordinators serve as 'champions' or internal field agents to facilitate local implementation of the recommended change agenda (e.g., Karlin & Cross, 2014). The primary task of such a team is to mould the various recommendations into a coherent vision, and to communicate that vision synergistically to all stakeholders. The efforts of this team must be supported by administrators in the form of structures that facilitate the changes and remove potential obstacles to implementing them.

Finally, the adoption of recommended changes can be greatly facilitated if one allows for, and even encourages, local adaptation of the recommended courses of action. Recommendations will have their greatest impact if changes are not only adopted locally, but also adapted locally (Berwick, 2003). That is, programme innovators must guard against the tendency to be too rigid in their insistence on exact replication of the recommended courses of action. Innovations and improvements are remarkably robust to modifications suggested by those who are ultimately responsible for translating them into the reality of practice. In fact, locally 'owned' adaptation is a critical and nearly universal property of successful dissemination of novel ideas and practices (Berwick, 2003). Such fertile reflection on the process, findings, and recommendations of an evaluation project is the essence of *continuing* quality improvement. It enhances capacity building by developing a culture of reflective practice and quality assurance. Moreover, local adaptation of evaluation outcomes stimulates the generation of new critical questions within the group of key stakeholders, which in turn sets in motion the wheels of subsequent rounds of programme evaluation. Good practice is reflective practice! Programme evaluation is the tool to ensure that reflective practice is happening.

A special case of local adaptation of recommended treatment guidelines occurs when empirically supported, manualized prevention and intervention programmes have to be adapted for use with different populations or to address the unique aspects and constraints of a particular local context. To ensure the validity and fidelity of the newly adapted manualized intervention, Goldstein, Kemp, Leff, and Lochman (2012) offer guidelines for a stepwise development and evaluation process. One begins by selecting a base manual for adaptation and determines its adaptability for the current situation. A very important principle at this stage is that one remains true to the underlying theory and change mechanisms that were empirically supported in the original manual. The essence of those core mechanisms must remain unaltered. In the next phase, one conducts focus groups with members of the new target population and makes initial revisions to the manuals based on the feedback received. This is followed by pilot testing of the initial revisions, collecting feedback from the facilitators of the new manualized intervention, and seeking consultation with experts. On the basis of staff and expert feedback, further rounds of more formal evaluation trials, or even a randomized controlled trial (resources permitting) may be conducted as part of the manual adaptation process.

In sum, empirically based outcome evaluation is the foundation of accountable clinical practice, both at the level of the individual patient and at the aggregate level of the service provider or agency. The mandate of accountability pertains to both the products of treatment and the procedures used to achieve these products. Regardless of which level of service delivery is targeted for quality improvement, delivering a high quality product requires good case management skills. In the next chapter, we will describe the key tasks involved in conscientiously managing all aspects of patient care from the first contact to termination of the therapeutic relationship.

Case management

The effective, efficient, and ethical delivery of psychological services requires good case management skills. Case management involves the integration of three interrelated tasks. In addition to the fundamental *conceptual task* of integrating evidence-based practice with practice-based evidence, which is the essence of the science-informed approach to clinical practice, treatment involves *management tasks* and *documentation tasks*. In this chapter, we will outline the key management and documentation tasks associated with specific phases of the treatment process, as well as some tasks that are important at all stages of treatment. Although many case management tasks have a purpose clearly linked to a specific treatment phase (e.g., a good intake report needs to be produced at the start of treatment), two particular tasks with respect to client data are relevant throughout the entire treatment process: keeping good records and maintaining confidentiality (see Figure 10.1).

Keeping good records

Professional practice guidelines stipulate that treatment providers must maintain adequate records of all contacts with clients or other persons involved in the treatment (e.g., family members, physicians), indicating date, time, and place of contact, persons present, and the nature of service provided or action taken. Good clinical records provide a clear picture of the patient and a clear account of what the therapist did, when and why. Documentation of these clinical activities serves several purposes (Luepker, 2003):

- *Records can facilitate communication between therapists and patients.* Jointly reviewing reports, test results, data on goal attainment, attendance patterns, etc. can help patients to gain insight into and become active partners in their change efforts, while building trust in the process and the therapeutic relationship.
- *Records document that a sound diagnosis, case formulation, and treatment plan have been generated.* This forms the basis for a purposive course of action and is essential for monitoring and detecting change, or modifying diagnostic impression and treatment strategies.
- *Records satisfy the accountability mandate.* Science-informed practice brings the attitude of a scientist into the clinical consulting room. This includes a commitment to showing 'proof' of what was done, when and how, to whom, and resulting in what outcomes. Contractual obligations with third party payers often require this information for reimbursement of services. Inadequate records may be interpreted by auditors as health care fraud, making practitioners vulnerable to criminal prosecution, civil penalties, or suspension of third party payments (Foxhall, 2000). From an

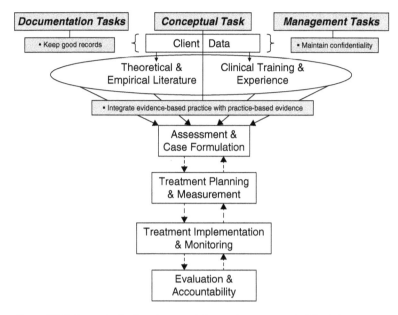

Figure 10.1 Conceptualization, documentation, and management of client data.

auditor's point of view, if a service was not documented, it did not happen; if it was billed, it constitutes fraud.

- *Records assist with continuity of care.* Good records of previous interventions can help facilitate treatment planning in the event a patient seeks help again, or needs to be transferred to a different therapist.
- *Records protect therapists and clinical supervisors against spurious allegations of harmful practices.* As in cases of alleged health care fraud, the lack of contemporaneous, detailed documentation makes it difficult for practitioners to prove that they acted in accordance with best practice standards. Keeping good records allows a therapist to document that decisions and actions were made in good faith and conformed to accepted professional practices.

Because of the multiple, simultaneous, challenging tasks that novice therapists must gain mastery over when learning the 'exciting' business of doing therapy, they may be tempted to view the seemingly mundane tasks associated with documentation as an additional burden of secondary importance. It should be clear from the above list of purposes of documentation that conscientious record keeping is an integral part of good case management, and that patient care will suffer without it. Trainees must be mindful not to neglect this important task, but they must also guard against the common tendency among beginning therapists to be overly detailed and comprehensive in documenting their every impression and each piece of information concerning their patients. We will review specific documentation tasks in more detail below, but will first present a few characteristics common to all 'good' clinical records that help to keep records concise, relevant, and accurate.

- *Good records are relevant.* They include only information germane to the presenting problem, treatment strategies, and outcomes. We will return to this point later, when describing strategies for keeping records (and presentations of client information) concise and relevant.

- *Good records are accurate.* They identify the sources of information. For example, if the patient says that her father 'was an alcoholic', it would be inaccurate to indicate in the record that 'the patient's father was an alcoholic', because the therapist has no objective information to confirm this as a fact. In this case, the record would be accurate if the therapist indicated that '*the patient stated that* her father was an alcoholic'. Similarly, if the therapist makes an interpretation based on information provided by the patient, this should be made explicit in the record (e.g., 'The patient clenched her fist and raised her voice, almost shouting; *she appeared* very angry with her husband's decision'). In addition to identifying unambiguously the sources of information, accuracy in records is achieved by checking and double-checking for errors. This is particularly important when recording test results and interpretations.
- *Good records are contemporaneous.* They are generated in a timely fashion, preferably immediately after a session or any action taken in relation to case management.
- *Good records are continuous.* They are recorded in a chronological order, each record is signed, and progress notes should be written in a continuous stream. This reduces the possibility of tampering and instils confidence in others that the records are complete.
- *Good records are consistent.* They reflect the course charted in the formulation and treatment plan. If, for example, the aim is to reduce a patient's fear of flying, a progress note stating that 'the session focused on an exploration of the patient's rivalry with her stepsister' would not be logical in the context of a treatment programme for reducing phobic anxiety, unless reducing distress associated with sibling discord was part of the agreed treatment plan.
- *Good records are legible.* Unless records are legible, they cannot serve the purposes outlined above. Illegible records have the same liabilities as no records at all. Typically entries are written in black ink to ensure that, when copied, any record continues to remain legible. When using electronic record systems, legibility is not an issue, but all other aspects of good record keeping apply regardless of format.
- *Good records are sensitive.* They avoid jargon, use simple language, and respect the uniqueness and complexity of each patient. A good rule of thumb for the beginning therapist is: if you would feel uncomfortable if the client were to read your report or notes in your presence, you should consider alternative ways of expressing the relevant passages.

Maintaining confidentiality

The second task that pertains to all aspects of case management (including record keeping) is the obligation to protect the privacy of the patient. Maintaining confidentiality not only requires attention throughout all phases of treatment, but remains a case management responsibility well after a patient's active file has been closed. The purpose of confidentiality between a patient and therapist is to create a safe therapeutic environment and to safeguard the patient from harm due to the unintentional disclosure of sensitive patient data. The establishment of trust based on a mutual understanding about confidentiality and its limitations is the foundation of an effective therapeutic relationship. To achieve the best health outcomes for patients, it is often necessary to share information between professional staff as part of multidisciplinary case management, as well as between patients' families and other carers. Maintaining confidentiality, then, involves maintaining a balance between the need to respect the patient's privacy and the need to consult with nominated people to optimize patient care, within the guiding parameters set by professional ethics codes and legal obligations. The parameters of confidentiality and its exceptions should be discussed with patients at the start of the first session. Likewise, if communication with families and other carers or professionals is desirable during treatment, an agreement about the purpose, nature, and extent of sharing information with others should be reached with the patient. This may require ongoing discussion and negotiation, and may entail the setting of very specific constraints, defining periods of time during which disclosure is permitted, and delineating precisely what may or may not be divulged to whom under what circumstances.

Talking about confidentiality with patients

Therapists have the responsibility of explaining confidentiality and its exceptions to patients when commencing a therapeutic relationship. A beginning therapist might worry that having such 'technical' discussions at the outset of the initial interview could be perceived by patients as uncaring and rigid, and hence interfere with rapport building. However, trust in the therapist, and the profession as a whole, will be undermined if total confidentiality is promised or implied without making patients aware of the limitations of confidentiality. Most patients will welcome the therapist's concern that they understand what is involved in the treatment process, and they are likely to experience this open and frank communication as reassuring. The brief focus at the start of the session on more innocuous procedures can even help to ease trepidations patients may have about the treatment process, before they talk about what is troubling them and what they are seeking help for.

Therapists in training will by definition consult extensively with supervisors and fellow trainees about their cases. Because supervision is typically aided by the routine review of videotaped sessions, and because the presence of a camera and microphone in the consulting room can be initially intimidating to patients, this special arrangement in training clinics should be explicitly addressed when trainees discuss confidentiality with their patients. The following example shows how confidentiality information can be communicated to a patient. This is not intended as a proscription of how it 'must' be said verbatim, but is meant to illustrate the level of detail and clarity needed to convey in a matter-of-fact yet warm manner what the patient needs to know:

'I'd like to take a few minutes to explain some of the clinic procedures to you and give you an opportunity to ask any questions you have about our services here.'

'First, you should know that in general everything we talk about in here is confidential. Of course, creating a safe place for talking about things that are often difficult to talk about and can make one feel very vulnerable is very important in our work together.'

'As you know, this is a training clinic, and so, information about a client is regularly discussed between therapists and supervisors. That is also why many sessions are videotaped. You should know that these video recordings are not permanently stored. They are only a tool to aid in ongoing supervision and ensure quality in care, and they are typically erased shortly thereafter or recorded over with subsequent sessions.'

'Do you have any questions about the video recording?' [pause for patient to respond]

'There are three circumstances that I need you to tell about, where I might be required by professional standards and the law to disclose information about our sessions to parties outside our clinic:

1. The first one is that, if you were to tell me that you intend to harm yourself or others, I would be required to take some appropriate action to prevent you from doing that and to help and assist you further in that situation.
2. The second circumstance relates to information about abuse or severe neglect of children or the elderly. In that case, I would have to notify appropriate authorities to provide assistance with that situation.
3. The third circumstance where I might have to release information is when I or the clinic gets a subpoena for client records from a judge or court.'

'Do you have any questions regarding any of these issues relating to confidentiality?'

The above discussion would typically take less than five minutes. This can be followed with a brief transition statement, outlining the goals and structure of this session, before 'turning it over' to the patient with a phrase such as: 'OK then, what brings you here?'

Negotiating confidentiality when working with minors

When working with children and adolescents, therapists need to balance the patient's need for confidentiality with the parent's or guardian's need for information. Therapists must be familiar with applicable laws and statutes governing the withholding of information from parents. Beyond the need to conform to any legal obligations, therapists should consider what level of information sharing with parents, guardians, and teachers is most helpful to achieve the best care and outcomes for their child and adolescent patients. Based in part on recommendations summarized by Luepker (2003), the following guidelines can help to determine whether or not to disclose information to parents or guardians:

1. Weigh the pros and cons of telling or not telling other parties. This includes determining if the recipient of the information would be in a position to protect the patient's privacy and to help with the treatment.
2. Discuss with the parents or guardians the importance of respecting the child's need for privacy for the success of treatment.
3. Explain to parents or guardians the importance of the therapist being able to make professional decisions, in accordance with professional ethics and applicable laws, about what is necessary for others to know.
4. Reassure parents or guardians that they will be informed of any risk which they can help to manage.
5. Limit discussions with teachers and principals to (a) information necessary for the child's safety, (b) general information about prognosis, such as when they might expect to see change in the child's behaviour, (c) assurances that the school's concerns are being addressed in treatment, and (d) things school personnel can do to assist the child's treatment.
6. Discuss with the child or adolescent the nature and extent of arrangements planned for the exchange of information with others.

Luepker (2003) further suggests having parents and guardians sign a confidentiality statement that acknowledges their agreement with the principles listed above in points two to four.

Controlling the scope of disclosure

When it is to the benefit of the patient to share confidential information with third parties, the type and extent of disclosure should be carefully controlled. The guiding principle is to restrict the information to be disclosed to the least amount necessary to serve a narrowly defined purpose, for a specified occasion or timeframe, involving a designated target person or persons. Different consent forms should be used that correspond to different types and levels of disclosure. For example, one type of form pertains only to *requesting information from others*. This deliberately restricts the information flow to one direction only (i.e., from others to the therapist), and does not release any current patient details to the other party (e.g., results from a medication evaluation by a general practitioner). Alternatively, another version provides consent only for *releasing information to others* (e.g., to the patient's lawyer in a custody case), but does not permit the other party (e.g., the lawyer) to divulge information to the therapist. Finally, the least restrictive type of consent form allows for the *exchanging of information with others*. That is, information may flow in both directions. Within each of those general categories of consent forms for disclosure of patient information, each one should be uniquely tailored to a specific purpose, clearly identify which person(s) are to provide or receive information, state the date or event when authorization expires, and document the patient's right to revoke consent at any time (Luepker, 2003).

As a general rule, when disclosing information to third parties, it is best to err on the side of caution and send too little rather than too much information. Recipients can always request additional information if necessary. Importantly, unless there are special circumstances defined by law or professional codes as discussed earlier in the chapter, therapists must seek consent of their patients before disclosing *any* patient information. Thus, when receiving phone calls or letters from third parties offering or requesting information about a patient, beginning therapists must be on guard to not even acknowledge that they know the patient, or that the patient is receiving services. For example, the simple confirmation of a patient being seen at a 'mental health' clinic could have harmful consequences for the patient, if the caller had sinister motives (e.g., a nosy employer or an ex-spouse involved in a custody battle). Therapists can respond to such requests for information that are not covered by prior signed consent agreements by saying: 'All information held at this clinic is confidential. I cannot tell you whether or not the person you are referring to is a patient here. If you want information regarding that person, you need to contact that person directly.'

Securing patient information

Therapists must ensure that all their patient records are stored securely and locked. Nowadays, information storage and transmission often occur in electronic format, which presents additional security risks that therapists must take care to minimize. Therapists have the responsibility of ensuring that no such materials are exposed in any way to the eyes of the innocent or interested. The following guidelines can help trainee therapists avoid the risks posed by some of the common threats to confidentiality:

- Return records (including USB sticks, portable drives, and video or audio tapes) to locked filing cabinets immediately after use.
- Do not leave any materials on which identifying patient information is visible on counters, desks, floors, or in unlocked furniture.

- Do not remove any files or patient records from the clinic or authorized premises (see also case example below). This applies to the files themselves as well as to electronic copies.
- Ensure that computers or workstations have appropriate security and that the security is operational (e.g., activate a password protected screensaver when leaving your desk). If the computer is networked, ensure that your files are not in a shared directory.
- Patient materials should not be duplicated for therapists' private records.
- Make it a routine practice to write in bold letters 'STRICTLY CONFIDENTIAL' at the top of all reports, faxes, and electronic or other similar communications.
- When writing or editing drafts of reports electronically, it is good practice to only use initials of the patient's name and disguise other identifying information, until you are ready to print the final version.
- When printing patient reports, test results, etc., collect printed materials immediately (e.g., do not stop on the way to the printer to chat with a colleague in the hall; an emergency call or other event can easily divert attention and result in the report being forgotten and left unattended in the printer tray).
- In the event of printer problems, always first delete your current print job before attempting to print again (e.g., having pushed the print button repeatedly in the belief it did not work the first time, can result in additional copies being printed and left unattended without the therapist being even aware of it).
- When faxing patient records, it is good practice to first call the recipient and ensure that authorized personnel are on standby to collect the transmitted materials. Conversely, when expecting a fax, ensure that incoming faxes are monitored and processed by authorized personnel only.
- Erase audio and video recordings of sessions immediately after their intended purpose (e.g., use in supervision) or in accordance with established agency policy.
- Do not discuss with others identifying patient information in hallways, reception areas, elevators, or similar environs that are open to the public or non-authorized personnel.

The following case example illustrates how the failure to follow these basic guidelines in securing confidentiality of patient information can lead to serious potential risk for the clients involved, as well as to serious repercussions for the trainee therapist responsible for the breach in security.

Case example. A student had taken various confidential case materials out of the treatment centre with the intention of completing several assessment reports at home. While the case materials were still in the student's car, the vehicle was stolen along with all the confidential case materials and some expensive testing kits. One of the serious implications for the affected clients was that the breach in security and the resultant failure to protect the clients' confidential details made them vulnerable to the risk of 'identity theft'. The repercussions for the student responsible for this security breach were appropriately severe. The student failed the practicum course, had to repeat an ethics course, had to purchase two test kits that had been stolen, had to recreate each of the clients' files, and had to inform the clients about the theft and the potential threat to their confidential details. Although most clients took the information well, one client expressed concern over becoming a victim of identity theft. In response, the training clinic offered the client a one-year membership to an identity theft company.

As this example illustrates, a breach of confidentiality resulted as a direct consequence of a student failing to adhere to established case management policies and procedures. It underscores the point made at the beginning of this chapter: there is no good treatment without good case management.

Protecting clients from unintended disclosure of confidential information has become more complex with rapid technological advances changing the ease by which psychologists create, transmit, and share electronic patient records. Trainees must learn how to understand and use the unique aspects of electronic record keeping in each of the settings they encounter during their practical training (American Psychological Association, 2007). Even beyond their current training environment, graduates must recognize the benefits and dangers inherent in the technological transformation of health care delivery and communication methods, anticipate how future advances will continue to impact practice, and prepare to embrace the opportunities it brings for improving patient care (e.g., Druss, Ji, Glick, & van Esenwein, 2014) while meeting new challenges to the security of patient information (Maheu, Pulier, McMenamin, & Posen, 2012). As the use of mobile smart devices and cloud computing spreads in health care delivery, it is imperative that psychologists provide protection against unauthorized access of sensitive patient records via the use of passwords and encryption methods (American Psychological Association, 2007).

A particular challenge to privacy and confidentiality arises from the unrelenting penetration of digital culture and social media for patients and treatment providers alike. Both psychologists and clients access personal information about each other via search engines and social networking sites (Kolmes, 2012). Trainees must be mindful how they want their private and professional identities in the virtual world to appear to their clients. When is finding this information beneficial or harmful to the therapeutic relationship? When does accessing information about a client on the internet blur the professional boundaries between therapist and client? There are many ethical pitfalls to be avoided when accessing internet data about clients. As a rule of thumb, Kaslow, Patterson, and Gottlieb (2011) warn that one should never seek internet information about a client simply out of curiosity, just as one would not be ethically permitted to pursue a sexual attraction. When in doubt, they recommend that the best course of action is always to consider how one would wish to be treated in a similar situation, and to keep the interests of the client paramount.

Tasks associated with the intake and treatment planning phase

In the following sections, we will review the key case management and documentation tasks associated with intake and treatment planning (see Figure 10.2).

Good management of the intake and treatment planning phase is essential for getting the treatment off to a good start. It facilitates early rapport building, generates momentum for change, and sets the tone for a goal-oriented working relationship with the client.

Getting treatment under way

The first case management task is to seek *informed consent* from the client prior to carrying out any assessment or intervention. Many clients sign informed consent forms as part of their application for services, others may wait until their first appointment to clarify any questions before signing. In either case, the parameters of the treatment process should be discussed before commencing therapeutic work. These include the limits to confidentiality (discussed earlier in this chapter), payment procedures, scheduling of sessions, and arrangements for consultation with third parties if applicable (e.g., monitoring medication by a psychiatrist, referrals for specialist testing, or periodic joint sessions with a spouse). When a client is accepted following a referral, the nature of the involvement (if any) of the referral

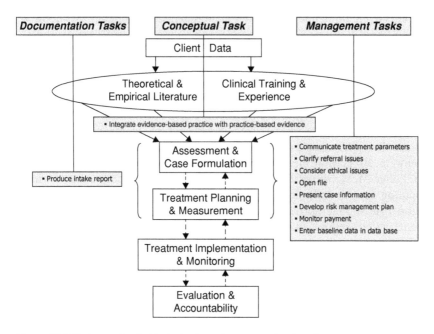

Figure 10.2 Tasks associated with the intake and treatment planning phase.

source needs to be clarified. Regardless of the extent of their continued involvement, referrers should be advised whether or not a referral has been accepted.

In addition to obtaining informed consent and clarifying referral issues, it is the therapist's responsibility to consider any *ethical issues* before providing services. For each client, therapists have a professional duty to make a judgement as to whether their abilities match the needs of the presenting case, or if other circumstances (e.g., prior acquaintance or relations with the client outside the therapeutic context) could jeopardize optimal client care. In those instances, clients should be referred to another professional.

Once a decision is reached to take on a client, a file needs to be opened that contains the signed consent form and any relevant referral information.

Presenting and documenting case information

An important aspect of good case management is the therapist's ability to communicate to others verbally and in writing who the client is, what the presenting problem is, what the factors are that cause and maintain the presenting problem, and how these factors can be influenced by the proposed treatment plan. Presentation of summary case information during the intake and treatment planning phase occurs in two main formats: brief verbal presentations at clinical staff meetings or rounds and succinct written intake reports. The operative words here are *brief* and *succinct*! Unfortunately, the aim of achieving brevity and succinctness in presenting case information tends to conflict with the novice's understandable anxiety over evaluation and their fragile confidence in knowing what details are germane to the case and should or should not be included when presenting a case. As a consequence, novices often test the patience of their colleagues and supervisors by indulging in meandering discourse about their patients' life journeys, only to end up rushing through what is

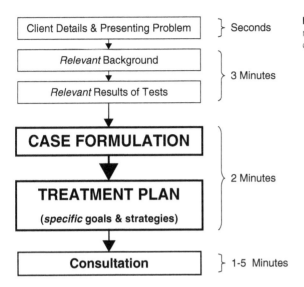

Figure 10.3 Schematic illustration of the relative importance of case presentation components.

the most important part of communicating case information – offering an integrative case formulation along with specific, measurable treatment goals derived from it. Unduly long presentations and reports also result from a tendency among novices to use templates of the structure and content of case reports inappropriately as a mandatory proscription to cover every point of the template, rather than using the template as a guide to be *selective* about which aspects of a case are the most germane for enabling others to understand the basis for the case formulation and treatment plan. What, then, is the cure from the novice's affliction to produce case presentations and reports that typically are too long to be useful in the fast-paced reality of modern clinical practice?

The first antidote to overly long case presentations and reports is to remember that clinical psychology services are delivered in a competitive health care market where time is a precious commodity. Put simply, there is no time for long presentations. Long reports do not get read and unread reports are not in the best interest of your client. The second antidote is to approach preparation of case presentations and reports not in the order in which they are eventually delivered (client details, presenting problem, background etc.), but by first writing out the case formulation and treatment plan. For example, presenting a formulation and treatment plan should take about two minutes. That means there are about three minutes left out of a finite total presentation time of circa five minutes. Thus, the number of background details that can be presented must be restricted to those that are the most relevant and that best illustrate the rationale for the formulation and treatment plan, while still fitting within the remaining three-minute time limit (see Figure 10.3).

The primary purpose of a case *presentation* is quality assurance. That is, an integrative case formulation and the treatment plan that follows from it are presented to colleagues for the purpose of feedback and consultation. Therefore, precious presentation time must be used wisely, with the components covering case formulation, treatment plan, and consultation with colleagues receiving the greatest weight (see Figure 10.3). The primary purpose of case *reports* is accountability. Similarly to case presentations, the emphasis in case reports should be on the case formulation and treatment plan, with details from background information, current interpersonal and social functioning, and scores on objective assessment measures serving as 'evidence' to support and *selectively* illustrate the rationale behind the case formulation and treatment plan. Because the complete test results are available in the patient's file for future reference, and because background details, if they were relevant enough to be recorded in the progress notes, can be retrieved at any time if necessary, it is sufficient for summary reports to only include illustrative key details supporting the formulation and treatment plan. This will ensure that case reports are succinct, focused on the presenting problem, and practical in day-to-day case management (see Chapter 3 for a comprehensive list of intake information from which key client data would be selected for inclusion in a case report). Notwithstanding the importance of succinctness in presenting and documenting case information, case reports do require greater detail when the assessment indicated that the treatment must also be accompanied by a risk management plan.

Assessing and managing risk

The burden of determining when clients are at risk to harm themselves or others weighs heavily on any therapist, especially on the inexperienced trainee. With respect to self-harming behaviours, the disconcerting fact is that they cannot be reliably predicted at the level of the individual (Fowler, 2012). Suicidal states are variable and usually time limited in nature, and they are modifiable in response to treatment. Therefore, the continual monitoring, assessment, and documentation of current risk level is an essential part of good case management and reasonable and prudent patient care (Bongar & Sullivan, 2013). Science can serve as an ally in the effective management of risk (Seligman, 1996a), because the burden of uncertainty can be allayed somewhat with the help of empirically derived practice guidelines on how to assess and manage suicidal clients.

A reasonable and prudent approach requires a multidimensional assessment incorporating both a thorough clinical interview asking about suicidal thoughts, plans, behaviour, and intent, supplemented by actuarial data from scales measuring relevant risk and protective factors. This information is used to benchmark risk, conduct a risk-benefit analysis of alternative courses of action, and inform an intervention plan to increase safety and reduce risk (Fowler, 2012). There are over 60 risk factors identified in the literature (APA, 2003), with the strongest empirical support for history of previous suicide attempts, mental disorders, social isolation, physical illness, unemployment, and family conflict (Bongar & Sullivan, 2013). There is emerging evidence that assessment of proximal risk factors arising from a sense of perceived disconnectedness from others and the belief that one is a burden on others, combined with an acquired confidence in being able to overcome one's innate fear of death and engage in lethal self-harm, should be part of a prudent risk assessment (Ribeiro, Bodell, Hames, Hagan, & Joiner, 2013). Particular emphasis is on those risk factors (e.g., social isolation, psychological distress, hopelessness, etc.) that can be modified as part of the intervention plan.

Although protective factors have received less attention in the literature, their protective counterbalancing role in strengthening resilience in the face of elevated risk may prove crucial in determining the outcome of a suicidal crisis (Johnson, Wood, Gooding, Taylor, & Tarrier, 2011). Protective factors can be external such as responsibility to loved ones or supportive interpersonal relationships, as well as internal such as strong reasons for living and zest for life (Harrison, Stritzke, Fay, Ellison, & Hudaib, 2014; Malone et al. 2000), a sense of meaning and purpose in life (Kleiman & Beaver, 2013), as well as good coping skills, frustration tolerance, and religious affiliations (Fowler, 2012). Scales such as the Reasons for Living Inventory (Linehan, Goodstein, Nielsen, & Chiles, 1983) can enhance the evaluation of suicide risk. One practical risk assessment framework that explicitly evaluates the counterbalance of protective factors is the Suicide Assessment Five-step Evaluation and Triage protocol (SAFE-T; www.stopasuicide.org/docs/Safe_T_Card_Mental_Health_Professionals. pdf).

Because suicide risk is fluid and can wax and wane rapidly, it is important to make a distinction between chronic and acute features of a suicidal crisis (Rudd, 2008). Those with a history of multiple suicide attempts should be considered at a higher baseline and chronic level of risk for suicide. That is, their risk is elevated even in the absence of acute risk factors, and their vulnerability to exacerbation in response to acute stress is greater than for those who are not multiple attempters. Taking this critical distinction as a starting point, an empirically grounded decision framework for determining the level of risk associated with suicidal symptoms, and what actions to take depending on the severity of risk, has been described by Joiner and his colleagues (Joiner, Walker, Rudd, & Jobes, 1999). According to this decision framework, the mere presence of some suicidal ideation is not very useful in determining risk status, because some suicidal thoughts are encountered routinely among treatment-seeking individuals and are not uncommon even in the general population. The most crucial variables determining suicide risk are history of prior attempts combined with the nature of current suicidal symptoms and the number of other known risk factors. Accordingly, the first step in the assessment of suicide risk severity is to determine whether the client can be categorized as a *multiple* attempter or *non-multiple* attempter, because the baseline risk for multiple attempters is always elevated compared to single attempters and mere ideators. Therefore, risk is assessed differently for multiple and non-multiple attempters (see Figure 10.4). The presence of at least one risk factor translates into at least a moderate risk level for multiple attempters, but not necessarily for non-multiple attempters, unless it involves *resolved plans and preparation* to commit suicide. Thus, the second step in assessing risk severity is to determine whether the client has a plan, how specific that plan is, if the means and opportunity to execute the plan are available, and if the client has made any preparations for the attempt. One should also consider here the duration and intensity (rather than frequency) of *suicidal desire and ideation*. The third step in suicide risk assessment is to identify any additional risk factors that can raise the level of risk beyond that associated with the domains of resolved plans and preparation or suicidal desire and ideation alone. These risk factors include, but are not limited to, (a) recent stressful life events (e.g., divorce, legal troubles), (b) diagnostic comorbidity (especially mood and anxiety disorders, alcohol use, and hopelessness), (c) chaotic or abusive family history, (d) impulsive behavioural style, and (e) limited social connectedness. Others such as hopelessness and perceived burdensomeness as mentioned above should be assessed.

Once the level of risk severity has been classified as either *low to mild, moderate,* or *severe to extreme*, different risk management strategies are called for depending on the level of risk. Table 10.1 summarizes the various risk management activities associated with each level of severity. It also provides example statements of how to discuss with clients the risk management activities at each level of intervention. It is recommended that patients at moderate risk be given a crisis response plan on a card that they can carry with them at all times (Joiner et al., 1999; Oordt et al., 2005). The card has a step-by-step list of what to do when thoughts about suicide occur, including phone numbers of alternative support services (e.g., *'If the thoughts continue, and I find myself preparing to do something, I call the clinic at: _____'*; or *'If I cannot reach anyone at the clinic, I call: _____'*).

Multiple Attempters

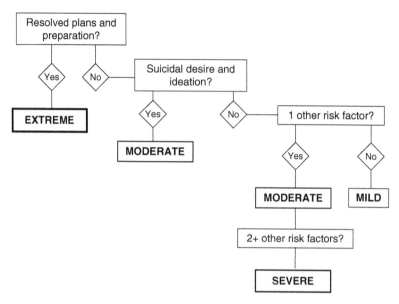

Non-Multiple Attempters

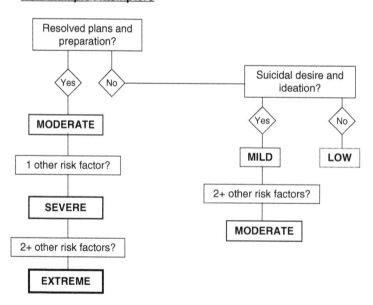

Figure 10.4 A decision framework for the assessment of suicide risk severity (based on Joiner, Walker, Rudd, & Jobes, 1999).

Table 10.1 Summary of what to do in response to different suicide risk categories

Risk severity	Risk management activities	Example statements
LOW to MILD	– continued risk assessment – document in progress notes	'In the event that you start feeling that you want to harm yourself, here's what I want you to do: First, use the skills for self-control we'll discuss, such as challenging your negative thoughts and seeking social support. If suicidal feelings remain, contact me or the clinic. If you are unable to reach anyone, or, if you feel you need assistance straight away, call or go to the emergency room – here is the number.' 'Have you had any thoughts of harming yourself since I last saw you?'
MODERATE	– increase frequency of sessions – involve supportive others – stay in touch via phone contacts – consider medication – provide detailed emergency plan – monitor changes in risk level – re-evaluate treatment goals – seek consultation – document changing risk levels – document clinical decisions – document actions taken – document risk resolution	'It is important that we put some strategies in place that keep you safe and help you gain control over your suicidal feelings.' 'One of the things that will help you is …' 'Until you feel things are under control again, I recommend that for the next [time period] we schedule more frequent visits.' 'I want you to carry this crisis response plan card with you at all times. It lists the steps you need to take when thinking about suicide. Do you agree to follow those steps when thinking about suicide?'
SEVERE to EXTREME	– accompany and monitor patient – evaluate for hospitalization – involve emergency services – involve family members – seek consultation – document risk status – document clinical decisions – document actions taken – document risk resolution	'At the moment you are not safe on your own.' 'Is there someone in your family that we can contact right now?' 'I am calling emergency services so they can assist us getting you to the hospital for evaluation and crisis care.' 'I am going to ask my colleague/supervisor [add name] to come and join us while we are waiting for your family/emergency staff to get here.' **Note:** If highest risk category becomes apparent during a phone contact, ask the following questions right away: 'Where are you? [do your best to determine the exact location] 'What is the phone number there, in case we get disconnected?' 'Are you alone or is someone with you?' 'Have you eaten or did you drink anything that is dangerous to your health?' 'Have you harmed or injured yourself?'

The importance of routinely documenting all decisions and interventions for maintaining the safety of clients until the suicidal risk has been resolved cannot be overstated (Rudd, Joiner, Jobes, & King, 1999). In terms of the characteristics of good records, more detail than usual is appropriate, because details are highly relevant in the context of risk management. In this instance, failure to be thorough can compromise patient safety, as well as the therapist's ability to prove that the level of care conformed to professional standards of empirically grounded practice and reasonable and prudent care. Trainees should note that the traditional widespread practice of using so-called 'no-suicide contracts' is not recommended (Rudd, Mandrusiak, & Joiner, 2006). Documenting in the file that a patient has 'contracted for safety' has no force in law and has little value in protecting therapists from malpractice liability (Bongar & Sullivan, 2013). Instead of a no-suicide contract, it is recommended, as mentioned above, to negotiate with the client a crisis response plan with the focus on an alliance for safety. Here the client is encouraged to make a commitment to living by agreeing to actively participate in the intervention and make use of the crisis response plan and any safety planning strategies agreed upon (for details see Rudd et al., 2006; Stanley & Brown, 2012). Finally, it is reasonable and prudent practice that when suicide risk increases, the level of documentation must increase to reflect this, and so should the amount of peer and expert consultation (Bongar & Sullivan, 2013). It is paramount for trainees to maintain meticulous, contemporaneous notes of the rationale for all critical crisis management decisions and to imagine when writing those notes that a lawyer is looking over their shoulder.

In addition to assessing and managing any risks to a patient's own safety, it may also become necessary to respond to situations where the patient's behaviour, or expressed intent to act, constitutes an imminent risk to others including the therapist. When such a crisis situation arises, the therapist must initiate *emergency procedures*. Although it is likely that a supervisor will be at hand to assist with or handle a crisis situation, every trainee has the responsibility to not only be aware of the emergency procedures pertaining to their training clinic or clinical placement sites, but to know them by heart. Once a crisis unfolds, it is too late to consult the procedures manual for guidance. Emergency procedures are usually tailored to specific demands associated with the locale, type of client population, availability of onsite staff, and proximity of support services such as police and psychiatric emergency response teams. Because these demands can vary considerably across sites, the onus is on the trainee to become thoroughly familiar with the emergency procedures specific to each training site. In general, all emergency procedures share the following core principles:

- Foremost, be aware of your own safety and that of others in close proximity.
- If necessary, get yourself and others away from the danger.
- Notify everyone in the clinic of the emergency situation (e.g., activate 'panic button' in the consulting room; alert the reception staff).
- Notify any available supervisors.
- Request intervention by security staff, police, or psychiatric emergency response units.

When it becomes necessary to involve specially trained emergency response personnel, the therapist needs to be prepared to tell them everything they want to know about the client and to listen to their advice on how the situation is to be handled. They are the experts, and once they are on the scene, they are in charge and the responsibility for the patient's well-being rests with them.

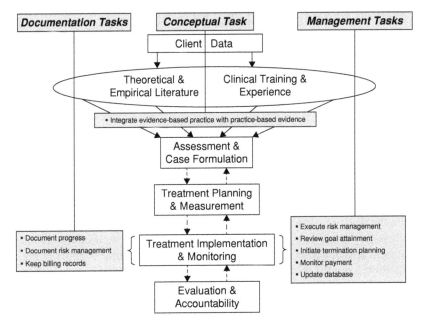

Figure 10.5 Tasks associated with the treatment implementation phase.

Finally, there are situations where the risk is not imminent, but where a client's behaviour nonetheless poses a potentially serious risk to others. For example, an HIV-positive patient might tell the therapist that he or she is engaging in unprotected sex with their partner(s) who are unaware of the patient's disease status. In many jurisdictions, therapists have a legal obligation to report infectious diseases to health authorities. In some jurisdictions, there are also provisions for health care providers to protect and notify identifiable others. In these situations it is good practice for therapists to seek legal advice on reporting infectious and potentially harmful conditions without the patient's consent (Luepker, 2003). As always, all activities associated with the risk management of such cases must be carefully documented in the client's file.

Tasks associated with the treatment implementation phase

Once an intake report has been filed, baseline assessment data have been collected for each treatment goal, and treatment has commenced, the focus of case management is to ensure that the therapeutic process unfolds in a manner consistent with the treatment plan. Thus, the key management tasks associated with the treatment implementation phase are (a) the routine review of progress towards goal attainment, which may necessitate adjustments to the treatment plan or diagnostic impression, and (b) the initiation of preparatory steps that will strengthen the client's capacity for independent coping upon termination of treatment (see Figure 10.5). If applicable, risk management activities need to be executed as planned and carefully documented, noting any change in risk status and any modifications to the risk management plan, and the reasons for those modifications. In the fiscal domain of case management, therapists must monitor the payment of services and keep accurate billing records which document the date, length, and type of services, the cost of the services, and in what form payment was received (e.g., cash, cheque, or credit card).

Documenting progress towards goal attainment

All events associated with the treatment of a client should be recorded in the progress notes. These provide records of every contact with the client (in person, by phone, email, text messaging, or post), or concerning the client (e.g., a phone call to arrange aftercare services), as well as an up-to-date summary of therapy sessions. Table 10.2 provides an outline and examples of how to write a typical progress note.

Initiating termination planning

The ultimate goal of treatment is to help clients to regain agency over their lives and emotional well-being in the shortest period possible. Thus, termination of treatment becomes an automatic goal as soon as the client walks through the door for the first appointment. In order for the client and therapist to know when treatment can be brought to a close, it is important for the therapist to consider this question jointly with the client throughout the treatment process as part of ongoing case management. Of course, thinking about the time *after* treatment and being on their own again without the regular support of the therapist may be furthest from the mind of clients who have just sought help because they felt helpless on their own. Similarly, beginning therapists understandably get preoccupied with the immediate demands of current treatment, rather than preparing simultaneously for the more distant time when they are not needed anymore by the client. Thus, the fear of the client of being 'abandoned' by the therapist before the client feels ready, and the inclination of the therapist to aim for the best possible treatment outcome before 'letting go' of the client, can conspire to overshoot the target and unnecessarily prolong treatment. That is, the failure to initiate termination planning early in treatment could lead to a bumpy ending of the therapeutic relationship, rather than a smooth transition towards closure and a return to life without therapy. Further, for individuals who require inpatient treatment, it is good practice to discuss possible discharge dates early in the hospitalization and subsequent plans for follow-up care so that patients have a clear concept of the treatment plan.

Routine termination planning during the treatment implementation phase helps the therapist to determine when treatment is 'good enough' (see also Chapter 15 on the concept of 'good enough treatment'). It also ensures that any distress associated with feelings of loss or abandonment that a client may experience as a result of terminating the therapeutic relationship can be dealt with in a gradual and supportive rather than abrupt fashion. There is a simple way of incorporating termination planning during treatment that is non-threatening and informative for both client and therapist. Early in treatment, the therapist can initiate termination planning by telling the client that *'therapy has a beginning, middle, and end'*, followed by the question, *'where do you see yourself at this moment in treatment?'* The simple opening statement raises the awareness of the client that treatment is time-limited and progresses towards a logical endpoint. At the same time, the use of an open-ended follow-up question reassures the client that the decision about ending treatment is reached collaboratively involving the joint input of client and therapist. The answers clients give to that question are often eye-opening for beginning therapists and serve as a reality check. Novice therapists are less experienced in picking up cues from clients that treatment gains have solidified, or have already generalized to domains in the clients' life that were not particularly targeted by the treatment. Consequently, novices tend to underestimate their clients' readiness for termination. The use of routine termination planning can help to correct for

Table 10.2 How to write progress notes

Order	Content	Examples from different clients
1.	A sentence describing the client's • appearance • moods and feelings • behaviour	*'Came on time, neatly dressed, sat stiff and tense the whole interview, occasionally fidgeting with things on the table; seemed anxious and angry.'* *'Came ten minutes late, unironed clothes, sat motionless staring at the floor, seemed deeply dejected.'*
2.	A sentence or two on what the client told the therapist about • changes in symptoms and behaviour • changes in life situation • new insights • thoughts on previous session or treatment goals	*'He said he was working more, but still unable to sleep and the quarrels with his wife were getting worse.'* *'She said that the children were getting along better at daycare and she wasn't so irritable at work anymore and that she and her husband seemed to be talking better. Now that communication within the family has improved, she wants to focus more on her goal to take up again some non-family related activities.'*
3.	A sentence stating what the primary goal(s) was (were) for the session	*'The primary goal of the session was to examine X's catastrophic thinking in response to her recent worries about her upcoming promotion to head one of the regional company offices.'*
4.	A sentence or two on the overall content of the session, and a statement of to what extent the session goal(s) was (were) met, or to what extent overall treatment goals were successfully addressed	*'He began by complaining about his wife, but towards the end of the session was talking more about how he may be contributing to what went on. This insight represents significant progress towards him taking more responsibility for his part in the ongoing distress and frustration he experiences in interpersonal interactions. The conflict with his wife served as an example for continuing with the assertiveness module and practising alternative approaches to communicating with his wife.'*
5.	A sentence indicating goals for the next session or any changes or innovations in the treatment plan	*'In the next session, we will again emphasize behavioural training in social skills via role-plays, now that trying to gain insight into the reasons for her shyness seems to have led to little change in the level of social interactions for the client.'*
Throughout	If applicable, important statements by the therapist or client should be recorded verbatim	*'I said that at this point it would be best for her to participate in the group programme offered at GetWell Hospital.'* *'He described his boss as a "liar and womanizer", and he believed that he had no chance of promotion despite his boss promising he "was next on the list".'*

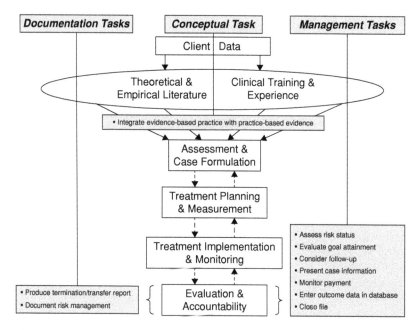

Figure 10.6 Tasks associated with the evaluation and termination phase.

this bias and ensure that the focus of valuable session time at the latter stages of treatment matches the client's increasing readiness for moving on.

Tasks associated with the evaluation and termination phase

Ideally, goal attainment signals the end of treatment. Therefore, the key case management tasks during the evaluation and termination phase are to collect final outcome data, examine the change from baseline values, and evaluate the clinical significance of the change in relation to the goals specified in the treatment plan (see Figure 10.6). If there is only partial change, or no change at all, or a worsening of symptoms in some areas targeted by the treatment, then the therapist should consider follow-up services. If it is clear that the client would not benefit from simply extending services, a referral to alternative treatment providers should be considered. Analogous to brief case presentations during the intake phase, where therapists share case information with colleagues for consultation on treatment decisions and planning, therapists often present a brief update or termination summary to their colleagues, who can provide reflective feedback on aspects of the treatment or suggestions for follow-up strategies if applicable. In terminating relationships with clients, therapists must have the best interest of the client in mind and show regard for the client's ongoing well-being. In the event that therapists must terminate treatment prematurely due to personal reasons (e.g., illness, change of employment, extended leave of absence), they should provide clients with an explanation of the need for such early termination and take all reasonable steps to arrange for alternative care.

If a risk management plan was in place during treatment, an important case management responsibility is to reassess risk status immediately prior to termination. Readiness for termination is contingent upon resolution of the circumstances that had put the client at a heightened level of risk at the start of treatment. Resolution of risk status needs to be carefully documented in the termination report. Should the assessment of risk status indicate any residual level of risk for the client, the therapist must document carefully what preventative steps have been taken to ensure the client's safety after the end of the therapeutic relationship.

A major documentation task at the end of treatment is for the therapist to produce a succinct *termination or transfer report*. A termination report should contain the following information:

- *Introductory summary:* A brief statement about the presenting problem(s), the number of sessions, and the time period over which services were provided (e.g., Ms P self-referred to the clinic for depression and relationship problems. She was seen for eight sessions between 16 November 2013 and 29 March 2014).
- *Focus of treatment:* A brief paragraph on the treatment plan and the strategies used to address goals of the plan.
- *Progress and goal attainment:* A paragraph stating what goals have and have not been achieved with direct reference to objective outcome measures (including a statement on risk resolution if applicable).
- *Concluding recommendation(s):* A brief statement about the reasons for termination and whether termination was mutually agreed upon, any specific arrangements for continuing care, and recommendations for relapse prevention and/or follow-ups if applicable.

The final case management task is to close the client file in a timely manner and ensure that it is stored securely in accordance with ethical guidelines and applicable legal obligations.

The processes of case management may appear difficult, and the prospect of juggling these management responsibilities alongside the many tasks associated with conducting therapeutic interventions may seem daunting. However, this is where availing yourself of competent and experienced supervision can be of real benefit. Clinical supervision will be the topic of the following chapter.

Supervision

Making the most of supervised practice

Supervised practice is paramount to the teaching and learning of psychotherapy (Watkins, 1997). The novice therapist in a university training programme typically receives formal supervisory feedback at least once a week, and often benefits from additional ad hoc and informal guidance by readily available supervisors. After graduating, therapists move on to positions where their contracts stipulate and guarantee them the accumulation of a required minimum number of supervised practice hours for accreditation. Once accredited, however, supervision is often harder to come by. Reviews of clinical supervision in various mental health professions (Spence, Wilson, Kavanagh, Strong, & Worrall, 2001; Strong et al., 2003; Townend, Iannetta & Freeston, 2002) concluded that the realities of high case loads, higher priority of crisis management, poor access to supervisors, and lack of clear policy guidelines are cited as reasons for many practitioners receiving little or infrequent supervision. For example, in a sample of 170 cognitive behavioural therapists in the UK, the mean number of supervision hours received was just over two hours per month for 52 hours of direct face-to-face client contact (Townend et al., 2002). Thus, the intense level of supervision available during the initial training of psychotherapists is a time-limited privilege! Moreover, in a survey of over 4,000 psychotherapists with different professional backgrounds, career levels, theoretical orientations, and nationalities, getting formal supervision was rated as the second most positive influence on their career development, after the experience of working directly with clients (Orlinsky, Botermans, & Rønnestad, 2001). With that in mind, novice supervisees should be highly motivated to be actively engaged in their supervision, and to make the most of this important and valuable aspect of their training.

Goals of supervision for science-informed practice

Supervision is an interpersonal intervention that is both collaborative and evaluative. It has the simultaneous goals of developing in supervisees the skills for science-informed practice, monitoring the quality of the treatments delivered, and providing a safeguard that prevents a supervisee who puts clients at risk from entering the profession (Bernard & Goodyear, 2004). In addition, by encouraging self-efficacy in supervisees (Falender & Shafranske, 2004), and by supervisors serving as role models, supervision provides a supportive learning environment for supervisees to develop their own professional identity.

Figure 11.1 illustrates how these four primary goals of supervision map onto the processes of the science-informed practice model introduced at the beginning of this manual. The development of skills and competencies focuses on the specific clinical tasks involved in

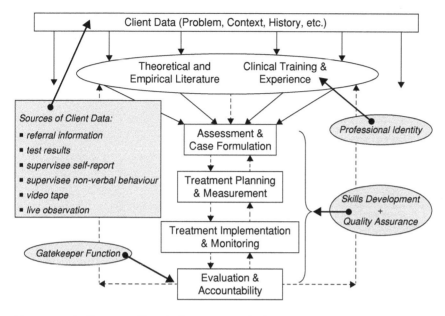

Figure 11.1 An illustration of how the four primary goals of supervision map onto the treatment process highlighting the sources of client data available for supervisory input.

linking client data to case formulation, treatment planning, implementation, and outcome evaluation. As such, 'supervision provides the structure and framework for learning how to apply knowledge, theory, and clinical procedures to solve human problems' (Falender & Shafranske, 2004, p. 6). The aim of enhancing the professional functioning of the supervisee in these essential clinical tasks goes hand-in-hand with the supervisor's primary ethical responsibility of monitoring client care. The supervisor must assure that the quality of the services delivered by the supervisee meets appropriate standards and achieves optimal outcomes for the client. In cases where formative feedback has failed to enhance the supervisee's competence and readiness to assume the role of an independent practitioner, the supervisor's summative assessment serves a gatekeeper function to protect the welfare of clients, the integrity of the profession, and society at large.

In addition to enhancing professional functioning and monitoring quality of client care, supervision serves the function of socializing supervisees into their professional discipline (Bernard & Goodyear, 2004). That is, the personal growth experienced by supervisees during training, as they gain experiences and mastery in clinical practice, occurs in close association with the role models provided by senior members of the supervisee's own professional discipline. This collaborative process allows supervisees to develop a professional identity, along with a clear sense of the unique contribution they can make within the context of health care delivery systems that are increasingly multidisciplinary.

Good supervision must achieve a delicate balance in meeting the four goals discussed above. This poses quite a challenge, because the relative weight assigned to each goal varies depending on the stakeholder involved. Figure 11.2 shows how the supervisor needs to consider the welfare of three principal stakeholders: the client, the clinician, and society at large. For example, quality assurance is of utmost importance to the client as well as society and supersedes educative and training goals of the clinician. At the same time, beginning

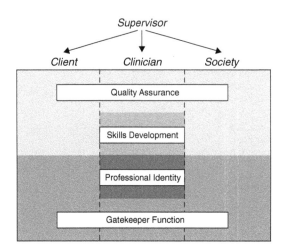

Figure 11.2 The relevance of the four primary goals of supervision for three classes of stakeholders.

therapists are expected to make mistakes and will need to hone their skills. This may result in some delays and detours before treatment strategies, with the benefit of formative supervisory feedback, are successfully implemented. The integration of the dual tasks of providing supervisees with practical experience in learning how to apply their knowledge and skills to the provision of clinical services, and ensuring that client welfare is not compromised in the name of training, requires careful consideration of the sources of data available for supervisory input and oversight (see Figure 11.1). Some client data (e.g., test results, video-recorded verbal and non-verbal behaviour) are directly available for inspection by the supervisor, but much data (e.g., supervisee self-report of session content or process) will first pass through the selective and interpretative lens of the supervisee. It is therefore important that supervisees learn to present supervision data in a way that maximizes their utility for skills enhancement, professional growth, and quality assurance. Before we discuss what supervisees need to do to achieve this, we will explain how the conceptualization of supervision goals within a science-informed model of practice as illustrated in Figure 11.1 is consistent with current competency-based approaches to supervision.

A competency-based approach to supervision

A scientist-practitioner looks for valid theoretical models to guide his or her professional activities. In the case of supervision, there is no shortage of available models, but empirical support for most of them is scarce, and many simply present personal views and anecdotal accounts of various aspects of supervision (Spence et al., 2001). Another significant problem with many current models of supervision is that they lack the specificity to tie the primary supervision goals to particular supervision strategies and processes, which in turn target the key components of clinical practice (Gonsalvez, Oades, & Freestone, 2002). Traditionally, several models were developed as a direct extension of a particular psychotherapy theory. Proponents of such *psychotherapy-based approaches* emphasize that supervision practices should reflect the particular theoretical orientation a supervisor holds with respect to treatment. For example, whereas 'cognitive behavioural' supervision is highly structured, emphasizes exploration, conceptualization, and modification of thoughts and beliefs, and uses didactic teaching and homework assignments to enhance skills (Liese & Beck, 1997), 'Gestalt' supervision is less skills-oriented, avoids didactic instruction, and instead aims to provide supervisees with 'conditions' that will help them to implement the therapeutic 'attitudes' necessary to affect therapeutic change in clients (Patterson, 1997). One would expect supervisory practices to greatly differ for such different schools of thought, but when one examines what supervisors actually *do* in supervision sessions (see Watkins, 1997), it is apparent that 'irrespective of professional and theoretical background, supervisors engage in very similar supervisory practices' (Spence et al., 2001, p. 138). This should not be surprising, because the aims of supervision, while they map onto the treatment process, are not equivalent to the aims of treatment, nor are treatment knowledge and skills readily transferable to the supervisory context (Falender & Shafranske, 2004). Moreover, contemporary models of psychopathology and treatment are multidimensional and integrative rather than based on a single theoretical model (Barlow & Durand, 2015). Hence, a useful model of supervision is one that embraces explicitly the need to be adaptable in light of current advances in the literature. In fact, a rigid adherence to a single, narrow, theoretical orientation early in training can lead to stagnation and impede the further professional development of supervisees (Neufeldt, 2003).

There are also supervision models that are not based on a particular theory of psychotherapy. For example, *developmental approaches* to supervision assume that supervisees change as their training progresses from novice to advanced status, and that supervisory practices should be matched to the supervisee's needs at a given level of experience and expertise (e.g., Stoltenberg & McNeill, 1997). These models highlight that a large part of a therapist's development occurs *after* formal training has ended (Neufeld, 2003). This broad perspective of novice-to-expert development extends well beyond the scope of the time-limited, formal training period most relevant to the beginning therapist. Further, there is much variation within and across developmental training levels. For example, an advanced trainee may need the type of supervisory input more typical of a novice trainee when faced with a crisis situation, or when transfer of skills to new clients and situations proves very challenging. As with the psychotherapy-based approaches, empirical support for developmental models of supervision is limited, although there is some support for the notion that inexperienced trainees benefit most from structured and directive methods (Spence et al., 2001).

Finally, *process-based approaches* to supervision emphasize that supervision is a unique professional praxis that involves specific roles, tasks, and processes within a supervisory relationship with the aim to facilitate the teaching and learning of specific competencies (Bernard & Goodyear, 2004). As illustrated in Figure 11.1, these competencies are evaluated against the measurable outcomes of supervisees' clinical interventions. The explicit articulation of supervision components that are linked to the primary supervision goals provides the framework for initiating, developing, implementing, and evaluating the processes and outcomes of supervision (Falender & Shafranske, 2004). That is, a *competency-based approach* to clinical supervision is goal-directed and accountable to stakeholders (Falender & Shafranske, 2012). Therefore, the development of competencies requires deliberate practice, rather than simple experience (Neufeldt, 1999). This means that supervisees must fully engage in the supervision enterprise and apply to their own learning the self-critical and reflective attitude that is the hallmark of scientific enquiry, hypothesis testing, and outcome evaluation (Shakow, 1976).

The reflective supervisee

Reflectivity in clinical practice is the deliberate process by which practitioners frame problems, modify their behaviour to test solutions, evaluate the outcomes of these tests, and then decide how to proceed in their work with clients in light of these insights (Neufeldt, 1999). Supervision aims to instil in supervisees this reflective approach to practice. The process of reflectivity is initiated when the supervisee encounters a situation in which she or he is puzzled or feels stuck and is unsure how to proceed. That is, 'the trainee's feelings of uncertainty signal a problem ripe for reflectivity' (Neufeldt, Karno, & Nelson, 1996, p. 6). Supervisees must learn to tolerate this ambiguity and use it constructively to guide their clinical thought processes and decision-making. They must resist the inclination to 'cover up' with defensive impression management arising from an understandable desire to not appear incompetent. Reflectivity in supervision is only complete if it results in supervisees changing their behaviour in subsequent sessions. We will draw on the integrated model of reflectivity described by Neufeldt and her colleagues (1996) to illustrate with an example what the supervisee's role, tasks, and responsibilities are throughout the sequential and iterative process of engaging in, and learning from, reflective supervision.

The trigger event

Consider a novice supervisee who is experiencing considerable frustration in her first couple of sessions with a new client, because the client 'does not provide much detailed information and seems reluctant to respond to follow-up questions when asked to elaborate on points'.

Following the trigger event

A reflective supervisee reacts to the trigger event as follows: She (a) is puzzled or feels stuck and unsure how to proceed, (b) knows that feelings of uncertainty signal a problem ripe for reflectivity, (c) takes responsibility for learning and professional growth, (d) avoids defensive self-protection, tolerates a sense of vulnerability, and is prepared to take a risk, and (e) is proactive and presents the trigger event in supervision.

Prior to supervision

A reflective supervisee understands that most of her learning occurs *between* supervision sessions. Therefore, she engages in several preparatory activities: she (a) uses self-assessment and selects valid information about the trigger event (e.g., relevant video segment of a typical incident of the client not responding to supervisee's questions), (b) considers own actions, emotions, and thoughts during the incident (e.g., How did I feel during the silence? Am I getting anxious to 'do something' during silent moments with the client? What was I thinking? Was I worried about getting through all my questions I had prepared? Did I give the client enough time to answer?), (c) considers the interaction between the client and self during the event (e.g., What am I doing? What is the client doing? Did my follow-up questions interrupt the client's thoughts? Would the client have answered had I shut up for just a little longer? How would I respond myself to rapid-fire questions from someone?), and (d) formulates a summary statement about the event and any insights or questions gleaned from the self-assessment to take into the next supervision session.

During supervision

The reflective supervisee brings a stance to supervision that is characterized by intent to understand what has occurred, and by an openness to accept and try solutions generated with the guidance of the supervisor. Hence, she (a) is open to new ideas, (b) critically examines supervision data such as a pre-selected video clip (e.g., Client appears to be contemplating answer.

Client shifts body and begins to open mouth, but then stops and listens to my next question.), (c) entertains alternative explanations (e.g., Client is not reluctant to answer. Rather, I am impatient, and the client is polite and/or not assertive enough), and (d) formulates alternative explanations as hypotheses and plans how to test these new ideas with the client in the next session (e.g., I will sit back after asking a question to rein in my impatience and to signal to the client it is her turn. I will tell myself that silence is OK. I will wait for the client to answer. I will attend to and observe outcomes of this deliberate change to my behaviour).

During subsequent session with client

The reflective supervisee understands that an event becomes 'reflective' only if the supervisee changes behaviour as a result of the reflective process. Consequently, she (a) puts into action her plan to 'experiment' and test the new ideas developed during supervision, and (b) uses reflection-in-action, that is, she attends to and evaluates what is happening while it is happening during therapist–client interactions (e.g., Client answers after a delay. Silence does not feel so uncomfortable after all. Let me try this again with the next question. Yes, it works again. Now look what happens, the client becomes talkative. I relax. I am getting somewhere with this client).

Following subsequent session with client

The reflective supervisee contemplates the consequences of her 'experiment'. She (a) evaluates outcomes of having used new behaviours and strategies (e.g., What worked and what did not work? Does the client provide more detailed information and respond to follow-up questions when asked to elaborate on points?), (b) selects valid information to document conclusions drawn from the above evaluation (e.g., relevant video passage(s) of attempts to use new strategy), and (c) goes through the routine steps of considering own actions, internal experiences, and dynamics of the interactions with the client, and then prepares a summary statement to take to the next supervision session.

During subsequent supervision session

The reflective supervisee takes responsibility for following up with her supervisor on any treatment decisions and plans suggested to her during the previous supervision session. She (a) updates her supervisor on outcomes of previously recommended changes to her in-session behaviour, (b) critically examines supervision data (e.g., pre-selected video clip of events that were targeted with newly adopted strategies), (c) considers the need for further refinement or alternative strategies, and (d) plans to consolidate new skills, transfer new skills to other situations, or test alternative ideas.

Setting an agenda

As we have highlighted in the first part of this chapter, a science-informed, competency-based approach to supervision requires that the supervisee is an active participant in supervision. There are a number of simple strategies that further assist supervisees in harnessing the anxiety they inevitably experience in their initial work with clients, so that they can make the most of the guidance provided by their supervisors. Evidence suggests that inexperienced supervisees benefit from directive and structured supervision methods (Spence et al., 2001). One such method is setting an agenda for the supervision sessions. Coming to supervision without a plan of what issues demand the most attention is the least productive way to utilize precious supervision time (Bernard & Goodyear, 2004). In contrast, developing a tentative agenda for their supervision sessions is empowering to supervisees (Pearson, 2004). At the beginning of each supervision session, supervisees should be prepared to do the following:

1. State what client contact has or has not occurred since last supervision.
2. Identify which issues with what clients need to be attended to.
3. Prioritize the importance of these issues. This includes estimating and requesting specific periods of time for each issue keeping in mind the total available time.
4. State how this time is best to be used (e.g., I like us to review and discuss about six minutes of videotape with Client A, and for Client B, I like to know whether I need to shift greater focus on the third goal of the treatment plan, and how I should go about doing that; this probably shouldn't take more than 10 minutes, since we already touched upon this last time).
5. Clearly identify your most immediate needs. As you set the tentative agenda, let your supervisor know what you definitely need to take away from this particular supervision session. One might call this stating your 'conditions of satisfaction'. That is, what is the absolute minimum you need to achieve during this supervision session, so that you can be satisfied that you have a plan and a reasonable degree of confidence for going into your next client sessions?
6. If supervision occurs in a group format, agenda setting may involve some negotiation and 'tradeoffs' between supervisees within and across supervision sessions in light of perceived urgency and complexity of all issues deserving attention.

Agenda setting and time management do not only enhance the effectiveness of supervision, but in this era of accountability in clinical service delivery, they are essential skills for optimizing quality of clinical services within the constraints of limited budgets and staff resources.

Learning from (audio-) video recordings
Video recordings are the technology of choice in supervision (Bernard & Goodyear, 2004), although audio recordings may serve as back-up. The capacity to directly examine what actually occurred during supervisee–client interactions provides an important tool by which quality assurance can be achieved. Supervisees can be coached and validated with respect to specific therapist behaviours in the context of specific situations, rather than receiving feedback that is only as good as the general 'picture' that is generated in the supervisor's mind through the lens of the supervisee's self-report. While the advantages for all stakeholders are obvious, supervisees tend to feel, at least initially, anxious and vulnerable when using video recordings, as 'there is no hiding from the stark reality of one's picture and voice being projected into the supervision room' (Bernard & Goodyear, 2004, p. 219). However, evidence suggests that after repeated exposure to being video recorded these initial aversive effects dissipate quickly (Ellis, Krengel, & Beck, 2002). There are three simple steps that supervisees can take to get the most out of using video recordings, while guarding against any inclination to engage in avoidance behaviours for the short-term gain of reducing their sense of vulnerability.

Selecting segments of tape
The first step involves the pre-selection of segments of tape that would be most productive to review. Although supervisors may at times review an entire tape prior to supervision,

Table 11.1 Impression management checklist

Impression management checklist:	Yes	No
1 Did I forget to bring my video recording to the supervision session?	☐	☐
2 Did I forget to press 'record' on the video equipment?	☐	☐
3 Did I forget to turn on the camera?	☐	☐
4 Did I record over the relevant session by mistake?	☐	☐
5 Was part of the session missing because of a technical glitch?	☐	☐
6 Did I bring the wrong recording with a different client's session?	☐	☐
7 Did I 'run out of time' before I got to show the tape?	☐	☐

supervisees are encouraged to become actively involved in this process from the outset (Bernard & Goodyear, 2004). In deciding which segment to select for supervision, the supervisee can consider the following questions:

1. What part of the session seemed to be particularly productive?
2. What happened when I attempted to direct the session towards a specific goal as planned in supervision?
3. What part was I particularly struggling with?
4. Was there a part that I was confused about?
5. Was there a part that raised a particularly important issue or recurrent theme?
6. Was there a part during which I felt a strong emotional reaction?
7. Was there a part during which my client expressed or showed signs of a significant emotional reaction?
8. Was there a part where something occurred that made me change my plans for the session?

Setting the stage

The second step involves succinctly introducing each video segment so that the supervisor is primed for what to expect and look for. Bernard and Goodyear (2004) recommend the following procedure for supervisees when presenting their pre-selected video segments:

1. State the reason why you want to discuss this particular segment in supervision
2. State briefly what transpired up to that point
3. Explain what you were trying to accomplish at that point in the session
4. Clearly state the specific help desired from your supervisor.

Guarding against impression management

The third step involves making a continuous commitment to contain counterproductive levels of evaluation anxiety. Consider the checklist in Table 11.1.

If you find yourself answering 'yes' to any of the listed items more than once over the course of two or more supervision sessions, there is a strong possibility that you are engaging in counterproductive avoidance behaviours designed to reduce your fear of being vulnerable. If so, it is important to address this issue with your supervisor. The benefits of learning from moment-to-moment analysis of video recorded client–supervisee interactions far outweigh the concerns.

Accounting for supervisory activities and outcomes

Standards of practice in most mental health disciplines stipulate that written records be kept of supervisory contracts and supervisee evaluations (Falvey & Cohen, 2003). In addition, there are at least four reasons why it is good practice to document activities and outcomes of supervision sessions. First, documentation of supervisory decision processes, recommendations, and outcomes affords some protection for supervisors who may be held liable for a supervisee's harmful actions. Second, it is a structural tool that brings into focus the deliberate nature of science-informed, reflective practice. Third, it provides the data for a proactive model of monitoring client progress, which can be used to modify treatment plans that appear to be ineffective (Lambert & Hawkins, 2001). Finally, the process of systematic and regular documentation reduces the risk that supervisees feel overwhelmed with the complexities of their cases, fail to implement key interventions in a timely manner, or overlook critical aspects of case management (Lambert & Hawkins, 2001).

Various templates have been developed for documenting supervision activities and outcomes (e.g., Bridge & Bascuc, 1990; Falvey & Cohen, 2003). An example of a Supervision Record Form is presented in Figure 11.3. The form begins with a section to record the supervisee name, client ID, date of supervision session, and information on frequency and type of client contact. The next few sections document the activities central to a goal-directed, reflectivity-enhancing, competency-based approach to supervision. First, the supervisee's specific agenda items are listed, along with previous session goals and progress on achieving them. The next item adds context (or the 'big picture') in terms of overall progress on the primary treatment goals. Then any relevant new issues that have arisen in the work with the client are recorded. This is followed by an explicit statement of what is planned for the next session. Finally, a separate section focuses attention on risk management issues and the steps taken to address them. Of course, risk assessment, crisis management, and safety planning decisions must be documented in greater detail than there is room for in this form (e.g., Rudd, Cukrowicz, & Bryan, 2008). Likewise, some of the other sections on goals, progress, and treatment planning would often require more details in the progress notes. The value of this succinct form is not in providing an exhaustive record, but in serving as a 'shorthand' tool to organize and focus the supervisee's thinking about the key aspects of the case at that point in time. This helps the supervisee to make the potentially complex and overwhelming task of preparing for and benefiting from supervision a more structured and manageable process.

Group supervision

The proactive, structured, and goal-oriented activities associated with agenda setting, purposeful examination of supervision data, and documentation of supervision interventions and outcomes are equally applicable whether supervision is delivered in an individual or group format. One often cited potential limitation of group supervision (Bernard & Goodyear, 2004), that individuals may not receive sufficient time to address all their individual concerns, is a case in point. There is little risk that supervisees who turn up to

SUPERVISION RECORD FORM

Supervisee: _____ Client ID: _____ Date: _____

Client Contact: ☐ Yes ☐ No   If YES, indicate:
   ☐ Face-to-Face   ☐ Phone   ☐ Correspondence ☐ Other
   Date(s): _____ Date(s): _____ Date(s): _____ Date(s): _____
   Duration: _____ Duration: _____

Agenda/ issues/ request(s) for feedback: _____
_____
_____

Previous session goal(s): _____
_____
_____

Progress on previous session goal(s): _____
_____
_____

Progress on main treatment goal(s): _____
_____
_____
_____

New issues: _____
_____
_____

Plan for next session: _____
_____
_____
_____

Supervisory activities: _____
_____
_____

Risk Management
   (a) Issues: _____
_____
   (b) Action(s) taken: _____

Figure 11.3 Supervision record form.

group supervision prepared, who have prioritized the issues that must be attended to before supervision ends, and who routinely document feedback and recommendations for these issues, will get less of what they need during group supervision than during individual supervision. Likewise, although there may be more opportunities for confidentiality concerns and unhelpful personal interactions to emerge when several individuals are involved rather than just two (Bernard & Goodyear, 2004), these problems can arise and require resolution in both formats. Moreover, when a supervisee experiences discomfort in a particular interaction with a supervisor, the presence of peers in the same room can be comforting and reduce supervisee dependence on the supervisor, and peers can be helpful in validating the supervisee's perspective during or after the event. In addition, there are a number of other advantages of the group format, including opportunities for vicarious learning, exposure to a broader range of clients, increased diversity of feedback, and greater resources to use action techniques. The modelling literature emphasizes that models of coping are better than models of mastery, and therefore, watching one's peers and senior students can be beneficial. Therefore, the assumption that individual supervision is inherently superior is not only a myth (Bernard & Goodyear, 2004), but the efficiency and advantages of group supervision may soon make it the format of choice as demands for enhanced efficiency and flexible formats in a competitive health care market increase (Milne & Oliver, 2000).

The challenge to advance beyond the familiar

The ultimate goal of supervised practice is for the supervisee to achieve competency as a clinician and readiness to assume the role of a colleague who independently contributes to the community and the discipline (Falender & Shafranske, 2004). The rate at which beginning supervisees increase the proficiency with which they apply complex therapy procedures and facilitate internal therapeutic processes varies considerably across individuals. The novice typically experiences high anxiety, is self-focused, is preoccupied with performance of techniques and following guidelines, and worries about evaluation (Stoltenberg & McNeill, 1997). Supervisory guidance during this period is therefore highly supportive, structured, and prescriptive. It focuses on consolidating basic strategies rather than challenging supervisees to quickly expand their repertoire of techniques beyond the trusted and familiar. As client contact increases and supervisees experience some successes in implementing planned interventions, their initial sense of incompetence gives way to a sense of accomplishment and even pride. At that point, supervisees must guard against getting stuck in this comfort zone, where a set of rudimentary skills may help a client or two and stave off disaster, but is inadequate for functioning within the full scope and demands of independent clinical practice. Indeed, early adoption of only one particular therapeutic approach or a rigid set of skills can lead to frustration with situations not fitting that narrow range of skills, and ultimately to professional stagnation or failure (Neufeldt, 2003). The challenge for supervisees is to remain flexible and open when prompted by their supervisors to use each increase in their competence as a platform for pushing off towards the next level of professional development. Venturing into unfamiliar territory will temporarily revive feelings of insecurity, but this is a small price to pay for the rewards associated with gaining mastery over an advanced repertoire of complex skills.

Formative and summative evaluation

Bernard and Goodyear (2004) described evaluation as the 'nucleus' of clinical supervision, because it simultaneously supports the learning process, case management, and quality client care. *Formative* evaluation is ongoing and involves direct feedback on the supervisee's professional growth and effectiveness in performing clinical services. This may take the form of formal reports at certain intervals (e.g., at the end of each rotation or period of working with a given supervisor), or informal, frequent feedback during each supervision session. In contrast, *summative* evaluation refers to 'the moment of truth when the supervisor steps back, takes stock, and decides how the trainee measures up' (Bernard & Goodyear, 2004, p. 20). Anticipatory anxiety about receiving summative evaluations can be quite distressing to supervisees. However, supervisees should bear in mind that the criteria used during summative evaluation are the same as those that were introduced at the outset of supervision as learning objectives, and that were used to provide intermittent formative feedback throughout their supervision. That is, if there was no clear indication during formative evaluation that a supervisee's performance was consistently below standard, then the supervisee should rest assured that summative evaluation will not be suddenly negative. Supervisors have an ethical obligation to apply due process procedures before a supervisee is given a negative final evaluation (Bernard & Goodyear, 2004). This involves providing the supervisee with sufficient prior warning, specific remedial advice, and a reasonable period of time to improve.

The more supervisees get actively involved in the formative evaluation process, the less daunting summative evaluation becomes. For the reflective supervisee who established a habit of self-scrutiny and responsibly documenting their supervision activities and outcomes, it is only a small step to also self-evaluate their own work using the same criteria as the supervisor. Not only will that prepare the supervisee for the summative evaluation process, but the skill of accurately assessing one's own strengths and weaknesses is critical for ongoing professional development and could be regarded as a prerequisite for anyone engaging in the supervision and evaluation of others.

Learning supervisory skills

Novice therapists are likely to give little thought as to what skills are needed to shift from the role of direct service provider to the role of supervising someone else to become the best service provider they can be. Yet, their experiences as 'consumers' of supervision combined with the modelling by different supervisors function as tacit training in the practice of supervision itself (Falender & Shafrankse, 2004). Until recently, such implicit models of 'training' supervisors were the norm, with a substantial proportion of supervisors having received no formal education and training in supervision (Johnson & Stewart, 2000; Spence et al., 2001; Townend et al., 2002). It is now increasingly recognized that training programmes should include and enhance formal training in supervisory skills (Gonsalvez & Milne, 2010; Hadjistavropoulos, Kehler, & Hadjistavropoulos, 2010). Novice therapists, of course, are not expected to already undertake hands-on supervisor training while their energies are still directed towards making their own fledgling steps as therapists. However, some basic supervisory skills are already relevant even to novice supervisees (for example, if they are involved in group supervision), and certainly to more advanced trainees who are involved in peer- or co-supervision under the guidance of an experienced supervisor.

When thinking about what it takes to become a supervisor, it is helpful to start by clarifying what a supervisor is not. First, the supervisor is not the therapist of the client. That is, the supervisee is not a surrogate for the supervisor as clinician. Second, the supervisor is not the therapist for the supervisee. The supervisee's personal issues are only addressed to the extent that they bear directly on client–therapist or therapist–supervisor interactions. Consider a trainee who is getting very emotional during a session with a client who relates feelings of guilt and distress regarding her indecision to abort her unborn child or to keep it. If reflective enquiry reveals that the supervisee's strong discomfort was related to her own past experience of an unplanned pregnancy, then the supervisor would focus on helping the supervisee figure out how she can be helpful to her client (from her client's perspective!) without letting her own emotional reactions get in the way of that task. In contrast, if it becomes apparent that the supervisee struggles to separate her own distress and needs from those of the client, and that she might benefit from personal therapy to better cope with the personal issues raised by this event, then it would be unethical for the supervisor to act as her therapist. Thus, when making the transition from clinician to supervisor, the focus shifts from exploring the meaning of an event to the way in which this event might affect the supervisee's work with the client (Neufeldt, 2003). In sum, the acquisition of beginning supervisory skills involves getting past being a clinician and attending to (a) the supervisee's learning, (b) one's own managerial competence to facilitate (a), and (c) the ethical obligations that arise when advanced trainees contribute to the supervision of more junior peers.

Advanced trainees can facilitate the learning of more junior supervisees by applying supportive, reflective, and prescriptive strategies:

Supportive strategies
- Provide praise and encouragement. Highlight any aspects that the trainee did well. Acknowledge that doing things for the first time is difficult. Help shift the focus from what went wrong to how to do better the next time.
- Be respectful and tactful when commenting on things that did not go well.

Reflective strategies
- Examine the trainee's behaviour. Ask the trainee to explain how a given behaviour does or does not serve the intention of the trainee at the time, the goals for this particular session, and the overall treatment goals.
- Ask the trainee to generate hypotheses about the client's behaviour, thoughts, or feelings. Consider a client who informs the therapist that her 16-year-old son is going to leave her in the near future to live with his father in another state, and then remarks quickly that she is 'OK with this'. Encourage the trainee to suggest several options as to what the client might be feeling about the upcoming event (e.g., does 'it is OK' mean 'it is not very painful' for the client, or does it mean it is very painful, but 'I will manage', or does it mean 'I am *not* OK', 'I will be lonely', 'I am afraid, my son won't talk to me anymore'?)
- Explore the trainee's feelings during client and supervision sessions. Ask in what ways these feelings can hinder or help working with the client.
- Help the trainee to plan ahead. Encourage the trainee to make predictions about which hypotheses about the client are most likely given what the trainee already knows about the client's circumstances and history. Then suggest testing that prediction in the next session.

Prescriptive strategies
- Offer alternative interventions or conceptualizations for the trainee to use.
- Explain and/or demonstrate how to use intervention techniques.

Bernard and Goodyear (2004) noted that one particular benefit of receiving feedback from fellow advanced trainees is that they are closer to their own recent experiences as novices than the senior supervisor is. Therefore, their explanations may at times be easier to follow than those of the expert.

In addition to facilitating novice supervisees' learning, advanced trainees can increase their managerial competence by taking an active role in structuring the supervision session, facilitating good time management, and keeping records of their supervisory activities.

Finally, advanced trainees must be aware of their ethical obligations when they participate in the supervision of more junior peers. This includes maintaining a professional distance from the junior colleagues they are supervising, which can pose a challenge within the small community of a training programme where students interact in classes, research teams, and social activities. However, dual relationship problems can be avoided by observing a few simple guidelines. Neufeldt (2003) recommends that (a) role obligations are clarified from the outset, (b) supervisory activities remain confidential and there should be no 'gossip' about supervisors or supervisees, and (c) advanced trainees should not supervise a peer who is a roommate, close friend, or romantic partner. In general, when considering dual relationships between a supervisor and trainee, the supervisor's needs are subordinate to the needs of the supervisee and the needs of the supervisee's clients (Falender & Shafranske, 2004). Any benefits derived from such relationships must be weighed against the imperative to minimize the potential for harm. A useful decision-making model by Burian and Slimp (2000) raises awareness of the issues and circumstances to be considered when contemplating the merits and risks of engaging in social dual-role relationships between supervisors and trainees. The first question to consider is the reasons for engaging in the relationship. A dual relationship may have merit if there are *professional benefits* to the trainee or supervisor. For example, conducting workshops together may involve planning meetings, lunches, or a social gathering with workshop attendees for a drink at the end of the day. As long as the purpose of the social activities remains focused on workshop-related activities and associated professional benefits for both persons involved, the risk of harm is minimized. In contrast, a social relationship should not proceed if it only has *personal benefits* to the supervisor, and should only proceed with caution and after careful consultation if it is primarily of personal benefit to the trainee. The second question to consider is the degree of power the supervisor has over the trainee. A possible social relationship is best postponed until a time when the supervisor has no evaluative role, either directly or indirectly, with respect to the trainee. The third question to consider is where this social relationship takes place. If the social contacts are in the context of the work site and are not exclusive of others who may wish to join the social interaction, the potential for harm, such as the perception of favouritism, is reduced. In addition to considering these three basic questions, before deciding to pursue a social dual-role relationship, it needs to be established that the trainee has the ability to leave the social relationship or activity without repercussions, and there is no negative impact on uninvolved trainees or staff members.

However, supervision is not the only context where difficult situations arise. More often than not, tricky situations arise within the course of consulting with a client. Supervision is a key component in responding effectively to problems during therapy. One such common problem is treatment non-compliance or therapeutic resistance, and it is to this topic that we now turn.

Chapter 12

Managing ruptures in the therapeutic alliance

Consider a client with depression who has intense fears of abandonment. After a period of therapy the symptoms of depression have begun to decline and she comments:

CLIENT: Do you think I am depressed?

PSYCHOLOGIST: I am not sure it is helpful for us to get tied up in labels. What is important is that when you began therapy you were very distressed, but now you have got to a point where you have a greater understanding of the issues in your life. Have you noticed a change in how you can manage these issues?

C: If it hadn't been for you I don't know how I would have coped. You have been a life-saver and I mean that literally. I might have killed myself if it hadn't been for our therapy.

One possible explanation for the client's responses is that they are worrying about the possible termination of therapy and beginning to test the psychologist. The tests involve seeking reassurance that the psychologist still sees the client as having a problem that deserves treatment and highlighting the potential risks of discontinuation. For a client who fears abandonment, the prospect of the termination of therapy will be scary. How would you manage the potential rupture to the therapeutic alliance now that symptom improvement has been achieved?

Now consider beginning a treatment session with an anxious client, who you had given the task of completing a diary with a 'fear thermometer' (i.e., rating anxiety on a 0–100 scale) along with a record of any anxiety-provoking situation, any unhelpful thoughts, and subsequent feelings. The session opens like this:

PSYCHOLOGIST: How have things been going this past week?

CLIENT: Pretty good. I've been doing what you asked me and I've noticed that the anxiety is a lot less than it was.

P: In terms of the 'fear thermometer' that you were using each day to rate your anxiety as homework, what sort of ratings did you get?

C: Well I didn't put them in my diary, but I thought about it each day and I've remembered my ratings.

P: That's OK. But it would be really good if you did it next week instead because it might show something useful.

C: Yeah, no problem at all.

In subsequent sessions, if this pattern continues, it will become entrenched with the client not ever bringing any homework to the sessions. Ultimately, the client may terminate therapy leaving you to lament that if the client had been more motivated, treatment would have had a more positive outcome. Could anything have been done differently to increase compliance with treatment?

While it perhaps seems self-evident that repairing alliance ruptures is necessary for the successful conduct of therapy, it is useful to note that there is a sound evidence base

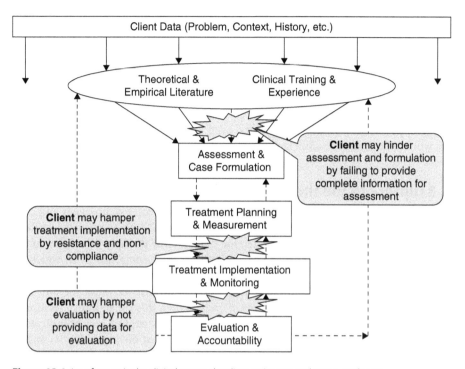

Figure 12.1 Interference in the clinical process by client resistance and non-compliance.

for the practice (e.g., Strauss et al., 2006). In a meta-analytic review Safran, Muran, and Eubanks-Carter (2011b) found that there was a moderate (r = 0.24), but significant, correlation between the repair of alliance ruptures and overall outcome. Furthermore, they showed strong correlations between the provision of training and supervision in rupture-repair and therapy outcomes, supporting the idea that the ability to repair ruptures is an important therapy skill, which can be learned and refined (see also Safran et al., 2014).

A model of ruptures to the therapeutic alliance

Reviewing our model of clinical practice (see Figure 12.1), it is apparent that in normal circumstances there is a flow of information from one element within the model to others. However, when these links are broken, clinical practice has the potential to break down. Some of these links can be affected by actions that are more under the control of the psychologist than the client and many of these have been considered in previous chapters. For instance, failing to conduct an adequate assessment or case formulation can undermine effective treatment planning. Poor treatment planning can in turn result in the implementation of potentially inappropriate, ineffective, or inefficient therapies. Likewise, failing to monitor progress towards treatment goals or to measure outcomes can lead to unnecessarily long persistence with an ineffective or counterproductive therapy. However, there are other points at which psychological practice can be disrupted by activities that appear, at first glance, under more control of the client than the psychologist. The client may fail to disclose all the relevant information, thereby hindering case formulation and weakening the value of pre-treatment assessments. A client may also be non-compliant with therapeutic suggestions and exhibit resistance within psychotherapy. Such non-compliance with the treatment strategies will hinder implementation and reduce the ultimate success of any intervention. The therapeutic alliance can be ruptured during treatment and the psychologist will need to work to restore the relationship.

The focus of the present chapter will be twofold. We will discuss client behaviours that can have a negative effect of treatment outcomes, and we will review strategies as to how the psychologist can deliberately exert influence over the therapeutic relationship to minimize the hindering impact of these client behaviours, even though many of the relevant client behaviours will not be under the clinician's direct control.

What is a rupture to the therapeutic alliance?

The therapeutic alliance describes the working relationship between psychologists and clients (Barber, Muran, McCarthy, & Keefe, 2013; Horvath & Bedi, 2002). As reviewed earlier, the stronger the therapeutic alliance, the better the outcomes of therapy. When the quality of the alliance is strong, psychologists foster a safe, trusting environment in which a shared purpose forms a means to working towards common goals. Therapist empathy and collaboration, as well as the use of progress monitoring and feedback build the alliance (Norcross & Wampold, 2011). An alliance rupture occurs when this collaborative relationship breaks down or becomes strained (Safran & Muran, 2006). The rupture may be indicated by confrontation (where the client exhibits hostility or criticism of the psychologist) or by withdrawal (when the client disengages from the therapeutic process or begins to express negative feelings and attitudes about the therapy or therapist in an indirect manner).

Broadly speaking, alliance ruptures can be addressed in a sequential process (Safran, Eubanks-Carter, & Muran, 2010). First, the psychologist identifies the marker of the rupture (e.g., refusal to complete homework). This marker is then disembedded from the psychotherapy process and explicitly attended to by the psychologist. This provides the foundation for the third step, in which the psychologist explores the experience of the rupture with the client. Finally, the psychologist explores any avoidant behaviours and any reasons for the behaviours that the psychologist has observed. As you work through the remainder of the chapter, you will see how these steps can be addressed for different instances of alliance ruptures.

One example of an alliance rupture involves therapeutic resistance. Resistance is defined differently depending on whether the source of the client's resistance is construed as residing within the client or as being triggered by something the therapist does or fails to do. Lazarus and Fay (1982) suggested that the notion of client 'resistance' is 'the most elaborate rationalization that therapists employ to explain their treatment failures' (p. 115). These writers place the responsibility for the non-compliance in the lap of the psychologist. Accordingly, the non-compliance may be illusory and an interpretation by the psychologist to rationalize therapeutic failures, or it may reflect the fact that client and psychologist have disagreed about the outcomes. In contrast, other writers place the responsibility with the client. For instance, Wachtel (1982) defines resistance as occurring when 'the sincere desire to change confronts the fears, misconceptions, and prior adaptive strategies that make change difficult' (p. xix). Implicit in this latter definition is the notion that 'ambivalence' towards treatment lay at the heart of client behaviours that manifested as resistance and non-compliance. Later in this chapter, we will review strategies that help clients shift from being stuck in a state of ambivalence by enhancing the value of changing relative to the benefits of not changing.

Reflecting upon these different approaches to defining resistance in therapy, it is evident that they are not mutually exclusive. It is conceivable that a therapist may rationalize a failure or unintentionally act in ways that impede therapeutic progress. It is also plausible that a client may fail to engage in the activities designed to bring about therapeutic change. Thus, it is not very helpful to debate in the abstract who is to 'blame'. It is more fruitful to consider how to manage resistance and non-compliance when it becomes a hindrance to achieving positive treatment outcomes.

We suggest that the clinical psychologist should take responsibility for dealing with resistance (without necessarily taking the blame for poor therapeutic outcomes). That is, the psychologist is a professional who is providing an expert service and part of that service is being able to deal with hindrances to a positive outcome. By way of analogy, consider a school teacher trying to teach an uncooperative 14-year-old. Good teachers will not blame the child, but see the situation as a problem to be solved and they will accept responsibility for attempting to find a solution. It will not help the student to blame him for not learning, or just to give up and accuse him of being uncooperative (even if this is true). Good teachers will look for ways to help the child to learn by overcoming the resistance rather than using resistance as a reason or an explanation for a failure to learn. Thus, we view therapeutic resistance as an issue to be addressed in the overall treatment plan, not as an explanation for therapeutic failure. In taking a problem-focused approach to resistance, we are also adopting a transtheoretical approach to resistance and non-compliance. The transtheoretical perspective is important because psychodynamic and family therapists may view the exploration of resistance as a critical ingredient for intervention, whereas cognitive and behavioural therapists tend to view resistance as a problem that must be dealt with so that therapy can return to its primary objectives. Our approach is a pragmatic one; the goal is the amelioration of the client's problems, and the clinician's job is to help the client achieve this goal. To the extent that alliance ruptures interfere with this goal, they need to be addressed during treatment.

Managing alliance ruptures during different phases of the therapeutic process

During the assessment phase

During the initial assessment there are a variety of ways that a psychologist can reduce the probability of therapy-interfering behaviours arising. First, contacting the client before the first session will increase the probability that the client will attend for the initial contact. Second, it is important to establish your credibility as a competent professional who can create the context for change. At first glance this presents a dilemma to the novice psychologist who will dread the question from their initial clients, 'How many people have you treated with problems just like mine?' How do you establish credibility in the absence of years of experience? One way to enhance credibility is by preparing thoroughly and drawing on the collective expertise of the setting within which you are working (e.g., you might respond, 'I have not treated anyone with this problem before, but we have been using these treatments with success in this clinic for many years'). Your credibility will also be conveyed in the professional manner in which you interact with your client, such as dealing with the referral promptly and efficiently, having relevant materials to hand, and so on. In maintaining a credible demeanour, it is important to remember that although you may feel inexperienced, you have had many years of training in psychology and your knowledge base of normal and abnormal behavioural patterns will be substantial. Therefore, try to focus on what you do know, rather than worrying about the things that you might not yet know. Finally, credibility is enhanced most by honesty and integrity in communication. Communicating accurately your expertise and experience in response to an enquiry will facilitate the therapeutic relationship more than trying to bluff your way through.

A third way to reduce the probability of therapy-interfering behaviours is to begin treatment by rapidly establishing good rapport with clients using the techniques outlined in Chapter 2. Fourth, alliance ruptures can be reduced by modelling good listening behaviours. Allow your client to finish each statement and reflect back both the informational and the emotional content. In so doing, ensure that you permit your client to express emotions fully. Fifth, when you are ready to use assessment procedures, take time to provide a clear rationale for the tests and give strong encouragement about completing the procedures. When the assessment process is finished, reward the clients for their efforts put into completing the assessments by providing them with clear and informative feedback. Sixth, employ strategies that increase the engagement of the client in therapy. It is possible to increase the engagement by gaining an explicit commitment to complete assessment, then treatment, and finally follow-up. These commitments or contracts are obtained in a sequential manner, so that you are just asking the client to commit to the next phase in the process of therapy. Seventh, if appropriate, engagement can also be enhanced by maintaining contact with the client between sessions with the aim of asking how things are going, checking that there have not been any difficulties with the homework assignments, and gaining a commitment to attend the next session. Finally, given the important role of homework compliance (Kazantzis, Deane, & Ronan, 2000; Kazantzis, Deane, Ronan, & L'Abate, 2005; Kazantzis & L'Abate, 2007), it is necessary to reinforce the completion of any assignments, a point that will be discussed in greater detail below.

During the implementation phase

Once treatment has begun, the psychologist can continue with many of the strategies described above and some other strategies can be added. First, articulating a clear, shared formulation of the problem and an explicit rationale for treatment is likely to increase the engagement of a client (but cf. Chadwick, Williams, & Mackenzie, 2003). This rationale may need to be repeated to repair a rupture, so do not think that, just because it has been articulated once, the client will continue to remember, agree with, or continue to find relevant the initial rationale (Safran et al., 2011b). Sometimes, the issue can be a simple misunderstanding that, once cleared up, allows therapy to proceed more smoothly. Second, client engagement can be fostered by conveying optimism about change, which can be achieved by citing data on the probability of success and by identifying the factors that predict improvement. For instance, you might comment, 'We know that two thirds of clients are improved to the point that they no longer meet diagnostic criteria for the problem that they sought help for. However, you might be thinking to yourself, "I bet I'm in the one third of therapy failures." But we know from research the reasons why people find themselves in the one third of people who don't succeed so well. One of the main factors is not complying with the treatment. Thus, the good news is, the harder you work in the programme, the more likely it will be that you will be one of the two thirds who succeed.' In addition to citing research evidence, optimism about change can also be enhanced by establishing a collaborative set. For instance, you might add: 'Also, I don't see therapy as a process where I sit on the sidelines watching you succeed or fail. I see my role as working with you all the way, overcoming obstacles, and doing everything I can to ensure that together as a team, we can collaborate to help you overcome this problem.' Third, client engagement can be enhanced by anticipating possible obstacles to treatment. The process of case formulation described in Chapter 5 provides a mechanism for identifying a client's weaknesses that may adversely impact on outcomes, as well as the client's strengths and resources that may be drawn upon to attenuate any adverse effects. Fourth, when resistance or non-compliance is blocking the process of treatment you may decide to raise the issue with the client explicitly (perhaps preferring to use less judgemental descriptions, such as 'something appears to be blocking our progress' or 'we seem to be encountering some difficulties in taking the steps we agreed would be helpful at this stage'). Work with the client to identify the meaning and function of the resistance, and then respond accordingly. Some examples of resistance are outlined below:

- The psychologist might describe a therapeutic technique and the client refuses to comply, claiming that she does not understand what to do. This problem may have arisen because the therapist has miscommunicated or the client has difficulty comprehending. The response would be that the psychologist would represent the technique, using different words than before, drawing upon examples and metaphors to assist comprehension.
- The client might appear unmotivated due to a lack of expectation of success. The psychologist could identify the reasons why the client has formed this view, clarify any misconceptions or unrealistic expectations, and then identify the probability of success and demonstrate which of the predictors of a favourable outcome the client possesses or are present in the environment.
- The client might be making unusually slow or erratic therapeutic progress. This could arise from any number of causes and so the psychologist should review the case to ensure that all the problems have been identified, and that the treatment is appropriate for the problem and the particular type of client. If these possible causes are not reasonable explanations, then the psychologist could consider other explanations, such as that the client's problem serves a function or meets a need that would remain unmet if the problem was ameliorated. For instance, the client's familiar problem may maintain an uneasy but reassuring balance within a family structure, whereas change in the client would disrupt this balance, and the need to adapt to this unfamiliar situation may be perceived as 'too hard' or distressing. Consider a client who after making successful progress in overcoming her agoraphobic avoidances reported that her partner was complaining that he did not like her new-found freedom. He was no longer sure that she was at home and hence worried that she might be forming relationships with other men. He did not like the fact that his dinner was no longer on the table when he walked through the door because his partner had been busy with other activities during the day. In this case, these issues did not necessarily cause the problem in the first instance, but interfered with progress by weakening the client's resolve (albeit temporarily) to overcome the agoraphobic avoidances. It is also possible that a client is slowing down progress deliberately to test the psychologist. For example, a client with a fear of abandonment may observe the psychologist's reaction to his failure to progress, waiting to see if the psychologist will 'dump him, just like all the other shrinks'. In

these cases, the reasons for non-compliance need to be explored as possible causes or maintaining factors in the problem and dealt with accordingly.

- Another scenario is when the client presents with a meaningful behavioural pattern or sequence that is a manifestation of avoidance behaviour. A client may behave in their relationship with the psychologist in a manner that 'acts out' some aspect of their presenting problem. For instance, a client who fears negative evaluation in performance settings could well view therapy as a social performance within which he is required to behave in a certain way, and if he fails to do so, then the psychologist will judge him negatively as a 'bad patient'. In this case, the psychologist would address the client's fear of negative evaluation and could use the manifestation as an opportunity to bring the problem into the therapy room and deal with it as the behaviour unfolds.

It is also important to consider that there may be a need to change or to renegotiate the clinical tasks or goals (Safran et al., 2011b). For instance, while CBT encourages the psychologist to challenge thoughts and beliefs, within DBT a psychologist may focus more on validating a client's experience. Hence, shifting strategy when challenging thoughts is not working may prove beneficial. It may also be that it is helpful to shift from a problem focus, to explore the relational themes associated with the rupture. As in the earlier example about the client with abandonment issues, Safran and colleagues (2011b) note that it is sometimes necessary to clarify the relational factors leading to an alliance rupture. They cite the example of a client who may not do homework assignments because the client feels to do so would be submitting to a dominant or controlling person. Evaluating the reasons behind the client's characterization of the relationship in terms of a power differential may be helpful. Sometimes these relational patterns can be new and at other times, they may reflect the emergence in the therapeutic relationship of patterns that are common to the client's life. In the latter case, the psychologist can investigate the situations in the client's life that have triggered similar responses to those observed in therapy and try to understand the triggers and the meaning the client attributes to the triggers.

Finally, confrontational ruptures to the alliance can occur when a client deliberately challenges the therapist. When this occurs, it is wise not to be defensive, but to make the concern explicit, and to deal with the challenge by addressing it. Sometimes the situation can be defused through humour (although this has the potential to backfire if the client interprets a humorous retort as belittling them or their concern). At other times the concern can be dealt with by matter-of-factly citing appropriate data. If a client's challenging style continues to a degree that a cooperative working relationship cannot be maintained, it might be appropriate to refer the client to another therapist.

During the termination phase

Considering termination there are a number of ways to increase alliance ruptures with the preparatory steps to facilitate an end to formal therapeutic contact. Addressing termination in an explicit manner is important. This allows the client to plan for termination, to deal with any grief and loss which may be experienced, and to raise any further matters which should be dealt with before termination is complete. Phasing the last treatment sessions so that they are spaced at greater intervals can be beneficial, as can scheduling a formal follow-up session (so that the client does not feel abandoned at the end of treatment). It is also useful during the latter phases of treatment to reinforce independence and discuss relapse prevention strategies. This will help to develop the client's self-efficacy that they are now able to continue to implement and apply the lessons and skills learned in therapy even after therapeutic contact has ceased. Clients who are confident that they will be all right after completion of therapy are not prone to show non-compliant stalling behaviours as the end of therapy approaches.

Sometimes the client's confidence can be undermined by unhelpful cognitions they hold. Cognitive behaviour therapists have suggested that the clinician can engage in a 'search & destroy' (Jacobson, 1984) approach. During the 'search' phase, the psychologist tries to identify cognitions that may be impeding termination planning. Once possible cognitions are identified, the clinician proceeds to construct behavioural experiments to test the validity of these cognitions, with the ultimate goal of disputing them. For example, one of us saw a client who became distressed at the prospect of termination, despite having made substantial progress. Careful interviewing revealed that the client was concerned that if he lapsed back into problem drinking, then there would be no way to access therapeutic assistance. Therapy then shifted to address these beliefs; examining the nature and consequences of termination, reviewing the skills attained, practising relapse prevention strategies, and clarifying ways to access future therapy if required.

For the beginning psychologist it may be a daunting prospect to think about identifying and managing alliance ruptures. Fortunately, there are some good psychometric instruments that may assist therapists in describing and characterizing problems with the therapeutic relationship (e.g., California Psychotherapy Alliance Scale; Marmar, Weiss, & Gaston, 1989). One such measure is the Working Alliance Inventory (WAI; Horvath & Greenberg, 1989); of which a shorter version is now available (i.e., the Working Alliance Inventory-Short Revised; Munder, Wilmers, Leonhart, Linster, & Barth, 2010). The WAI examines the tripartite components of alliance, namely bonds, goals, and tasks. Since the scale is completed by the client, it provides the psychologist with a formal way to characterize the client's perception of the alliance and can help guide a consideration of issues in therapy.

Managing withdrawal alliance ruptures by enhancing motivation

The therapeutic alliance may be ruptured as the client withdraws or disengages. Often it is useful to not label the withdrawal as 'resistance' and identify it as a problem as such, but instead to reframe resistance and withdrawal as understandable processes common in many people seeking treatment. The psychologist could identify benign explanations for 'resistance' and seek to sidestep a direct confrontation. For instance, instead of treating ambivalence about continuing in treatment as an absence of motivation, the psychologist could discuss how ambivalence is a natural response to the simultaneous presence of approach and avoidance motivations. When either approach or avoidant motivations dominate, then the behavioural outcomes will be clear, but when approach and avoidance motivations are similarly strong, ambivalence will occur. This can be reframed as a 'good state to be in', because it is evidence that the client still sees enough value in treatment to not have simply dropped out. The focus of therapy can then shift towards an evaluation of the twin motivations and seek to 'tip the balance' in favour of continuing to engage in treatment (cf. Breiner, Stritzke, & Lang, 1999).

Arguably the most helpful and readable book on this topic is Miller and Rollnick's *Motivational Interviewing* (2012; see also Arkowitz, Westra, Miller, & Rollnick, 2007). One of the important contributions that this book makes in the present context is the

acknowledgement that motivation is not an issue that is constrained to the initial assessment, at which time the psychologist judges to what degree motivation for change is present
or absent. Instead, motivation is to be recruited at all points throughout therapy to get and to
keep the client engaged with treatment. In particular, motivational interviewing is especially
relevant to clients who are ambivalent about treatment. Clients with substance use problems
typically fall into this category, but many other clients are ambivalent too. For example,
anxiety-disordered clients often begin treatment highly motivated, but once the prospect of
confronting feared situations emerges, the client can become scared and ambivalent. In addition, clients may have participated in failed treatment attempts and hence are ambivalent
about the value of the present intervention, especially if it is similar to one that has already
been tried. Clients may also be ambivalent about treatment if their relationships are threatened by the prospect of successful treatment or if undesirable consequences follow amelioration of the problem. For instance, clients may derive social support and reassurance as a
consequence of having problems and recovery may put an end to such secondary 'benefits'
of the status quo.

To counter the negative impact of these hindrances on treatment compliance, the task
of the clinician is to ensure that the person's motivation for treatment is maximized and
remains sufficient to propel the individual to a successful completion of the treatment
programme. To this end Miller and Rollnick (2012) identified five general principles of
motivational interviewing which can be applied fruitfully to a broad range of presenting problems, not just addictive behaviours. The five principles are expressing empathy,
developing discrepancy, avoiding argumentation, rolling with resistance, and supporting
self-efficacy.

Expressing empathy

People who suffer with psychological problems frequently complain of being misunder-
stood. For instance, a person suffering from Obsessive-Compulsive Disorder may finally
bring themselves to describe their uniquely terrifying experiences to another, only to be
frustrated with the responses. Trite advice may be forthcoming (e.g., 'You must be uptight,
why don't you just relax?'), or even worse, sympathy is offered (e.g., 'I check too. When I
leave my car I check I haven't locked my keys in. I really understand how you must feel').
Therefore, it is imperative that the individual feels from the psychologist's first utterance that
their complaint has been heard.

An empathic response responds to the meaning and emotion expressed in a communication, all the time accepting the validity of the person's experience. For instance, a person
describing the experience of a panic attack is usually trying to communicate an occurrence
of fear which is perceived to be qualitatively different from any anxiety, worry, tension, or
fear which they have experienced before. In addition, they often conclude on the basis of this
experience that the event must be unique and an indication of a serious physical or mental
problem. By extension, the person is communicating that, although they have previously
been able to manage anxiety in all its forms using various coping strategies, this is different; these attacks of panic are uncontrollable. An accurately empathic response accepts the
validity of the person's experience, leaving the person with the perception that the listener
has heard what has been said. These principles which underlie empathic communication are
illustrated by contrasting two client–therapist interactions, where one does not include an
empathic response (Psychologist 1) and the other does (Psychologist 2).

CLIENT: Panics are the most terrifying experience I have ever had. Have you ever had a panic attack?

PSYCHOLOGIST 1: Yes, I think I have. It was during the war when we were under enemy fire …

PSYCHOLOGIST 2: I've been anxious before, but it sounds as if you have found panic attacks to be quite different from the anxiety that you used to feel.

The first response is less helpful because the therapist fails to identify with the client's experience. The client is testing to see if the therapist understands the uniqueness of their experience of panic, but the therapist does not respond to this theme. Instead, the psychologist moves to relating personal experiences that may or may not be relevant, thereby shifting the focus from the client to the therapist. The second psychologist draws attention to the qualitative difference sufferers perceive between anxiety and panic. Such a response is preferable because it draws attention to the uniqueness of the experience and returns the interview to the client's concerns.

CLIENT: When I'm having a panic all my rational thoughts go out the window and I think I AM going to die of a heart attack.

PSYCHOLOGIST 1: But you have had many clean ECGs, your cholesterol is low, and you are young. Everything points against you actually dying of a heart attack.

PSYCHOLOGIST 2: It makes it difficult to stop the panic when the worry about dying becomes so overpowering.

The first psychologist jumps in to offer premature reassurance. But the client is not saying that she really believes that she is dying, only that the panic appears to rob her of her rational powers. The second psychologist responds to this comment by reflecting the meaning conveyed. It is the second response which will lead to the client continuing the interaction with the accurate perception that the psychologist has heard the communication.

CLIENT: I've had this problem for ten years, I've been to so many different psychologists it is not funny, and I haven't got better so far.

PSYCHOLOGIST 1: Well, we use a cognitive behavioural programme which is very successful and I'm very experienced in delivering the technique. You should improve quickly.

PSYCHOLOGIST 2: Having failed before, it must have been hard to bring yourself along to the clinic. What made you decide to try again?

The first psychologist responds to the client's implied doubt about whether psychological treatment works for her by presenting therapeutic credentials. In contrast, the second psychologist perceives the deeper issue and draws the person's attention to the motivation which was recruited in order to re-engage in treatment. Having done so, the psychologist will be in a position to build upon the person's existing motivation to engage in treatment. Importantly, the second psychologist implicitly acknowledges that ambivalence about treatment is normal and models that building on existing motivations is a useful therapeutic strategy.

In summary, expressing empathy involves accurately responding to the meaning and emotion in a communication in such a manner that the other feels understood.

Developing discrepancies

Accepting the validity of a person's experiences does not necessarily involve accepting that clients stay as they are. To the contrary, the purpose of offering empirically validated treatments is to modify maladaptive cognitions and behaviour. But encouraging change should not involve vigorous confrontation, as this can lead to alienation of the client (Miller

& Rollnick, 2012). That is, while the goal may be to produce an awareness of the need for change, direct verbal challenges may not be the best way to achieve this goal. A better strategy is to focus on developing a discrepancy between the person's current behaviour (and its consequences) and future goals. Every client presents to treatment with some degree of ambivalence. The task is to ensure that the rewards of recovery outweigh the benefits associated with maintaining the status quo.

By drawing attention to where one is, in relation to where one wants to be, it is possible to increase awareness of the costs of a maladaptive behavioural pattern. Importantly, it is necessary to focus upon costs that are seen as relevant to the client rather than the psychologist. For instance, one of us mistakenly suggested to a person with agoraphobia that her child might be pleased and proud when she could be taken on the train into the city, only to face the response, 'I know I should want to get better for my kids, but I don't. Everyone says I should, but I can't seem to care.' Instead, for this client the most salient motivation was the freedom to be able to go to the local shops while unaccompanied. Once this goal was identified it was possible to use it as leverage to further enhance the value of personal freedom relative to the value of anxiety reduction during shopping outings that is contingent upon reliance on others. The greater the discrepancy is between these competing values, the greater is the motivation for change.

One way to develop discrepancies between current behaviour and future goals is to enquire about what the person would most enjoy doing when unshackled from their panic disorder or agoraphobic avoidance. When this image has been developed, it can be contrasted with the person's present state. The resulting dissatisfaction with the status quo can then be used to motivate the person to engage in therapeutic activities.

In summary, all clients are ambivalent about treatment to varying degrees. To enhance motivation it is useful to develop a discrepancy between clients' current behaviour and their desired state. By increasing the perceived value of changing relative to the perceived benefit of staying the same, the balance can be tipped towards greater treatment compliance.

Avoiding argumentation

Once a person initiates treatment and begins to comply with the components of the programme setbacks invariably occur. An unsatisfactory way for a psychologist to respond is to harass the person to complete an exercise or berate the person's non-compliance (quietly cursing the client's passive aggressive personality disorder). Miller and Rollnick (2012) suggest that it is more profitable to avoid argumentation. They encourage the view that therapeutic resistance is not so much a signal of client failure, but a signal for the psychologist to shift strategy. Resistance is a problem which the psychologist must take the responsibility to solve. The shift towards problem-solving enables the psychologist to avoid argumentation and 'roll with resistance'.

Rolling with resistance

Therapeutic resistance may signal a lack of understanding of the purpose of part of the programme or it may indicate a lack of success with one of the treatment components. Resistance may also indicate a weakening of resolve, indicating the need to develop a discrepancy to once again enhance motivation. Whatever the case, the psychologist must back-track and solve the problem. Regardless of the origin of the difficulty it is necessary to avoid argumentation and roll with resistance. Rather than pushing against the resistance, the therapist can extract from the complaint or refusal a foundation of motivation upon which to rebuild the treatment. Consider the following examples of therapeutic interactions.

CLIENT: I'm having a bad day with my agoraphobia. I don't think that I can do today's assignment.

PSYCHOLOGIST 1: You have to face your fears. Remember, avoidance makes fears worse. You will just have to go out and catch the bus.

PSYCHOLOGIST 2: When we agreed to the assignment yesterday you felt that it was achievable. What do you think it takes for you to achieve the task?

Both psychologists have the same goal in mind; they want to motivate the person to complete the agreed assignment. The first psychologist pursues this goal by reinforcing good reasons for attempting the assignment. Even though the reasons are valid, they are suboptimal for two reasons. First, they encourage refusal from the client, leading to a possible confrontation. Second, the response indirectly encourages dependence upon the psychologist for the recruitment of motivation necessary for task completion. When treatment is terminated the client will no longer have the psychologist's support and therefore, the aim is to encourage client autonomy. In contrast, the second psychologist encourages the client's autonomy by asking the person to find a solution. While the psychologist would obviously provide assistance, the goal is for the client to identify why the task is no longer achievable and how these obstacles can be overcome.

As part of rolling with resistance it is useful to implicitly convey the expectation that the client has the resources necessary to achieve the task. For this reason the second psychologist did not ask how the task could be made more simple (which may implicitly convey that the task is too difficult), but shifts attention towards how the task can be achieved. While the latter approach may involve breaking the step into a series of graded easier steps, the psychologist conveys an expectation that the task is achievable.

CLIENT: I did everything right, but I still find myself having panic attacks. Your treatment just isn't working.

PSYCHOLOGIST L: We know the treatments are effective, what do you think you did wrong?

PSYCHOLOGIST 2: Even though you battled hard to manage your anxiety, the panic still breaks through. Are there any lessons that you can learn to help you have greater success next time?

The client is expressing frustration that despite their best effort, the treatment techniques appear to be ineffective. The first psychologist responds by drawing attention to the person's possible poor conduct of the technique. Although clients may have difficulties because they fail to use the treatment techniques appropriately, it rarely helps to direct blame towards the client. Instead, the second psychologist empathically acknowledges the frustration but directs attention to the future. Implicitly the psychologist is communicating that setbacks are not a reason to throw in the towel, but an opportunity to learn. The second psychologist also implicitly assumes that the client is going to continue to work towards managing panics. Probably both psychologists would identify the same problems in performance. However, the second does not oppose the resistance. Rather, the psychologist rolls with the resistance, arriving at a position where motivation can be evaluated and practical strategies to attempt the next assignment can be identified.

In summary, argumentation can be avoided if one rolls with therapeutic resistance. In doing so it is helpful to respond to resistance with a shift in strategy to problem-solving. The psychologist always implicitly conveys the knowledge (based on clinical experience and the empirical literature) that the disorders can be managed more effectively using the techniques being taught.

Supporting self-efficacy

Resistance in therapy can often follow a setback. At such times self-efficacy decreases as the person feels that successful mastery of the problem is no longer an achievable goal. In working with a client, it is particularly important to reverse decreases in self-efficacy. Low self-efficacy appears to be a predictor of the development of fearful avoidance, the exacerbation of depression, and substance use. Therefore, if self-efficacy fails to increase, or even decreases during therapy, it is highly probable that the problem behaviours will return and therapeutic progress will be hindered.

Central to supporting self-efficacy is conveying the principle that change is possible. This has already been alluded to in the context of rolling with resistance but it is important that the belief that change is possible be conveyed throughout therapy. In addition, there are three critical times when the likelihood of change needs to be explicitly communicated. First, at the start of therapy it is essential to communicate a positive and realistic expectation of therapeutic change. For example, in our group programme for agoraphobia it is common to begin with a comment such as:

We have seen how fearful avoidance is driven by panic attacks and we have discussed how life would be different if you could be free from panic attacks. We know from past groups that around nine in ten people, just like you, become free from panic attacks. Free from panics not only in the short term, but we have followed these people for up to two years after treatment and they remain panic free. Although you may find this difficult to believe, our results are no different from other similar centres around the world.

However, I suspect that even though I have told you that people can learn to master panics you are thinking, 'I bet I'm the one in ten who doesn't get better.' Therefore, the more important question is not how many people are panic free, but how do you move from being the one in ten, to being one of the nine in ten? The simple answer is, you will need to work hard.

The techniques that we will teach you are effective and this is demonstrated by the high success rates. Our experience has shown us that those people who do not improve (i) do not put in the effort necessary to learn the techniques, (ii) do not practise the techniques, or (iii) give up and go back to using the strategies which they have used before to partially manage anxiety and panics. We will teach you new techniques which will enable you to control your panics. It is up to you to learn and practise the techniques, working hard to conquer the panics, because when you do, you can be free of panic.

The second time when self-efficacy must be supported is during setbacks. At these times, when the client is demoralized and possibly resistant to therapeutic interventions, it is necessary to solve any problems while conveying the belief that change is still possible. The third time when self-efficacy must be particularly supported is at the termination of treatment. At these times clients are often worried how they will fare without the support of the psychologist, and if treatment has been in a group context, without the support and encouragement of other group members. This difficulty can be tackled by reminding clients that the gains during treatment were due to their efforts. In addition, it can be helpful to offer follow-up sessions. Clients are invited to attend follow-ups if they suffer setbacks or need some extra encouragement. Clients often say that they feel comfortable knowing that there is a 'safety net' should they need one, and they feel that they can use the resource on an irregular basis.

In summary, low self-efficacy is related to failure to progress in many problems. Therefore, it is helpful to foster and support a belief in the possibility of change. Then the psychologist can provide the effective treatment techniques which make long-lasting and self-initiated change possible.

Summary

Ambivalence about treatment is common among clients. There are both gains and losses associated with recovery and it is the psychologist's role to ensure that the former always outweigh the latter. It is possible to achieve this goal by expressing an empathic understanding for the client's condition and experience while developing a discrepancy between current functioning and the desired functioning. Conflict or resistance in therapy is best handled by avoiding argumentation (and subsequent polarization) as the psychologist rolls with the resistance, seeking to solve any problems and restore motivation, rather than 'pushing' the client towards recovery. Implicit in all of this is that the psychologist must keep uppermost in mind the knowledge that the treatment techniques are effective and that change for the better is within the person's capability. Conveying the attitude that change is possible will not in and of itself cure the client's problems, but it will bring the person to the point where effective change is possible.

Managing homework compliance

In addition to the broader issues of motivation, there is a specific behaviour in therapy that hinders progress, namely, a lack of compliance with homework assignments (Shelton & Levy, 1979, 1981a, 1981b). This is not an insignificant problem because homework assignments play an important role in outcome (Burns & Auerbach, 1992), such that clients who are less reliable in completion of these exercises demonstrate worse outcomes (Kazantzis et al., 2000). For instance, Kazantzis and colleagues in their meta-analysis found that setting homework accounted for 13% of the variance in outcomes ($r = 0.36$) and homework compliance accounted for 5% ($r = 0.22$) in therapeutic outcomes. The extent of these effect sizes can be used to support a number of points. First, it is important and worthwhile to encourage clients to conduct homework assignments, especially given that this is a factor that is potentially under therapist control to some degree (Bryant, Simons, & Thase, 1999). Second, it is worthwhile reflecting upon the amount of time that should be allocated to homework, given that these activities only predict a relatively modest amount of variance in outcomes. If you find yourself struggling in vain to encourage a non-compliant client to complete homework assignments, there is still a substantial portion of the variance in therapeutic outcome to be explained by other factors. Therefore, if compliance with homework is becoming contentious, it is better to build upon the client's strengths and focus more on those aspects of treatment that the client does engage with. However, most of the time, homework is an important component of therapy and there are a number of non-confrontational ways to increase compliance.

In addressing the problems of non-compliance with homework instructions, Birchler (1988) has produced a number of recommendations. First, only provide homework assignments once a satisfactory level of rapport has been established. The rationale behind this is that the more your client values you and your opinions, the more likely they are to comply with your requests (see also Linehan, 1993a). Second, any homework that is prescribed should correspond to the therapeutic goals. Accordingly, the psychologist needs to create an expectation that completing homework will alleviate presenting problems. Third, the client should be involved in planning the homework. By maximizing the perception of control and willing participation, the likelihood of compliance will increase. Fourth, check that the assignment does not exceed the client's present motivational levels. In this regard, consider factors such as time, energy, and cost. Fifth, ensure that the task does not exceed the client's level of competence. One way to achieve this is to observe the client practising within the therapeutic session. Sixth, reduce any threatening or anxiety-provoking aspects of homework. The aim is to achieve goals by using small, attainable steps. Seventh, make sure that tasks are specific and clear. Asking a client to repeat or to paraphrase instructions can assist this process. Giving written assignments and reminder notes can also help. Further, Birchler (1988) suggests that the psychologist considers any possible secondary gain if the client does not comply. Think about the impact of the assignment on the client's family system and any supportive or sabotaging effects that others may have. If any can be anticipated, identify the potential problems and setbacks, and normalize these experiences. Finally, review all homework assignments. During the review the therapist should provide support for the client, help to shape early attempts into correct behaviour, and acknowledge positive efforts. It is easy to extinguish homework compliance through non-attention.

Thus, when giving homework it is important to allocate time to the process. Typically novice therapists will underestimate the time taken and will try to cram it into the last few minutes of a session. If you consider that the prescription of homework assignments will involve (i) explaining why you are asking the client to do the homework, (ii) getting the client's involvement and commitment, (iii) describing the homework in detail, (iv) requesting that the client paraphrase and then practise the exercise, it is apparent that a reasonable amount of time will need to be allocated to the exercise (especially initially). Our experience suggests that 10 minutes will not underestimate the time required to assign homework, although the time reduces as therapy progresses and the client is more familiar with the process.

In addition, homework must be essential to therapy. If the assessment or the task is not essential and linked to specific therapeutic goals, then why are you wasting the client's time with it? If the homework is essential, then it follows that you must review the homework exercise at the next session. In addition, if the homework is essential to the progress of the next session, then it is problematic if the client does not comply. Some have even suggested that if homework is not completed, the therapist should consider cutting the session short and postponing the sections of the sessions that required the homework until the following week. The strength of this approach is that if we are convinced that homework is a central component to the satisfactory completion of treatment, then cutting the session short will convey clearly the value of homework to the client, and this may increase compliance. And note, while this is a direct and firm attempt by the therapist to encourage compliance with homework assignments, it avoids argumentation and rolls with resistance by adapting the course of scheduled session times without abandoning the objective to get the client to engage in treatment.

Engaging the client with therapy so that it stands the best chance of success is an important clinical activity. During the course of ensuring compliance, it is not unexpected that client-related factors may become of importance and these will require sensitive handling on the part of the therapist. It is to some of these issues that we will now shift our discussion.

Chapter 13

Respecting the humanity of clients: cross-cultural and ethical aspects of practice

Individuals function within a complex array of familial, social, historical, political, cultural, and economic influences. Consideration of these influences draws attention to individual-specific matters such as cultural and ethical issues. In addition, we need to be cognizant of those factors that pertain to the broader social systems and structures within which both our clients and we are located. Clinical psychologists must deal sensitively with these issues in a manner that respects each client's uniqueness and humanity while being mindful of the socio-cultural context.

From Figure 13.1 it is apparent that there are a variety of ways that social, cultural, and legal issues may influence the relationship between the psychologist and the client. Running through all these facets is a central theme, in which the psychologist seeks to afford the client the dignity that is warranted by virtue of being a member of the human race. Recognizing our humanity requires acknowledging our individuality as well as our social nature. We are individuals who live in social structures and as such we both act upon and are acted upon by our environments. This means that clients will present for therapy as unique individuals, who have been shaped by particular social, cultural, historical, and political forces. The clinical psychologist needs to understand and respect how these forces can both constrain and enrich the therapeutic relationship. Like their clients, psychologists will be influenced by their own social, cultural, historical, and political contexts, and they must strive to minimize any negative or constraining impact that may have on the client.

If the broader social context of the practice of clinical psychology is not considered, unforeseen problems may arise. For example, MacIntyre (2001; MacIntyre & Petticrew, 2000) has drawn attention to circumstances where the provision of a well-meaning health intervention may exacerbate health inequalities because a socio-economically advantaged person's greater resources may offer that person greater access to the health intervention. Some of these resources will be financial, but other less obvious ones may include education, coping skills, as well as the chance or ability to take up the health opportunities. Thus, an intervention can have the greatest effect among those who need it least. For instance, Schou and Wight (1994) examined the effectiveness of a dental health campaign in Scotland. They found that mothers of caries-free children were better educated, had better awareness of the campaign, and engaged in better dental hygiene than mothers of children with caries. This is not to say that the campaign overall was not a success, but that the intervention was differentially successful depending upon socio-economic factors. Similarly, in our own work one of us was examining the extent to which exercise was being taken up by people with intellectual disabilities living in group homes. In general, the picture was positive, but the degree of activity was strongly correlated with independent ratings of ability, such that the

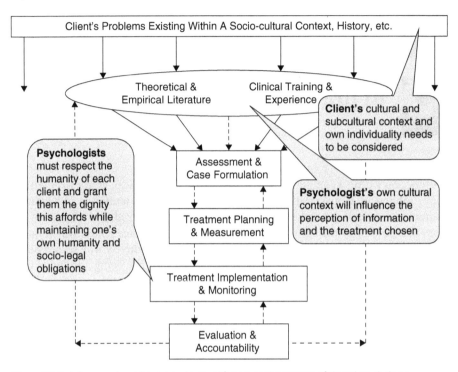

Figure 13.1 Influence of social, legal, and cultural factors on the practice of clinical psychology.

more active lifestyles were more common among those with higher ability levels. Now while it is predictable that individuals with greater abilities will be more likely to hear and respond to messages about increasing physical activity, in an ideal world, a health intervention would be uncorrelated with ability. The practical implication is that clinical psychologists need to carefully consider each client as an individual and examine all the factors that may impinge upon a particular intervention. In the remainder of this chapter, we will examine first some of the challenges and parameters associated with conducting clinical practice in a culturally sensitive manner. Then we will present a structured problem-solving approach that can be applied when relating to clients as unique individuals while bearing in mind cultural as well as ethical issues that may arise within the therapeutic relationship.

Culture-sensitive practice of clinical psychology

Acknowledging that each client is a human being entails a recognition that each person must be treated with the dignity that they deserve. This will involve appreciating the unique qualities of each person and the cultural influences that shape them (Kazarian & Evans, 1998; Ryder, Ban, & Chentsova-Dutton, 2011). Before we review some principles of culture-sensitive practice (Sue & Sue, 2012), it is necessary to consider several caveats. First, a focus on culture as a specific topic in clinical psychology could unintentionally lead to the neglect of other important qualities of an individual when planning treatment (such as their socio-economic status, social class, gender, sexual orientation, and so forth). These attributes will vary in their perceived importance among individuals and will vary according to the social context in which they live. For example, sexual orientation may be seen relatively unimportant to a middle-aged heterosexual client living a white, middle-class, suburban lifestyle, but a young gay man living in the same suburb, who has been socially ostracized during his schooling, may perceive his sexual orientation to be a core attribute of his self-definition. Second, the focus on large cultural differences (e.g., white American versus black American versus Hispanic American) may overshadow important but less obvious differences. For instance, two Christian clients may present for treatment with obsessional guilt about their sinful thoughts, but if one is Roman Catholic and the other is Lutheran, the theological frameworks within which they would conceptualize guilt and forgiveness are fundamentally different. Third, the literature on cultural psychology itself suffers from a cultural bias, with the vast majority of it being based in North America and Europe. For instance, in an edited book on cultural clinical psychology only one author was working at a university outside North America. This is unfortunate since there is a risk that the literature itself will reflect a particular cultural emphasis. As residents of Australia we notice this because rarely is there any mention of the indigenous peoples of Australia and New Zealand, and there is less coverage of people likely to migrate to Australia. Although relevant research is accessible, the difficulty for the individual clinical psychologist is that there is still an insufficient empirical base for guidelines that cover each of the myriad cultural groups and subgroups whose members may present for treatment. For these reasons, we advocate a structured problem-solving approach to organize a culturally sensitive understanding of each individual client.

That is, the application of the culturally relevant knowledge will be so varied that it is more helpful to focus on broad principles of application rather than the specifics of each culture. In so doing, it is important to acknowledge that mainstream clinical psychology tends to reflect Western values, such as individualism. The treatments outlined in Chapter 6 all emphasize the individual as the central organizing feature. Thus, the treatments tend to give implicit assent to values such as self-reliance, self-determination, self-understanding, self-awareness, and self-initiated action (Toukmanian & Brouwers, 1998). These attributes contrast with values of family kinship and community membership, and a sense of self embedded within the needs and norms of a particular group, that are emphasized in many non-Western cultures. In order to develop a problem-focused approach to address these biases, it is first necessary to appreciate the ways that cultures differ.

Parameters of culture-sensitive practice

One context to culture-sensitive practice for a science-informed practice is to examine the data on outcomes. Ryder and colleagues (2011) conducted a meta-analytic review and drew three conclusions. First, clients had a moderately strong preference for a therapist from their own ethnic group and second, they tended to perceive them more positively than therapists from other ethnic groups. Together these data suggest that it is important to be sensitive to client's preferences and be aware of the potentially less favourable impression that you might make when treating a person from a different ethnic group. However, the authors did not observe evidence of beneficial or harmful effects in terms of treatment outcomes when there were ethnic differences between client and therapist. Thus, be aware of the clients' preferences, but there does not yet seem to be widespread evidence that outcomes will be adversely affected by any differences (see also Lambert, 2010).

Given the concerns that clients have, it is important to be as sensitive to differences as possible. Kluckhohn and Stodtbeck (1961) identify a variety of parameters of relevance when considering the values implicit and explicit in different cultures. The first parameter is the orientation to human nature, which describes the ways that different cultures may view the nature of persons. People may differ with respect to the views about *human character*; whether humans are considered to be basically good, bad, neutral, or a mixture of both. They may vary in terms of what is considered to be innate to the human character, how character is produced, and what makes a human a person.

A second parameter is *relational orientation*, which can be lineal, collateral, or individualistic. That is, a key issue for any individual is how to relate to others, and one's culture provides guidelines for doing so. Within a lineal culture a person relates to others on the basis on their lineage. People may be of a higher or lower social standing dependent upon the lineage into which they are born and therefore relationships are 'vertical' in that they extend vertically through time. Another way to address the issue of relationships with others is collateral, where society is divided into 'us,' who may be trusted and collaborated with, and 'them', who are not to be trusted. In contrast to a lineal and collateral group orientation is an individualistic approach to others, in which others in society are dealt with in a manner determined by their perceived individual merit. Relationships are 'horizontal' in that one's lineage through time or group membership is much less relevant. Society in the US tends to be individualistic, whereas some Middle Eastern countries are lineal and collateral.

The next parameter is the *relationship between people and the natural world*, such that people are regarded as in subjugation to nature, are in harmony with nature, or seek to master nature. Is life determined by external forces beyond personal control? Within this category we can also include the perceived relations between the person and their internal (emotional) environment. Thus, cultures may vary in terms of value placed on mastery of emotions.

The fourth orientation refers to *preferred mode of activity*, and the orientation can be one of being, being-in-becoming, and doing. This orientation will express itself in terms of the degree to which life is valued in itself, the extent to which development of the inner self is valued, and the extent to which rewards in life are seen to be self-determined and obtained through individual effort.

Cultures may also vary in terms of the *relationships between people*. Individuals in different cultures may differ with respect to the extent to which they believe in individual autonomy, independence, and competition versus leadership, helping, cooperation, and interdependence. These perceptions will also influence the way that friends and families are perceived, such that some cultures may view friends and family as the primary means of problem-solving, whereas other cultures may emphasize autonomy and independence in problem-solving.

Finally, there is an *orientation to time*, where the focus can be on the past, present, or the future. Cultures within which people tend to focus on the past may emphasize tradition and focus on history, whereas people from present-focused cultures emphasize living for today, and people from cultures with a future focus will be more inclined to live in such a way that sacrifices are made with the aim of creating a better future. For example, Western culture tends to view human nature in a negative or neutral manner, possesses an individualistic focus, perceives the need to exercise mastery over nature, evaluates individual worth in terms of what one can do, and emphasizes the future more than the past or present.

Awareness of the parameters of cultural differences allows clinical psychologists to articulate their own beliefs, values, and attitudes so that they can recognize differences and respond appropriately. Conducting a self-evaluation will assist a psychologist to be aware of the extent to which they are able to accept differences and the need to learn about other cultures. Learning about other cultures involves deliberately taking opportunities to expose oneself to other social groups, cultures, and subcultures. This may include partaking in cultural events and activities, as well as seeking insights through media such as books and film.

With the benefits of a self-evaluation regarding the relevant cultural parameters, the psychologist will be in a better position to assess whether any of these parameters are relevant to the treatment of a particular client. Most often this assessment will need to be made by the therapist, because values tend to be implicit and therefore clients may not be able to articulate key issues. The aim is to evaluate the extent to which the attributes of the individual affect the therapeutic communication and process of treatment. In so doing, be aware that as a clinician both your verbal and non-verbal messages are congruent and culturally appropriate. For instance, Eastern cultures tend to be more reserved than Western cultures and therefore it can be inappropriate to engage with the client in an open and frank discussion about problems related to themselves and their family in ways that might be appropriate with a client from a Western background. In terms of the therapeutic process, it is important to consider that the therapeutic goals are culturally consistent or that the method of intervention includes the relevant individuals. For example, certain behavioural changes may meet with the approval and support of key family members while other changes may bring about cultural disapproval or sanctions. O'Leary, Curley, Rosenbaum, and Clarke (1986) found that training women in assertiveness was associated with increases in domestic violence; therefore a clinician needs to be mindful of the social and cultural context within which a person resides. When a few possible courses of action or methods of proceeding are enumerated, the clinician can specify the possible consequences, both positive and negative, of the different options. Once articulated, a decision can be made, implemented, and evaluated. If the evaluation indicates a negative outcome, then an alternative action plan is initiated. Thus, the process once more is akin to structured problem-solving in that the stages are: define the problem, develop alternative courses of action, evaluate and then choose an action, and evaluate the outcomes. Before articulating the problem-solving technique in detail, we will review some of the issues that arise when considering the role of clinical psychology among older adults.

Clinical psychology and older adults

The number of older adults continues to grow and the population is becoming increasingly diverse. These two demands put pressure on the profession of clinical psychology to ensure that its practitioners are able to meet the challenge (Karel, Gatz, & Smyer, 2012) and the American Psychological Association has provided helpful guidelines (2014) which serve to illustrate the application of the general ethical principles to the particular instance.

For example, one ethical principle is respect for the dignity of persons. That is,

the belief that each person should be treated primarily as a person or an end in him/herself ... (i)n so doing, psychologists acknowledge that all persons have a right to have their innate worth as human beings appreciated and that this worth is not dependent upon their culture, nationality, ethnicity, colour, race, religion, sex, gender, marital status, sexual orientation, physical or mental abilities, *age*, socio-economic status, or any other preference or personal characteristic, condition, or status. (Canadian Psychological Association, 2000, p. 7; italics added)

In terms of older persons this means that it is necessary to ensure that your practice is not clouded by stereotypes. Some stereotypes of elderly people are that they are frail, depressed, in cognitive decline or dementing, socially isolated, and stubbornly inflexible. In addition to the cognitive error of assuming that characteristics of some individuals must apply to all members of a defined group, Knight and Poon (2008) distinguish negative and positive maturation. Even though ageing is associated with some negative maturation, such as physical decline and reductions in some facets of cognition (e.g., fluid intellectual abilities may decline while crystallized intelligence may remain intact; Dixon, 2003), the detrimental effects are not universal. In addition, positive maturation can be observed in areas of cognitive complexity. That is, adults demonstrate improving performance across the lifespan in tasks that involve information, vocabulary, and mathematical skills. The wisdom that comes from the accumulation of knowledge, both factual and procedural, means that older adults can exhibit superior performance in some areas relative to younger adults. Likewise, older age tends to be characterized by greater emotional complexity than younger adults and better emotional regulation and more positive emotion (Urry & Gross, 2010). Falling prey to the negative stereotypes may lead to a style of therapy that is overly paternalistic, which arises from a misperception that the older person is weak, frail, and needs protection. However, we know that paternalistic attitudes in psychotherapy tend to undermine the therapeutic relationship and foster dependency (Knight, 2004). Thus, when working with older clients it is important to be mindful of stereotypes and seek information to ensure that they do not impede your ability to work effectively with clients.

Another couple of principles that clinical psychologists abide by are to keep

up to date with a broad range of relevant knowledge, research methods, and techniques … in order that their service … will benefit and not harm others [and they need to evaluate] how their own experiences, attitudes, culture, beliefs, values, social context, individual differences, specific training, and stresses influence their interactions with others, and integrate this awareness into all efforts to benefit and not harm others. (Canadian Psychological Association, 2000, pp. 16–17)

Therefore, it behoves clinical psychologists to familiarize themselves with the dynamics of ageing. Developmental theories identify social and psychological factors that influence the individual and the life trajectory they are on. Retirement, relationship losses, and life changes will affect the social and occupational environment for an older person (Sterns & Dawson, 2012). Age-related physical changes, health concerns, and disability all have the capacity to impose restrictions on a person's life and functioning (Aldwin, Park, & Spiro, 2007). For a trainee clinical psychologist these life events may seem distant and may require investigation (see Craik & Salthouse, 2007; Lichtenberg, 2010; Schaie & Willis, 2011; Scogin & Shah, 2012). However, when faced with an older client it can be challenging to know how to proceed. One helpful strategy can be derived from reminiscence-based approaches to therapy (Bornat, 1994; Gibson, 2004). The approach uses music, photographs, and archival recordings to prompt memories and to stimulate a discussion about past events. While more research into the therapy is needed (Woods, Spector, Jones, Orrell, & Davies, 2005), the process can be helpful for a junior clinician in getting to know an older client. By asking about a person's favourite music it can help you to start a conversation and get to know a person better. The relatively neutral topic can serve as a way of engaging with the client and building rapport. Furthermore, reminiscence is a mechanism used by older adults to process and integrate experiences in a way that builds well-being (O'Rourke, Cappeliez, & Claxton, 2011) and may assist in fostering a positive relationship for therapy.

There are also specific areas that clinical psychologists will need to be mindful of because they are associated with issues that arise due to the client's stage of life. These issues moderate the clinical presentation and can determine the life events that impact upon a client. Older clients are more likely to experience loss of friends and family members. The older they become, the more likely it will be that they are the last of their common-aged peers and this brings with it social ramifications as well as practical issues of care (Wrzus, Hänel, Wagner, & Neyer, 2013). Older clients may also require additional care, for both physical and psychological well-being. In addition, there is also the caregiving responsibility that may fall upon friends and family members. For example, a spouse might become the primary caregiver for an infirm partner or for younger family members.

As well as these factors, the clinical presentation may differ among older adults. A common issue is the differential diagnosis of depression and dementia, since not only can these conditions be comorbid, they share overlapping symptom profiles. Awareness of these conditions and the methods of disentangling the separate contributions against a backdrop of normal ageing requires additional skills and careful practice (Fiske, Wetherell, & Gatz, 2009). Similarly, anxiety disorders, while less prevalent, may also have a different profile. Panic disorder, for example, may be characterized more by intrusive cognitions and memories than physiological arousal (Lauderdale, Cassidy-Eagle, Nguyen, & Sheikh, 2011) and worries may be more health-related. Certain assessment requests (e.g., competence to manage one's affairs) may be more common than in younger clients (Moye & Marson, 2007).

By way of summary, while there are many nuances in the delivery of psychological services to older adults, there is good evidence that both individual (Scogin & Shah, 2012) and group (Burlingame, Strauss, & Joyce, 2013) psychological treatments are effective with older adults and so clinical psychologists can be confident that the well-being of clients can be improved with the provision of appropriate services. Clinical psychologists need to familiarize themselves with these nuances when working with this client group as they will need to do with every client group. We will now turn to a consideration of structured problem-solving as a clinical technique and its application to the practice of culture-sensitive clinical psychology.

Applying structured problem-solving to culture-sensitive practice

Structured problem-solving was developed by D'Zurilla (1986) and it can assist clients to identify problems, recognize resources they possess, and teach a systematic method of overcoming and preventing problems. Structured problem-solving recommends moving through a sequence of steps (see Hawton & Kirk, 1989).

The first step is to *define* the current problem. If there are multiple problems, these can be dealt with sequentially after an order for dealing with them has been chosen. The second step is to *brainstorm* all the possible solutions. Once a list of possible solutions is written down, then the therapist and client can evaluate the pros and cons of each and in so doing *select* what they think will be the best solution. This option is then *implemented*; a step that will involve preparing a plan of action in which the necessary steps are clearly articulated and then enacting that plan. Sometimes cognitive or behavioural rehearsal (e.g., role-plays) can be useful in preparing the client, for anticipating difficulties, and building a sense of self-efficacy among clients. Finally, the implemented solution is *evaluated*, by asking whether the solution did indeed solve the problem, and by assessing the success and failure against some pre-agreed criteria. If it failed to redress the difficulty, the clinical psychologist and client can select the next best solution, brainstorm some other solutions, or even check that the problem has been correctly identified and fully articulated.

Table 13.1 Analogies between structured problem-solving, the process of research, and the conduct of clinical practice

Problem-solving	Research	Clinical practice
Problem definition	Research question	Presenting problem
Brainstorming	Hypothesis generation	Preliminary formulations
Choose solution	Select hypothesis	Choose intervention
Implement solution	Conduct study	Implement treatment
Evaluation	Analysis/interpretation	Evaluation

Table 13.1 outlines these five stages of problem-solving, by drawing parallels with two activities familiar to psychologists. The central column identifies a series of stages in the process of conducting research. Research begins with identification and selection of the research question, which in turn will lead to hypothesis generation. Of the possible hypotheses, the research will select a subset. These steps of research are analogous to problem definition, brainstorming, and selecting a solution. A researcher then conducts a study to test between hypotheses and analyses the data to determine the fate of the hypothesis, which is analogous to implementing and evaluating a possible solution to a problem. Thus, the structured problem-solving approach is one that is familiar to a psychologist trained in research. Furthermore, the parallels also extend to the model of clinical practice we have been outlining. The clinician identifies a presenting problem, generates a formulation, which in turn will guide the choice of an intervention. After implementing the intervention, the clinical psychologist will measure the effectiveness of the treatment by conducting an evaluation.

This same approach can be extended to situations where cross-cultural matters need to be considered and responded to. The strength of the approach is that it is possible to take into account some general principles or theories about culture, even though each situation is unique and will require a considered individual solution. For example, López (1997) describes a couple who migrated to the US from north Mexico. They presented with marital difficulties which had reached a point at which the couple had settled into a pattern of silence interspersed with verbal hostility. Initially, the husband only agreed to attend treatment separately from his wife. Therapy was soon abandoned when he indicated that his wife was to blame for their problems. He believed that he fulfilled his role as a husband (by working hard and providing financially), but that she failed to fulfil her role as a wife (by failing to cook meals, wash clothes, and be available for sexual relations). Later they attended as a couple but one problem arose when the therapist offered the interpretation that perhaps the husband felt hurt that his needs were not being considered by his wife. He responded that no one could hurt him, but that if they did then he would make sure that they knew it. He indicated that he was a strong man and that the efforts on behalf of his wife and daughters to make him a wimp would fail. The case study highlights a number of problems which could be addressed by taking a problem-solving perspective. In reflecting on the case, López notes that his suggestion was problematic in that it elicited a vehement response from the client that did not facilitate change. Thus, the therapist could reconsider the way this suggestion was offered by re-evaluating the impact of the cultural context from which the couple came, issues that may have arisen concerning acculturation to life in the US, possible discrepancies between the husband and wife's views of the problem and the person responsible of

change, and perceptions of the purpose of therapy. In so doing, the problem-solving provides a framework for addressing potentially difficult cultural issues in therapy. The same
holds true when considering how ethical principles (such as those articulated in the codes
of ethics developed by each country's psychological society) apply to a particular situation
or therapeutic relationship.

Applying structured problem-solving to ethical decision-making

Consider a client who seeks counselling after receiving a positive HIV test result. He is unsure how he became infected but thinks that it followed a homosexual encounter while he
was exploring his sexuality. A typical session would involve outlining his prognosis as well as
describing 'safe sex' and what he could do to protect sexual partners from infection. Consider how you would respond if the client informed you that he was soon to marry his fiancée
and settle down. He did not want to inform her that he was HIV-positive in case it affected
his marriage plans.

A practical way to handle ethical situations such as the one just described builds upon
a structured problem-solving approach (see Keith-Spiegel & Koocher, 1985 and Eberlein,
1987). It identifies ethical dilemmas as problems that require solutions and rather than prescribing answers, it provides a problem-solving framework within which to seek a set of
possible solutions.

Keith-Spiegel and Koocher (1985) suggest that the place to begin is by describing the
parameters of the situation. In the preceding example, these would involve his HIV infection and the relationship with his fiancée. The second step is to expand on the problem by
identifying the key ethical issues. Redlich & Pope (1980) suggested the following principles
to guide ethical decision-making. They noted that psychologists (i) should do no harm,
(ii) should practise only within competence, (iii) should not exploit, (iv) should treat people
with respect for their dignity as humans, (v) should protect confidentiality, (vi) should act
(except in extreme cases) only after obtaining informed consent, and (vii) should practise
(as far as possible) within the framework of social equity and justice. These principles highlight the need to protect the client's confidentiality, but also to take into account the need to
avoid harm to the client's fiancée in the example above. However, what is needed is an organizing framework to decide when there are conflicts among principles.

The Canadian Code of Ethics for Psychologists (Canadian Psychological Association,
2000; see also Truscott & Crook, 2013) remains a model for ethical thinking about psychology and it has isolated a set of principles and organized them into a hierarchy to assist
ethical decision-making. One of the strengths of the principled approach to ethical practice
is that they can be applied to situations that were not in the minds of the people framing
the guidelines (e.g., how the principles can be used to examine online personal information accessibility, web-based advertising, and electronic data storage; Nicholson, 2011). The
hierarchical organization implies that the principles are considered in order and greater
weight is given to those higher in the hierarchy. The first principle is respect for the dignity
of persons. Except when a person's physical safety is under threat, assuring people's dignity
should be the most important ethical principle. Responsible caring is the second principle
and implies the caring should be carried out competently while respecting dignity. The third
principle is integrity in relationships. The Canadian Code of Ethics notes that on certain
occasions the values of openness and straightforwardness might need to be subordinated in
order to maintain the respect for human dignity and responsible caring. Finally, it highlights

responsibility to society and suggests that this principle be given the lowest weight when it is in conflict with others. The CPA Code suggests that

When a person's welfare appears to conflict with benefits to society, it is often possible to find ways of working for the benefit of society that do not violate respect and responsible caring for the person. However, if this is not possible, the dignity and well-being of a person should not be sacrificed to a vision of the greater good of society, and greater weight must be given to respect and responsible caring for the person. (Canadian Psychological Association, 2000, p. 4)

As an aside, the reader will notice that this last point makes explicit a cultural position on the parameter of the relationships between people in which individual autonomy is valued over interdependence and therefore it will be necessary to be sensitive to the cultural sensitivities of clients who may not hold this view. However, when considering the preceding example, it would be clear that the possible specific threat to another person may take ethical precedence.

The next step is to consult any available professional guidelines to see whether these might assist in the resolution of each issue. Most professional guidelines for psychologists share a similar structure. There are guidelines relating to professional practice, the conduct of research, issues that are specific to working with humans or animals, and regulations relating to the professional society. The ethical guidelines cover matters related to general professional conduct, maintaining and working with professional competence, obtaining consent, and confidentiality. Considering the preceding example, the British Psychological Society's 'Code of conduct, ethical principles and guidelines' notes that

in exceptional circumstances, where there is sufficient evidence to raise serious concern about the safety or interests of recipients of services, or about others who may be threatened by the recipient's behaviour, take such steps as are judged necessary to inform appropriate third parties without prior consent after first consulting an experienced and disinterested colleague, unless the delay caused by seeking this advice would involve a significant risk to life or health. (British Psychological Society, 2005, pp. 3–4)

Similarly, the Canadian Psychological Association (2000) recommends:

Do everything reasonably possible to stop or offset the consequences of actions by others when these actions are likely to cause serious physical harm or death. This may include reporting to appropriate authorities (e.g., the police), an intended victim, or a family member or other support person who can intervene, and would be done even when a confidential relationship is involved. (p. 22)

Thus, professional guidelines provide some direction about how to proceed.

With this information, Keith-Spiegel and Koocher (1985) suggest that the next step is to evaluate the rights, responsibility, and welfare of affected parties. In the present example these issues relate to the client's right to privacy and the fiancée's right to safety and protection. After describing these rights, the next step is to generate the alternative decisions possible for each issue and enumerate the consequences of making each decision, considering any evidence that the various consequences or benefits resulting from each decision will actually occur. When this has been done it will be possible to make a decision and evaluate its success, which in the current example would identify the need to inform the fiancée. Having made a decision, the best way to implement the chosen course of action will need to be determined. For example, the clinician could boldly inform the client that regardless of his wishes the therapist is going to contact his fiancée or, alternatively, could decide to spend time in therapy considering the consequences for the client and fiancée of his proposed course of action. The hope of the latter discussion would be to bring the client to a realization of his responsibilities as a fiancé and a fellow human being and the possible outcomes

Table 13.2 Worksheet for assessing ethical dilemmas

Worksheet for assessing ethical dilemmas
Describe the parameters of the situation
Define the potential issues involved
Consult guidelines, if any, already available that might apply to the resolution of each issue
Evaluate the rights, responsibility, and welfare of affected parties
Generate the alternative decisions possible for each issue
Enumerate the consequences of making each decision
Present evidence that various consequences or benefits resulting from each decision will occur
Make your decision and evaluate the outcome

of different actions. The principle of respecting the client's confidentiality and individual dignity must be weighted against the risk of delaying disclosure to the fiancée, who would remain at risk of being seriously harmed if the therapist chooses to not inform her immediately.

Thus, ethical decision-making is like structured problem-solving in that the stages are: define the problem, develop alternative courses of action, analyse courses of action, choose the course of action, and evaluate it. This process is depicted in the Table 13.2. You may find it helpful to use this worksheet as you consider how the model would apply to situations you might encounter in your training.

Confidentiality

Having described a general problem-solving strategy for addressing ethical issues, it is relevant to consider some specific ethical issues. *Confidentiality* is an issue that arose in the context of discussing case management. To reiterate, the term acknowledges that when a client enters therapy they inevitably relinquish a degree of personal privacy, by providing the therapist access to normally private information. However, the client has the reasonable expectation that any information disclosed to the therapist remains confidential. Thus, confidentiality refers to legal rules and ethical standards that protect clients from the unauthorized disclosure of information that has been disclosed in therapy or has arisen in the course of therapy. Ethical guidelines require clinical psychologists to maintain client confidentiality and in so doing reflect the principle that confidentiality is the prerogative of a client not a therapist. That is, a client can choose to take a therapist into their confidence by providing that information, but the client still retains control of that information. The client may permit the therapist to communicate the confidential material to a third party (e.g., give written permission to include the material in a referral letter to another mental health professional), but the decision in almost all circumstances lies with the client.

One aspect of confidentiality that has arisen with the increase in popularity of social media is the ability of psychologists to obtain information about their clients online, but it is also possible for clients to access information about you … and they do. Therefore, it is wise to be prudent about information that you display in public forums and social media sites. It is advisable to ask yourself four questions before posting information online: First, what costs and benefits accrue? Second, what is the probability that clients will be negatively affected? Third, how might this disclosure affect my relationship with my clients? Finally, does the disclosure threaten my credibility or undermine the public's trust in clinical psychology? It is also prudent to give careful thought to who you accept as friends and the degree of privacy that you grant to others (Barnett, 2008). Be mindful that the online information may have impacts not only on you, but also on your employer.

The online environment also requires us to consider the ethical issues associated with seeking out information about your client from social media sites. Avoid obtaining information on your client without their permission, not only because of the ethical issues involved, but also because it has the potential to undermine the relationship of trust that is foundational to psychotherapy.

Dual relationships

Having described a general problem-solving strategy for addressing cultural as well as ethical issues in respecting the humanity and dignity of individual clients, one aspect is worthy of specific attention. This concerns dual relationships. A dual relationship exists when a therapist is in another, different relationship with a client. Usually this second relationship is social, financial, or professional. For instance, if a professor of clinical psychology required students to enter into psychotherapy with him- or herself as part of their training in clinical psychology, a dual relationship would exist. In such an instance, the psychotherapeutic relationship coexists with an educational relationship where the professor grades the student's work. These other relationships have the potential to erode and distort the professional nature of the therapeutic relationship, create a conflict of interest, as well as potentially compromise the professional disinterest and sound judgement required for good practice. On the other hand, the existence of a therapeutic relationship means that a client or ex-client cannot enter into a business or secondary relationship with the therapist on an equal footing because there is the potential for a therapist to use confidential information maliciously. In addition, if a therapist is invited or compelled to offer testimony regarding some aspect of therapy, the existence of a dual relationship will undermine their credibility as a witness. Thus, as a general rule, it is best for psychologists to avoid dual relationships with clients altogether. Sometimes, though, clinical psychologists work in settings where it is not possible to entirely avoid dual relationships (see Chapter 14 for strategies on how to deal with dual relationships in a manner that does not compromise the well-being and dignity of the client).

One particular form of dual relationship that therapists need to be on their guard about is sexual relationships with their clients. For instance, the Canadian Psychological Association (2000) warns:

[The therapist should] be acutely aware of the power relationship in therapy and, therefore, not encourage or engage in sexual intimacy with therapy clients, neither during therapy, nor for that period of time following therapy during which the power relationship reasonably could be expected to influence the client's personal decision making. (p. 21)

If trainees find themselves in a situation where sexual tension or innuendo appears to be present during sessions with a client, the onus is on the trainee to immediately consult with a supervisor on how to resolve the situation and ensure that interactions with the client are refocused on the purposeful application of science-informed treatment strategies within the bounds of a caring and strictly professional relationship.

Although dual relationships are to be avoided, there are some situations in which avoidance becomes increasingly difficult. One such situation is in the context of clinical practice in rural or remote settings. The luxury of restricting the relationship between the clinical psychologist and the client to a purely professional one is often not possible in small rural towns, and therefore this special case will be examined in some depth in the following chapter.

Chapter 14

Working in rural and remote settings

Psychological practice in rural and remote settings involves several unique personal and professional challenges. Generally, very few psychology trainees are formally prepared for those challenges because curriculum components and supervised practice experiences tend to be focused on urban and metropolitan settings. Yet, in Australia, the proportion of relatively inexperienced psychologists with one to five years of experience who work in remote locations is twice that of more experienced psychologists (Mathews, 2011). Perhaps not surprisingly, historical shortages of speciality mental health professionals are a persistent problem in most rural communities (DeLeon, Wakefield, & Hagglund, 2003). For example, in Australia, nearly one third (31%) of the population lives outside major cities (Australian Bureau of Statistics, 2011), but only about 14.6% of all Australian psychologists work in those areas (Mathews, 2011).

Mental health services in rural communities

There is no consensus regarding the definitions of *rural* or *remote* as opposed to *metropolitan*, but a common characteristic of rural and remote communities is that they are descriptive of areas where the population density is low (US Census Bureau, 2002) and geographic distance imposes restrictions upon accessibility to the widest range of goods and services and opportunities for social interaction (Australian Bureau of Statistics, 2001). Long distances and harsh environmental conditions constitute significant barriers for rural residents to access mental health services (DeLeon et al., 2003). Likewise, delivering services to where they are needed by consumers can be a daunting routine if a home visit by a psychologist means driving several hundred kilometres (Lichte, 1996). If hospitalization for severely disturbed individuals is required, the logistics of transferring a client to an inpatient psychiatric unit, usually located in the nearest regional centre or city, create a considerable burden for the referring clinician as well as for clients and their families (Lichte, 1996). There also exist economic barriers to health care utilization in rural areas, because rural economies are fragile. They often depend on a single industry and are at the mercy of the uncontrollable whims of nature such as floods, draught, wildfires, frost, and hail (Barbopoulos & Clark, 2003). As a result, financial stresses among rural residents are common and health insurance coverage may be suboptimal.

In addition to these geographic and economic barriers to mental health service utilization, help-seeking behaviours are influenced by social context. Rural residents may be reluctant to seek help for psychological problems because of prevailing attitudes in rural areas to being self-reliant and considering talking about one's problems a luxury (Boyd et al., 2008;

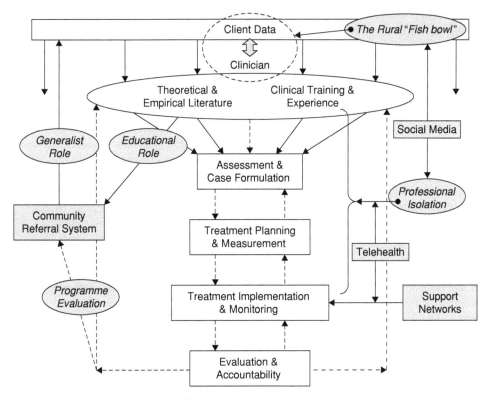

Figure 14.1 Applying the scientist-practitioner approach in rural practice.

Kennedy, Maple, McKay, & Brumby, 2014). The diminished degree of privacy in close-knit small communities can also heighten self-consciousness about seeking help for problems that are associated with social stigma such as mental illness, drug abuse, or domestic violence (Stamm et al., 2003). The high visibility and interconnectedness of individuals living in small communities is often likened to living in a 'fish bowl', which makes it impossible for anyone, including the local psychologist, to slip into anonymity (Dunbar, 1982). Psychology trainees who wish to gain experience in rural settings will need to learn to cope with a number of specific personal and professional challenges that living and working in the rural fish bowl present.

Maintaining professional boundaries in the rural fish bowl

The activities and associations of a small-town psychologist are under regular observation. Encounters with clients in the street, supermarket, post office, swimming pool, social clubs, school function, or any local event are inevitable, and those benign boundary crossings are a normal and healthy part of rural living (Malone, 2012). The highly visible public image of rural practitioners greatly curtails their personal privacy and affects the personal and professional lives of their families. Likewise, the opportunities for observing clients or potential clients outside the treatment context are enhanced, and the therapist may inadvertently learn more about a client from other clients since their social and professional lives are more intertwined in a small community (Hargrove, 1982). Figure 14.1 illustrates how this blurring of professional and personal roles affects the therapeutic process. The context of the rural fish bowl increases the likelihood that the client data available for inspection include information and affective reactions linked to the clinician's own personal and private life. This has the potential to both sharpen and blur the acuity of the expert lens through which the therapist filters client data for the purpose of case formulation.

Whereas urban-based ethical guidelines hold psychologists responsible for avoiding interactions with clients outside the therapy sessions, there are at least two reasons why 'rural practitioners must be careful *not* to ignore or avoid their clients outside of the therapy sessions' (Campbell & Gordon, 2003, p. 432, italics added). First, unlike their urban counterparts, rural psychologists typically do not have other colleagues to whom they could refer clients they personally know. Thus, avoiding dual relationships could mean depriving rural clients of the only specialist mental health service available to them. Second, to be effective, psychologists must first become part of the community (DeLeon et al., 2003). Their active community involvement is essential for lessening suspicion, increasing approachability, and ultimately gaining acceptance as the 'local' mental health expert (Schank & Skovholt, 1997). This is increasingly true if there are particular subcultures, racial minorities, or indigenous groups living in the area, and appropriate provision of services requires working as an ally with the community (Malone, 2012). Consequently, multiple non-sexual relationships in rural practice are not only expected, they are encouraged! (Campbell & Gordon, 2003). This blurring of professional and personal roles in rural practice requires that practitioners are particularly mindful of the ethical obligation to manage multiple relationships in a way that they do not impair the objectivity and effectiveness of the therapist or expose the client to exploitation or harm (American Psychological Association, 2002; Australian Psychological Society, 2003). The extent to which these ethical ambiguities are handled in a comfortable and competent manner may in large part determine the success of the rural practitioner (Hargrove, 1982).

Strategies for managing multiple relationships in rural practice

Because of the specific ethical demands that arise in rural settings, the standard principle of strict separation between personal and professional roles expected in urban practice cannot be applied automatically in rural practice. Several authors (Barbopoulos & Clark, 2003; Campbell & Gordon, 2003; Schank & Skovholt, 1997) have sought to address this ethical dilemma by offering a number of practical guidelines for how rural practitioners can manage multiple relationships in an ethical manner:

- *Compartmentalize roles and relationships.* This involves keeping different roles mentally separated when interacting with clients, and adopting a demeanour in line with the role relevant in a given instance. This allows the practitioner to be a professional helping expert one day, and a fellow parent at a school meeting the next. That is, in the latter situation, the practitioner can be warm and friendly while maintaining confidentiality, but will drop any air of the expert helper and will deliberately embrace a stance reflecting the situational context and purpose of the present contact. Relationships can also be separated in terms of degree of involvement. Shopping at a local grocery store where a client might be working constitutes less of a softening of boundaries than hiring a client (who may be the only electrician in town) to do some work in one's home. In the urban environment, boundaries usually are protected by the cloak of anonymity; in the rural setting, compartmentalizing private and professional roles means learning to wear the right hat for the right occasion.

- *Document overlapping relationships in case notes.* An important strategy to avoid the risk of boundary violations or the accidental disclosure of confidential information is to make explicit in the documentation of case progress the nature and details of overlapping relationships. This will help clinicians to keep original sources of information clear in their mind and minimize the risk of unintentional breaches of confidentiality.
- *Discuss out-of-therapy contact with clients upfront.* It is good practice to routinely discuss with clients at the start of treatment the high likelihood of out-of-therapy contact. Clients can be assured that every effort is made to respect their privacy during chance encounters and contacts that may even be predictable in a small community. Clients are given the opportunity to communicate how they feel about such encounters, how they intend to respond, and how they wish the therapist to respond.
- *Obtain informed consent.* As with explicit documentation of overlapping relationships in case notes, informed consent forms should include explicit mention of any multiple relationships and state that the client has been made aware of this issue when consenting to engage in treatment.
- *Educate clients about professional boundaries.* Clients should not be assumed to know what therapists mean by professional boundaries. It may be necessary to explain to some clients what a professional boundary is. This may take the following form: 'Because you are my client, you cannot be my friend. I listen to you, I care about you – but friends care about one another. But you don't come in so that I can sit down and tell you about my problems and my life. I don't call you when I am hurting or need a friend for support' (adapted from Schank & Skovholt, 1997, p. 47).
- *Stick to time limits.* Beginning and ending therapeutic contacts strictly within the designated appointment times helps to highlight the professional nature of the relationship.
- *Develop procedures that reduce accidental disclosures.* The exchange of information between professionals in a small community may require additional safeguards to protect client confidentiality. For example, files or reports sent to a physician in a hospital might be open to inspection by administrative or other staff who know the client or members of the client's family.
- *Monitor one's own comfort level.* If therapists experience discomfort with a dual relationship, that can compromise their objectivity and effectiveness. For example, a therapist might learn that her daughter is bringing a friend home after school who also happens to be a client of the therapist. The therapist has to weigh competing ethical choices: protect the client's confidentiality and cope with the personal discomfort, or break confidentiality by restricting whom her daughter can have as friends. Which choice is in the best interest of the client depends on the therapist's ability to compartmentalize the relationships and manage her level of discomfort while remaining therapeutically effective.
- *Put client's needs first.* Therapists need to reflect about their motives for maintaining dual relationships, so that clients are not used inadvertently for one's own gratification or exploitive purposes.
- *Imagine the worst case scenario.* In deciding whether or not it is in the client's best interest to maintain a dual relationship, it can be very instructive to consider the

possible harm that could stem from the relationship not only in the present but also in the future.

- *Monitor the 'slippery slope' phenomenon.* Boundary compromises that seem minor in isolation can have cumulative effects and lead to more substantial boundary violations.
- *Monitor warning signs of role–boundary conflicts.* It is essential to be aware of any changes in the nature of interactions in overlapping relationships. Is there more self-disclosure by the therapist? Is there greater anticipation of meeting with a client? Does the therapist feel a desire to prolong a session with a client or increase the frequency of meetings with the client? Is the therapist reluctant to terminate or refer a client? Does the therapist want to please or impress a client? Affirmative answers to these questions indicated an increased potential for role–boundary conflicts in multiple relationships.
- *Terminate overlapping relationships as soon as possible.* Prompt termination of multiple relationships following the conclusion of their primary purpose is in the client's best interest.
- *Seek consultation.* Because of the professional isolation of rural psychologists which limits the opportunities for ad hoc consultation with colleagues regarding ethical issues, the onus is on the psychologist to make special efforts (e.g., using telecommunication or internet tools) to maintain links with other professionals who can provide feedback on ethical decision-making.

Coping with professional isolation

Ethical decision-making is not the only aspect of rural practice affected by professional isolation. As shown in Figure 14.1, the rural psychologist must deliver the core clinical tasks of applying science-informed, up-to-date knowledge and skills to case formulation and treatment planning often without easy access to consultation from other mental health experts, state-of-the-art diagnostic and treatment resources, or continuing education (Stamm et al., 2003). It is therefore essential that rural practitioners learn to practise independently with minimal support from colleagues within their own discipline, and be comfortable with assuming ultimate responsibility for decisions concerning case management (Lichte, 1996). On some occasions this might mean working under conditions well beyond what they were prepared to do (Gibb, Livesey, & Zyla, 2003). As a back-up, rural practitioners must become familiar with what clinical services are available in the nearest metropolitan area and develop procedures for facilitating long distance referrals (Keller & Prutsman, 1982). Although working in relative isolation is demanding and can lead to professional burnout, there are also positive features associated with isolation including a greater sense of autonomy and opportunities to respond to community circumstances with a great deal of flexibility and creativity (Wolfenden, 1996). Moreover, as technological innovations and opportunities are continuing to advance, the impact of professional isolation on the ground can be at least in part overcome by seeking professional consultation via the internet.

Telehealth

The advent of sophisticated telecommunication technology is increasingly providing rural practitioners with alternative means to overcome some of the barriers associated with professional isolation. Figure 14.1 indicates how the application of telehealth facilities can moderate the impact of professional isolation in the delivery of psychological services. Telehealth refers to 'the use of telecommunications and information technology to provide access to health screening, assessment, diagnosis, intervention, consultation, supervision, education, and information across distance' (Farell & McKinnon, 2003, p. 20). Telehealth has improved the provision of care to underserved and isolated communities considerably, and its potential to do so will increase as the 'digital divide' between urban and rural areas continues to narrow in the immediate coming years (Comer & Barlow, 2014). For example, in Australia, the national Suicide Call Back Service (see www.suicidecallbackservice.org.au/) uses telephony and web-based technologies to provide professional, suicide-specific mental health care services available 24 hours a day, all year round.

As the opportunities for the practice of telehealth are rapidly expanding, there is an urgent need for professional organizations and regulatory bodies to catch up with the digital revolution (Comer & Barlow, 2014). Standards are needed to resolve legal and regulatory issues of providing care at a distance across state lines and different jurisdictions, as well as supervision for trainees without professionals licensed in their field being physically present (Stamm, 2003). In the meantime, it is incumbent upon psychologists to be aware of and comply with standards or practice for the jurisdiction(s) in which they engage in telepsychology activities. The Joint Task Force for the Development of Telepsychology Guidelines for Psychologists (2013) has recently published guidelines to assist psychologists in adapting to the new challenges arising from technology-based mental health service provision. Psychologists must consider patient preferences and assess and communicate any risks and benefits of services delivered via telepsychology, including those arising from issues related to privacy and safety of the remote environment in which the patient receives the services. New challenges also arise in protecting the security of patient data and information when relying on telecommunication technologies, and from managing professional boundaries in an ethical manner when the potential scope and reach of patient–therapist contact is not limited to the traditional consulting room and working hours. Avoiding boundary violations requires even more vigilance if psychologists use social media for both professional and personal purposes (Kolmes, 2012). In a practice environment where video-conferencing, smart mobile devices, cloud computing, and virtual applications are increasingly utilized, the challenge of today's clinical psychology trainees is to make themselves more relevant in the evolving technological health care marketplace (Maheu, Pulier, McMenamin, & Posen, 2012), while avoiding errors in judgement in their online professionalism which have led to serious disciplinary actions (e.g., Greysen, Chretien, Kind, Young, & Gross, 2012). Nonetheless, the telephone, email and web-based applications, and mobile communication devices are promising to ameliorate the isolation of rural mental health professionals and thereby improve direct patient care and opportunities for consultation, supervision, and continuing education (Miller et al., 2003; Wood, Miller, & Hargrove, 2005). Importantly, telehealth can also be instrumental in moderating the impact of professional isolation by facilitating the use of informal support networks and multidisciplinary collaboration (see Figure 14.1).

Incorporating natural support networks and multidisciplinary care

The relative scarcity of mental health resources in rural regions makes coordination with medical practitioners, social services, law enforcement agencies, educational institutions, religious communities, and informal support systems imperative (Stamm et al., 2003). As mentioned earlier, rural residents often feel reluctant to seek help for mental health problems. In one study, of those who had screened positive for depression, anxiety, and alcohol abuse disorders, and who had received education about the respective disorders and available treatment services, 81% failed to seek help because they 'felt that there was no need to' (Fox, Blank, Rovnyak, & Barnett, 2001). Of those who had sought help for mental health problems in the past year, most approached a friend or family member rather than a psychologist or physician (Fox et al., 2001). By tapping into such natural support networks during treatment planning, the isolated professional can extend the reach of continuing care. Of course, before family members and friends are co-opted in any treatment plan, it is important to determine to what extent the social group is creating or exacerbating the presenting problems of the patient (Dunbar, 1982). Similarly, paraprofessionals and volunteers for crisis counselling and similar adjunct services can be a valuable resource, but care must be taken in selection, training, and supervision of those informal helpers (Heyman & VandenBos, 1989).

Traditionally, most rural psychology is practised by professionals without expertise in advanced psychological skills, such as physicians, nurses, welfare workers, teachers, and clergy (Wolfenden, 1996). Developing partnerships with those established mental health service providers in rural communities is particularly important. By collaborating with established agencies and community referral systems (see Figure 14.1), the psychological expert can engage their familiarity and credibility to contribute quality mental health care to the community (Sears, Evans, & Kuper, 2003). Depending on available resources and local circumstances, such multidisciplinary collaboration may involve informal contacts or coordinated links between referral systems, or even integrated partnerships with sharing of resources, personnel, and responsibilities for development of service delivery systems (Lewis, 2001; Sears et al., 2003). Thus, the development of consultancy skills is an essential prerequisite for psychologists in rural settings. Rural psychologists need to educate the community about the unique expertise that psychologists bring to patient care, and they need to be prepared to provide consultancy services for a broad range of community needs and problems.

Rural psychologists have an important *educational role*. Community education involves expanding the appreciation of what psychologists have to offer, reducing the stigma and misinformation associated with mental disorders, and providing information on how to achieve and maintain optimal health (Lichte, 1996; Wolfenden, 1996). In addition, rural psychologists can address the relative lack of professional development opportunities in rural settings by offering information sessions and workshops for other mental health workers (Barbopoulos & Clark, 2003). Similarly, rural psychologists can help inform laypersons and self-help groups by organizing public presentations and community events related to mental health. They should liaise with community leaders and elders, including religious institutions, to promote psychological approaches for bringing relief to people who experience personal crises and suffering. Enlisting the sponsorship of these influential members of the community helps to gain the trust of rural residents and establish the psychologist as a valuable participant in addressing local needs.

Perhaps the best advertising for psychological services is first-hand experience of what the psychologist does (Wolfenden, 1996). One thing that psychologists are trained to do particularly well, and that sets them apart from most other mental health professionals, is applying research skills to applied problems such as the design and implementation of *programme evaluation* studies. For example, rural practitioners can play a critical part in developing prevention and outreach programmes or crisis response teams (Barbopoulos & Clark, 2003). Many rural mental health services have few, if any, staff resources in this area. By virtue of their training as scientist-practitioners, psychologists will be called upon to contribute their expertise in selecting the appropriate techniques from the programme evaluation literature and measuring the success of target outcomes (Sears et al., 2003). This important role of the rural psychologist as a programme evaluator is illustrated in Figure 14.1 by the additional feedback loop linking the 'Evaluation & Accountability' component of the model to 'Community Referral Systems'. Particularly in the present era of accountability, these evaluations will be useful in supporting efforts of a community to lobby for additional resources to support local health care services.

However, the specialist knowledge and skills of the psychologist are not sufficient for being a successful rural practitioner. In light of the scarcity of mental health professionals in rural settings, psychologists can achieve maximum utility with practical patient outcomes only if they are able to respond to a wide range of problems across people of all ages, types, and backgrounds (Sears et al., 2003). In addition to dealing with adult psychopathology, the clinical activities include relationship and family counselling, behavioural management programmes for children or individuals with disabilities, care of rape and domestic violence victims, critical incident management, and a host of other problems. Rural psychologists may also find themselves acting as social workers, housing advocates, or liaison officers between distressed individuals and other community agencies. In other words, the effective rural psychologist above all fulfils a *generalist role* (see Figure 14.1). Of course, it is desirable for a generalist to have a wide repertoire of skills, but more important is that 'the generalist has a method of intervention that can provide a guide and framework into most any situation' (Dunbar, 1982, p. 63). As we have illustrated throughout this manual, and again in Figure 14.1 in this chapter, a scientist-practitioner approach serves as a reliable framework for adapting one's practice to the particular professional challenges one might encounter in any situation or setting, including those presented by working in the rural fish bowl. A science-informed practitioner of clinical psychology is also well placed to extend their professional role beyond the traditional focus on 'mental' health into the broader domain of general health care. Thus, the final chapter will consider these newer frontiers of clinical psychology.

Chapter 15

Psychologists as health care providers

The role of psychology in health care delivery has undergone a dramatic sea change. Joseph Matarazzo's (1980) vision over three decades ago, that 'some of what is today called clinical psychology will soon be labeled health psychology' (p. 815), is now reality. Clinical psychologists today increasingly will need to be competent to function in the broader context of *health service psychology* (HSPEC, 2013). The core identity of clinical psychologists has broadened from the traditional focus on 'mental health' to a professional role that brings psychological expertise to the maintenance and restoration of 'health' more generally (American Psychological Association, 2005). In the second decade of the new millennium the pace of this change has further accelerated with major health care reform agendas being implemented in a number of developed countries such as the No Health Without Mental Health strategy in the United Kingdom (HM Government, 2011), integrated health care models in the context of the Patient Protection and Affordable Care Act in the United States (US Department of Health & Human Services, 2010), and the Better Access to Mental Health initiative in Australia (Australian Government Department of Health, 2013). These ongoing reforms mark the dawn of a new era in health care delivery where there is greater recognition that mental health issues substantially contribute to the burden of disease worldwide (Prince et al., 2007), yet the majority of affected individuals do not receive any treatment for their condition, and of those who do receive care, less than one third are treated by a mental health care professional (Comer & Barlow, 2014).

Among the ten leading causes of illness in industrialized nations are lifestyle behaviours such as smoking, poor diet, lack of exercise, alcohol misuse, sexual behaviour, and illicit drug use (Johnson, 2003). In addition to health threats associated with these behaviours (e.g., cardiovascular diseases, cancer, HIV/AIDS), health and illness are influenced by psychological factors such as stress, positive and negative emotional states, beliefs and coping styles, and social relationships (Compare et al., 2013; Salovey, Rothman, Detweiler, & Steward, 2000; Stowell, McGuire, Robles, Glaser, & Kiecolt-Glaser, 2003). It is now well documented that psychological interventions targeting these factors can make a significant contribution to the prevention and treatment of medical conditions, as well as the promotion of healing (Christensen & Nezu, 2013; Nicassio, Meyerowitz, & Kerns, 2004; Schein, Bernard, Spitz, & Muskin, 2003). As noted by Belar (2012), psychological service provision is relevant to each and every one of the health conditions listed in the International Classification of Diseases (ICD-10; World Health Organization, 2010). The essential role of mental health in achieving health for all people has recently been confirmed in the WHO's (2013) Mental Health Action Plan 2013–2020, which articulates a clear vision of 'parity of esteem' (HM Government, 2011, p. 2) between mental and physical health services. These comprehensive, global reform agendas for mental health care have major implications for the training of clinical psychologists. A clinical psychologist needs to be prepared to add value within a health care environment that will be increasingly characterized by integrated, patient-centred, accountable, and efficient systems of care, including a greater emphasis on health promotion, primary and secondary prevention (Belar, 2012), and economic incentives to keep people healthy (Kelly & Coons, 2012).

Evolving parameters of psychological service delivery

Towards integrated, patient-centred care

Prominent in the redesign of health care systems is the spread of integrated care models, where health care is comprehensive, continuous, coordinated, culturally competent, and consumer centred (Kelly & Coons, 2012). This includes a greater emphasis on mental health promotion, early intervention in crises, and accessible community-based care. At the heart of the integrated approach is the notion of 'one stop' care in settings such as Patient Centred Medical Homes in the United States (see www.pcpcc.org/) or Medicare Locals in Australia (see www.medicarelocals.gov.au/internet/medicarelocals/publishing.nsf#.Us4DQrSE71U), where primary and speciality service providers are co-located in the same premises providing team-based care. This goes beyond multidisciplinary care where diverse health professionals add their individual ingredients of expertise to a consultative meal. Integrated care involves interprofessional teamwork, communication, and team-based decision-making in all aspects of patient care. In such a care environment, patients encounter psychologists as members of the team, often in the form of a 'warm hand off', where a primary care provider introduces and transfers patient care to the 'behavioural specialist' while the patients present for their primary care appointment (Cubic, Mance, Turgesen, & Lamanna, 2012).

Evidence-based care and accountability are here to stay

Accountable health care is measured in terms of both the effectiveness of interventions to achieve optimal health outcomes, and the relative economic value of alternative interventions within the context of competing models of health care delivery, funding, and reimbursement.

Competitive health care is care that reliably improves health outcomes at a cost the market will bear, and that satisfies the consumer (i.e., the patient). The scientist-practitioner training, with its emphasis on science-informed practice, outcome evaluation, and ongoing quality improvement in service delivery, provides precisely the skills needed for clinical psychologists to add value to health care in the context of interdisciplinary care settings. However, for clinical psychologists to become established as health care providers on a par with medical professionals, they need to make adjustments to their traditional modes of delivering psychological treatments. This includes an understanding of the health care marketplace, a focus on good enough treatment, an investment in consumer education and marketing of services, and a willingness to embrace the culture and pace of integrated care settings (Kiesler, 2000).

To be competitive in the health care marketplace, providers – including psychologists – need to offer evidenced-based, cost-effective services with measurable outcomes (Kelly & Coons, 2012), increasingly in accordance with national guidelines for quality standards (e.g., NICE; see www.nice.org.uk/guidance/qualitystandards/qualitystandards.jsp), or in-novative reimbursement structures such as Accountable Care Organizations (AOCs; www.cms.gov/Medicare/Medicare-Fee-for-Service-Payment/ACO/index.html?redirect=/ACO). In the traditional fee-for-service model, practitioners tend to treat patients over an ex-tended period of time, without requirements to account for outcome or length of treatment (Sanchez & Turner, 2003). In such a system, there is no incentive for cost-effective treatment, because the more services are offered the higher the income for the provider. The resulting escalation of mental health care costs led to the emergence of various managed care systems. Although these systems vary considerably in the type of cost-control strategies used (e.g., limit number of sessions, reduce fees for services, provide financial rewards for efficient and effective care), and in the extent to which they have private or public sector involve-ment, they all involve some kind of *capitation*. That is, the demand for services by a specific number of patients (or potential patients) is predicted for a given period of time, and a fixed amount of money is allocated to meet that demand (Tovian, 2004). In contrast to a fee-for-service system, a pay for performance model includes financial penalties and rewards (Kelly & Coons, 2012). That is, the risk is shared between provider and payer, and simply offering more services does not generate more income for the provider. Instead, incentives are geared towards care that produces quality outcomes with high efficiency. Thus, cost containment strategies and capitation together with integrated care models are designed to rein in uncon-trolled escalation of overall health care costs by improving quality and efficiency of services for a greater number of people. From a public health perspective, this is desirable, but cost cutting must be balanced with optimal patient outcomes, because failure to adequately treat mental health conditions impacts service utilization and costs in every area of primary and speciality health care (Gray, Brody, & Johnson, 2005).

Competition for health care resources is therefore not so much an issue of who costs the least, but rather who adds value (Kiesler, 2000), where value is a function of optimal treatment outcomes achieved in a time-limited, resource-efficient manner for the greatest number of people. By virtue of their scientist-practitioner training, psychologists are par-ticularly well prepared to function in such an empirically based service system. The value of psychological services must be communicated via information feedback loops between the data generated by routine outcome evaluation and both the system managing health care costs, and the consumer determining demand (see Figure 15.1). The main difference to traditional outcome assessment is that psychologists must not only show that treatment works, but that it is cost-effective. *Cost-effectiveness* compares the costs of an intervention with the amount of improvement in health status (Kaplan & Groessl, 2002). Improvement is evaluated in relation to specified treatment goals and against standard criteria of normal functioning in a normative comparison group. *Cost-offset* compares the costs of an interven-tion with the costs saved elsewhere in the health care system as a result of that intervention, independent of the amount of improvement in health status (Kaplan & Groessl, 2002). For example, a programme to achieve weight loss may reduce a patient's number of visits to a hypertension clinic or eliminate the need for hypertension medication. If the reduction in visits and medication saves more money than it costs to run the weight loss programme, a cost-offset has been achieved. There is robust evidence that psychological interventions can produce medical cost-offset effects, especially in the context of surgical procedures (Chiles, Lambert, & Hatch, 1999). Although the demonstration of cost-offset can enhance the value of psychological services, the goal of treatment is not to save money, but to improve health. Indeed, if health status is unaffected by treatment, the cost of that treatment amounts to

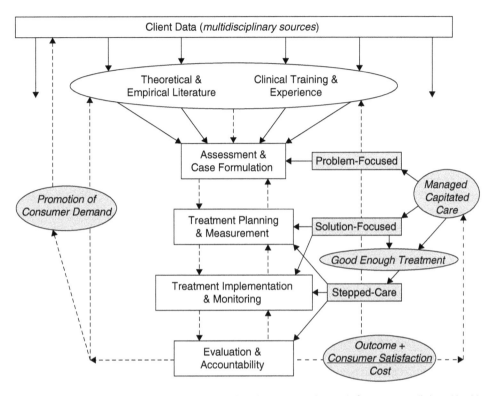

Figure 15.1 The scientist-practitioner approach to clinical practice is tailor-made for an empirically based health care system.

waste of limited health care resources. For example, in the US more than 650,000 arthro-scopic surgeries for osteoarthritis of the knee are performed at a cost of over three billion dollars annually, but carefully controlled trials showed that this intervention did not achieve any better pain relief or improvement in function than a placebo procedure (Kirkley et al., 2008; Moseley et al., 2002). This creates an opportunity cost problem (Kaplan & Groessl, 2002). The billions of dollars spent on ineffective surgeries for pain relief are not available to non-surgical interventions that may have a superior evidence base (e.g., Gatchel, 2005). In the competition for health care resources, the onus is on psychologists to build on their strengths as scientist-practitioners and demonstrate that their treatments provide value for money, and that they add unique value as part of multidisciplinary health care settings at the primary, secondary, and tertiary levels of care (Tovian, 2004).

Psychologists add value to integrated care

About three out of four mental health patients are treated by primary care physicians (Hickie, Groom, McGorry, Davenport, & Luscombe, 2005; Olfson et al., 2002), but evidence suggests that only a minority of patients receive adequate treatment at the primary level of care (Gray et al., 2005). For example, general practitioners fail to accurately recognize common mental disorders in 30–70% of patients who have a psychological problem (Coyne, Thompson, Klinkman, & Nease, 2002; Hickie et al., 2005; Sanchez & Turner, 2003), and they often fail to follow up or adjust treatment (Gray et al., 2005), or may even overprescribe psychotropic medications (Coyne et al., 2002). With the advent of new medications for depression such as selective serotonin reuptake inhibitors (SSRIs), there has been a dramatic increase in the percentage of primary mental health patients receiving medication (Medco Health Solutions, 2011), while the percentage of patients receiving psychological treatments declined (Gray et al., 2005). This is despite evidence that psychological treatments alone or combined treatments achieve superior treatment outcomes than pharmacotherapy alone, if one takes into account that psychological treatments are more effective at preventing relapse or recurrence of depression (Pettit, Voelz, & Joiner, 2001), and prolonged use of antidepressants can even worsen depression (Fava, 2003; Fava & Offidani, 2011). Thus, integrating mental health specialist services in primary care does not only add value by achieving better health outcomes, but integrated care is estimated to reduce health care costs by 20–30% (Gray et al., 2005). Importantly, when primary care physicians and mental health specialists operate as a team within the same setting, the number of referrals for psychological services that are followed through by the patient have been found to increase eightfold (Cummings, 1999). However, for psychologists to become valued players on integrated health care teams, they need to tailor their interventions and strategies to the needs and circumstances of general practice and hospital settings.

As indicated in Figure 15.1, it is important in the initial encounters with patients to be *problem-focused*, so that assessment information is relevant to the specific referral question within the context of other assessment data contributed by different members of the multidisciplinary team (Haley et al., 1998). Likewise, treatment planning and implementation must be *solution-focused*, because in medical settings results are expected far more quickly than in traditional mental health settings. Finally, the need to balance optimal care with efficient utilization of health care resources means that the modal form of treatment is guided by the concept of *good enough treatment.* As Kiesler (2000) noted, good enough treatment is guided by three principles: (a) no treatment is perfect, (b) more treatment might achieve better outcomes, but would do so at the expense of other patients who would miss out on care because the amount of available resources is finite, and (c) treatment to relieve acute distress and avoid relapse is sufficient under the circumstances. Moreover, not all patients need the same type and intensity of treatment. One way to ensure that patients receive all the care they need, but not more, is through the application of *stepped care* models. Davison (2000) described stepped care as 'the practice of beginning one's therapeutic efforts with the least expensive and least intrusive intervention possible and moving on to more expensive and/or more intrusive interventions only if deemed necessary in order to achieve a desired therapeutic goal' (p. 580). A stepped care approach is readily compatible with the purposeful planning, monitoring, and modification of treatment strategies inherent in the scientist-practitioner approach to clinical practice (see Figure 15.1). The psychologist simply needs to increase attention to the concept of good enough treatment to maximize efficiency of resource allocation (Haaga, 2000).

One example of how psychologists add value to integrated care by applying a focused set of treatment strategies within a stepped care framework is the treatment of hypertension. The first step in the sequential implementation of graded interventions involves the initiation of lifestyle modifications such as physical activity, weight loss, smoking cessation, and stress management (Blumenthal, Sherwood, Gullette, Georgiades, & Tweedy, 2002). For instance, a weight loss of as little as five to eight kilograms can produce clinically meaningful reductions in blood pressure (Blumenthal et al., 2002; Smith & Hopkins, 2003). If the lifestyle modifications fail to achieve blood pressure values within the desired range, adherence to the treatment regimen will be assessed, and care may be 'stepped up' by introducing a low dose of medications such as diuretics or beta-blockers. If response is still inadequate or side-effects are experienced, another drug might be substituted or a second drug from a different class might be added. Thus, ongoing treatment decisions of stepping up or stepping down care are directly informed by the degree of satisfactory progress a patient makes. Psychological interventions add value because they can reduce or eliminate the need for medications in some patients, and they can improve poor rates of treatment adherence at every level or type of treatment modality (Blumenthal et al., 2002).

Another example of how psychologists can add value to integrated care involves the stepped care approach to pain management. We mentioned earlier the poor outcomes of some very costly surgical procedures to alleviate knee pain (Kirkley et al., 2008; Moseley et al., 2002). In a stepped care approach, less costly and intrusive interventions should be attempted first. With respect to pain management, the first step is a brief, one-off psychological intervention addressing patients' fears and beliefs about their pain to help them adjust to and manage their pain while returning to regular daily activities (Otis, Reid, & Kerns, 2005). For patients who do not improve after a few weeks, care can be stepped up to include multiple visits to providers from different disciplines (e.g., psychologists, physical therapists, physicians) to initiate structured activity programmes, practise cognitive behavioural coping strategies, or prescribe pain medication to assist patients with resuming work and recreational involvement. Only if these less intense interventions fail to bring about improvement, or if the initial assessment indicates a high risk of becoming permanently disabled, Step 3 interventions should be considered. These may include surgical techniques and more intense speciality services often within multidisciplinary pain management centres (Gatchel, 2005; Otis et al., 2005).

Value adding to health care delivery based on a stepped care model is also increasingly achieved by implementing broad health workforce reforms such as the Improving Access to Psychological Therapies (IAPT) initiative in the UK (HM Department of Health, 2012). The aim is to increase availability of first tier treatment providers who require less training (and hence less pay) to deliver low-intensity, evidence-based interventions for the most common mental health conditions (i.e., anxiety and depression disorders). Only individuals who fail to respond adequately to the low-intensity interventions (e.g., guided self-help or computerized CBT) will be stepped up to higher intensity interventions such as face-to-face therapy sessions delivered by higher qualified (and hence more costly) service providers (Clark, 2011). The rationale is that allocating a larger share of limited health care resources to the broad dissemination of evidence-based treatments for the most prevalent mental health problems will improve health outcomes for a majority of treatment seekers. The initial outcomes of the IAPT programme are impressive. After the first three years, a competent workforce of nearly 4,000 new practitioners was trained delivering NICE-recommended treatments to over one million people, with recovery rates in excess of 45% and economic gains of over 45,000 people moving off sick pay and welfare support (HM Department of Health, 2012).

The British example of successfully initiating rapid growth of a large skilled mental health workforce delivering effective interventions with demonstrable economic benefits will provide added momentum to similar sweeping reforms to health workforce models under way in other countries (e.g., Health Workforce Australia, 2011). A substitute psychology workforce (Littlefield, 2012), requiring shorter training courses and less qualified to provide the full range of psychological services, will become preferred providers for less complex, manualized treatments within a structure of ongoing supervision and session-by-session outcome monitoring systems (e.g., Clark, 2011). These reforms constitute a seismic paradigm shift in a new way of thinking about sustainable health care design and planning to meet current and future health workforce demands, 'one that works backwards from outcomes for communities, consumers and population need, versus the current thinking that is generally focused on working forward from the base of existing professions and their interests and skills, demarcations and responsibilities' (Health Workforce Australia, 2011, p. 5). Clinical psychologists are well positioned to flourish in this new health care world and can add value to mental health care delivery. However, their role in reformed health care systems will be alongside a range of practitioners across and within professions, including an army of mental health workers less qualified but nonetheless effective within the scope of their targeted training and low-intensity service provision for certain mild to moderate conditions (Clark, 2011).

This push towards more integrated, generalist models of care means that clinical psychology training must be adapted to produce more generalists to match workforce demands. However, at the same time, there remains a vital need for those competencies that are needed to deliver speciality care for the more complex or less prevalent conditions (Comer & Barlow, 2014). That is, a practitioner workforce strong in generalist skills, or trained in focused skills targeted for providing front-line care to the less intense, common conditions, may not be sufficient to address the full spectrum of the burden of mental illness. Health service psychologists, therefore, encompass competencies as both primary care professionals and as speciality care professionals (Health Service Psychology Education Collaborative, 2013). Comer and Barlow (2014) envision a range of psychological stepped care options which at the initial level include low-intensity, technology-based options with minimal therapist involvement, followed by direct care from a generalist provider, and then direct care from a generalist provider with consultation from a specialist, and then at the highest step direct care from a specialist. As technological innovations are beginning to transform health care delivery, behavioural telehealth care models are likely to have a vital role at each level of stepped care in direct service provision, consultation, and supervision. The core scientist-practitioner training provides psychologists with a solid base from which to venture into this changing health care market. However, there are a number of specific, practical tips emerging from the evolving field of psychology as a broader health care profession on how psychologists need to adapt their repertoire of skills to provide quality services in primary care and other medical settings.

Psychologists need specific skills to adapt to integrated care settings

1. Psychologists need to provide effective interventions expeditiously

Focus on the presenting problem or referral question. Clinical psychologists traditionally have been trained to conduct thorough assessments by obtaining information from lengthy interviews and extensive psychometric testing. In medical settings, psychologists must be able to assess presenting problems far more quickly and offer practical recommendations immediately (Gatchel & Oordt, 2003). There may be no more than two treatment contacts in inpatient settings, and typically six or fewer contacts in outpatient settings (Cubic et al., 2012). Across OECD countries, the average length of inpatient admissions is about 7 days, and only 5 days in Australia or the United States (OECD Health Data, 2013).

Rather than working within a standard 50-minute session schedule, initial appointments rarely exceed 25 to 30 minutes, with follow-up visits typically lasting between 15 and

20 minutes (Rowan & Runyan, 2005). Moreover, the initial appointment is not all reserved for assessment, but swiftly moves towards the initiation of an intervention. Rowan and Runyan (2005) recommend five phases for conducting a highly structured initial evaluation appointment:

- *Introduction* (1–2 minutes). This is a well-rehearsed statement to clarify the psychologist's role on the health care team, the purpose of the appointment, and the nature of information that will be documented in the patient's medical record. A brochure with the same information may be handed to the patient at the same time for future reference.
- *Bridge to assessment* (10–30 seconds). The bridge usually is a sentence or two that serves to direct the patient's attention straight to the referral question or primary presenting problem (e.g., 'Dr. Morgan was concerned about the recent increase in your blood pressure and was wondering how your everyday behaviours and activities might contribute to it. What does a typical week look like for you in terms of physical activity, eating patterns, or daily stress?'). A purposely vague bridge (e.g., 'What brings you here today?') is less useful, because it is likely to invite responses that stray too much from the referral problem.
- *Assessment* (10–15 minutes). Assessment of the patient's symptoms and daily functioning is focused on the referral question. To identify possible avenues for appropriate interventions, it is important to also assess strengths and strategies that have helped the patient in the past to alleviate or manage the impact of the presenting problem, as well as any barriers that might render particular psychological treatments less likely to succeed.
- *Bridge to intervention* (1–2 minutes). This bridge is a brief summary of the most critical parts of the assessment information, how they link to the presenting problem, and what interventions have proven successful in treating this type of problem. Building on any helpful strategies the patient is already using well can enhance rapport and readiness to engage in change.
- *Intervention* (5–10 minutes). Intervention strategies should be concrete, practical, and easy to implement after minimal instruction. They should be aimed at producing tangible symptom reduction or improvement in functioning soon after treatment commenced. Because opportunities for in-session education and demonstration of techniques are only brief, therapists have an extensive array of sufficiently detailed, stand-alone handouts and 'self-help' materials ready for patients to take with them. They may also use 'behavioural prescription' pads to outline the treatment plan and associated patient tasks.

Follow-up appointments are variable in length and help to establish momentum for change. They can be as brief as five minutes, if progress and current presentation of the patient reveal no need for more intense intervention or consultation.

Be decisive with limited data. Sheridan & Radmacher (2003) noted that the great time pressures, the flood of information from multiple sources and people, and the distracting stimuli typical of medical environments may be stretching the health care provider's capacity to process information accurately and efficiently. Hence, the ability to arrive at a correct diagnostic impression and intervention plan under those circumstances requires that psychologists adapt to the rapid pace of medical settings and learn to make efficient use of the brief time available with each patient (Gatchel & Oordt, 2003). Just as psychologists need to be comfortable with the principle of good enough treatment, they need to be tolerant of gaps in the data guiding their decision-making during case conceptualization and treatment planning. This process can be greatly facilitated by the judicious use of brief, validated psychometric instruments relevant to the particular aspects of a presenting problem (Gatchel & Oordt, 2003).

Fill your toolbox with effective short-term treatments. Considering the practicalities of integrated care settings, the modal form of treatment will be solution-focused and brief (Kiesler, 2000; Sanchez & Turner, 2003). Hence, students should strive to develop an extensive repertoire of behavioural and cognitive behavioural short-term strategies. These include approaches such as Screening, Brief Intervention, and Referral to Treatment (SBIRT; SAMHSA, 2014) and the 5 A's model (e.g., Kaner, Newbury-Birch, & Heather, 2009). The five A's refer to *ask* about the problem, *advice* to change the problem using clear personalized feedback, *assess* willingness to change, *assist* to change, and *arrange* follow-up and support. Motivational interviewing skills are core components of these brief intervention approaches.

Become an expert in motivational interviewing techniques. Medical patients are often reluctant to engage in action-oriented lifestyle changes (Gatchel & Oordt, 2003). Brief motivational interventions can enhance a patient's readiness to make the recommended changes and become an active partner in their own treatment. As with other interventions in medical settings, the constraints on time and the limited number of patient contacts require that motivational interviewing is adapted to a briefer format, sometimes referred to as 'brief negotiation' (Resnicow et al., 2002). Whether it is the adoption of lifestyle changes or adherence to medication regimens, treatment compliance is a common problem. Sheridan and Radmacher (2003) list the following principles for encouraging treatment compliance:

- Interact with patients in a warm, empathic manner.
- View patient as a key partner in the treatment team.
- Be specific with your instructions and make sure they are understood.
- Explain why you are confident that the treatment plan will be effective.
- Provide skills training when appropriate.
- Arrange for social support when appropriate.
- Provide praise for effort and for actual compliance.
- Use at-home reminders.
- Anticipate barriers to compliance and help patients cope with them.
- Monitor compliance in a caring, respectful manner.

2. Psychologists need to be good team players

Accept all referrals. Good integrated care depends on good interprofessional collaboration (Cubic et al., 2012). In a team-based environment everyone needs to pull their weight. Psychologists in medical settings are expected to attend to all behavioural and psychosocial aspects of general health care (Gatchel & Oordt, 2003). To the extent that they are willing and able to meet those expectations, they will be regarded as a valuable asset to the team. In fact, psychologists should not just wait for patients to come to them, but they should actively promote their services and enhance the visibility of the broad range of interventions they offer (Haley et al., 1998).

Communicate clearly and frequently. As participants in interprofessional care, psychologists must be mindful of the formal and informal ways by which information is exchanged and documented (American Psychological Association, 2013). Communication occurs during onsite patient encounters, team meetings, phone or email consultations, and via medical record systems. Psychologists must understand and speak the languages of diverse care providers, and in turn communicate psychological concepts in a manner useful to other professionals. This also requires familiarity with using succinct technical terms which are routinely abbreviated for rapid communications based on Latin phrases such as 'PRN' for 'as needed' or 'PO' for 'by mouth' (Kelly & Coons, 2012). Psychologists must make sure that their interventions are in sync with the treatment objectives of other members in the team. According to Gatchel and Oordt (2003), good communication with medical colleagues involves (a) getting to the point quickly, (b) avoiding psychological lingo and jargon, (c) keeping documentation succinct, (d) giving feedback promptly, and (e) expressing one's perspective confidently, but not being offended if one's advice is not taken on board by other team members. It is also important to avoid ambiguity when responding to requests for input and always clarify what the specific referral question is (Haley et al., 1998).

Be sensitive to and tolerant of hierarchical team structures. Physicians typically have the final say in treatment matters. Medical appointments often take precedence over non-medical (even scheduled) activities. For example, patients participating in a small group session on stress management may be pulled out for medical tests without prior notice.

Be flexible and available. Psychologists need to establish ways of being reachable when not in the office and should be willing to respond to calls for assistance without delay whenever possible. This might also mean interrupting the 'sanctity' of the treatment session, which psychologists are accustomed to when working in traditional mental health clinics (Gatchel & Oordt, 2003).

3. Psychologists need to gain familiarity with 'all things medical'

Become knowledgeable about physical conditions, medical procedures, and medications. When working on the psychological components of a patient's treatment plan, it is essential that psychologists remain mindful of the patient's experience with physical disability and suffering (France et al., 2008; Haley et al., 1998). They should develop a basic understanding of the symptoms associated with common health problems and the procedures and medications to treat them (Gatchel & Oordt, 2003). Because patients presenting with psychological symptoms in integrated care settings may first be assessed by a psychologist, it is important that psychologists are able to obtain a brief medical history (Robinson & James, 2005). This is important because psychological symptoms can mask the presence of certain medical disorders. A brief set of questions can be incorporated into the interview asking about recent changes in health status, awareness of any medical conditions, family history of medical disorders, current medications, results of last physical examination, history of head trauma or loss of consciousness, and changes in weight, diet, sleep, or appetite (Robinson & James, 2005).

Become familiar with health policy, care systems and reimbursement structures and codes. In the last decade, progress has been made in the US towards establishing reimbursement codes for psychological services that do not require a mental health diagnosis but target physical health problems (Smith, 2002). Similarly, in Australia, psychologists became eligible to receive Medicare rebates for their services (Martin, 2004). These were significant milestones towards redefining 'health as a multidisciplinary enterprise rather than a medical monopoly' (Martin, 2004, p. 5). During this period of 'health-care reform exploration' (Ivey & Doenges, 2013) and proliferation of integrated health settings with a diversity of reimbursement structures, it is important that psychologists seek clarity on different contractual and financing arrangements operating in different care organizations (Kelly & Coons, 2012). Psychologists need to keep abreast of further developments in this arena, as these are likely to further smooth the path for psychologists practising in medical settings.

When in the medical world, do as the medicos do. A core component of interprofessional competence is to recognize and respect the competencies of other professions (Belar, 2012). Becoming part of the team means that psychologists, while maintaining their distinctive qualities, must adopt the pace and culture of their medical colleagues. This includes getting involved in the things that the other providers do, such as attending presentations by pharmaceutical representatives, staying informed about current medical issues by reading relevant medical journals, and participating in professional events and social functions (Gatchel & Oordt, 2003). Psychologists should also be willing to be trained and educated on issues that initially go beyond their expertise (Haley et al., 1998). Admitting ignorance is the first step towards acquiring the information necessary to become familiar with the local culture. Receptiveness to the complementary expertise offered by psychologists is highest if it comes packaged in the wrappings and trimmings familiar to medical professionals. This is not to imply that psychologists should 'disguise' their professional identity or not stand behind their perspective in the face of opposing opinions (Gatchel & Oordt, 2003). After all, it is their different training and expertise that adds value to the medical model of health care delivery.

4. Psychologists need to articulate their distinct roles and services

Although when in the medical world psychologists need to assimilate to the specific culture, language, and pace of those care settings, it is equally important that they foster reciprocal understanding by other professionals of the unique skills and potential contributions psychologists bring to collaborative care (American Psychological Association, 2013). This is done in the context of both routine communication and team meetings, but also by regularly participating as a presenter at information seminars or lunchtime talks. Likewise, psychologists should invest in enhancing psychological health literacy directly among patients to provide them with the knowledge and tools to make informed decisions about the psychologist's role in their own care (Karlin, & Cross, 2014; Santucci, McHugh, & Barlow, 2012). The strong scientific training and skills in practice-based research essential for programme development, evaluation, and quality improvement remain distinctive features in the core competencies brought by clinical psychologists to integrated care (Health Service Psychology Education Collaborative, 2013).

5. Psychologists need to be accountable for outcomes

Accountability requires good skills in database management. Kiesler (2000) noted that 'the database needed to track services is about the same as the database needed to do good research' (p. 486). Thus, psychologists with a scientist-practitioner background are well equipped to enhance the quality and utility of locally relevant data management systems. However, research-skilled psychologists must fine-tune their approach to documenting outcomes in line with the principles of time-efficiency, practical utility, and good enough treatment.

6. Psychologists need to attend to ethical issues

Adapting the delivery of psychological services to the pace and culture of medical settings raises some important ethical issues for psychologists. Perhaps foremost among those is the ethical obligation to provide services only within the boundaries of one's competence (American Psychological Association, 2013). In particular, the pressure to conduct consultations more rapidly and for a larger number of patients than is typical of the specialist mental health setting must be balanced with a calm and methodical approach to determining if more comprehensive psychological assessments and/or interventions are indicated (e.g., in cases of high suicide risk, substance abuse, or complex family problems). If necessary, psychologists must triage those patients and refer them to appropriate specialist care (Haley et al., 1998). It is important that psychologists are skilled in managing the ethical dilemmas unique to interprofessional care settings and avoid compromising their professional judgement in the face of systemic constraints or pressures by other team members (American Psychological Association, 2013). In this context, it is important that psychologists guard their professional integrity and are upfront with a patient about their particular role in the patient's overall care, so that they avoid making unwise commitments or raising false expectations (Gatchel & Oordt, 2003).

Confidentiality is an issue of heightened concern in settings where many staff members from different disciplines are involved in patient care and have access to patient records, and where the setting is dominated by the culture and practices of another profession (Ivey & Doenges, 2013). For example, for physicians it is common and acceptable to treat multiple members of a family or friends that come to the same practice, whereas psychologists strive to avoid such dual relationships in their work if possible. In care settings where many patients can be expected to know each other, it is important to balance ethical concerns about confidentiality and any potential harm to patients with the opportunity loss for patients to access vital behavioural health care. Ivey and Doenges (2013) recommend considering three dimensions in ethical decision-making to determine the risk for harm regarding multiple relationships in primary care settings: (1) What is the duration of the treatment contacts? (2) What is the chance of future contacts? (3) What is the level of intensity of the treatment contacts? If the intervention is brief (1–3 contacts), with a low chance of future contact, and the care is limited to consultation with or without the patient present, there is low risk of harm. If several contacts are required (4–10), with a medium chance of future contact, and the care involves brief interventions such as psychoeducation, skill building, and motivational interviewing, there is a medium risk of harm. If longer-term care is required (>10 contacts), with a high chance of future contact, and the care involves a therapeutic relationship with high level of patient disclosure and vulnerability, there is a high risk of harm. Decision-making can be guided by considering whether answers to the questions along these three dimensions for each of two patients predominantly fall in the lower or higher risk categories. The ultimate decision must take into account whether the potential harm from treating multiple patients that know each other outweighs the harm resulting from the loss of an opportunity to intervene. Sometimes the question might not just be 'Can I see this patient?' but rather, 'What services can I ethically provide to this patient to maximize benefits and avoid harm' (Ivey & Doenges, 2013, p. 222). As with all ethical decision-making in patient care, if in doubt, seek consultation.

Striving for prescriptive authority – a bridge too far?

For over two decades there has been vigorous debate as to whether clinical psychologists should strive to gain the right to prescribe psychoactive medications (Lavoie & Barone, 2006).

Some considered seeking prescription privileges for psychologists (RxP) as 'psychology's next frontier' (DeLeon, Fox, & Graham, 1991), whereas others have documented the lacklustre success of the campaign to promote RxP and view it as a misguided agenda (Robiner, Tumlin, & Tompkins, 2013). The rationale for seeking RxP was that the mental health needs of society were not being met, and by increasing psychology's scope of practice the underserved public would have increased access to qualified professionals who can prescribe. However, only a minority of psychologists is interested in pursuing the training and authority to prescribe (Fox et al., 2009), and none of the psychologists in the first jurisdiction (Guam) to pass RxP legislation in 1998, have gained prescription authority since then (Robiner et al., 2013). Moreover, while appropriately trained psychologists are eligible to prescribe in Louisiana and New Mexico and the United States military (American Psychological Association, 2011), this success in three jurisdictions is dwarfed by the 167 failed bills to enact RxP legislation between 1995 and 2012 in other jurisdictions (Robiner et al., 2013). Despite this paltry record of enactment of RxP legislation, combined with the general lack of enthusiasm among most practising psychologists, some national bodies such as the American Psychological Association (2011) view the further spread of RxP as inevitable and along with other professional bodies such as the Australian Psychological Society (Stokes, Li, & Collins, 2012) continue to lobby for it. But others such as the Canadian Psychological Association Task Force on Prescriptive Authority for Psychologists in Canada (2010) viewed the push towards prescriptive authority as premature and recommended against making it a priority goal or focus of professional advocacy. Instead, they recommended active collaborative practice with prescribing professions as the optimal standard for contemporary psychological practices.

Although some interest groups within psychology continue to hanker for RxP, the modest progress of the RxP movement appears destined to stall even further as the era of interprofessional care is gaining momentum amidst radical health care reforms aimed at incentivizing efficient team-based care. Interprofessional collaboration in co-located care settings is rapidly emerging as a compelling alternative to RxP (Robiner et al., 2013). Clinical psychology trainees have more to gain from pursuing training opportunities that enhance readiness for collaborative, team-based practice (HSPEC, 2013), than from investing additional years of training to achieve the standards necessary for prescriptive authority and thereby simply duplicate the competencies already represented by the prescribing members of the team. The future of psychologists as health providers is only bright if they can make a distinct contribution to collaborative care and are not seen as doing the same thing as other types of providers working in the team (Belar, 2012).

More so than ever the public interest is better served by access to mental health professionals who can offer effective alternatives to medication than by adding psychologists to the number of providers who already can prescribe (DeNelsky, 1991). There is no consumer demand from the general public for psychologists being granted prescription privileges (Lavoie & Barone, 2006), and for the most common mental health conditions (depressive and anxiety disorders), three in four patients prefer psychological treatments to medication (McHugh, Whitton, Peckham, Welge, & Otto, 2013). When patients do receive medication, adherence is poor (American Psychological Association, 2011). Of those initiating antidepressant medications, four in ten discontinued the medication within the first 30 days of treatment, and nearly three in four had stopped taking it after 90 days (Olfson, Marcus, Tedeschi, & Wan, 2006). Moreover, while pharmacological treatments dominate the mental health market, their burgeoning use over the past decades has proven ineffectual in stemming the worsening chronicity and severity of mental disorders or reducing stigma associated

Andersson, G., Cuijpers, P., Carlbring, P., & Lindefors, N. (2007). Effects of Internet-delivered cognitive behaviour therapy for anxiety and mood disorders. *Psychiatry*, 2: 9–14.

Andrade, J. (2001). *Working memory in perspective*. Hove, UK: Psychology Press.

Andrews, G., & Harvey, R. (1981). Does psychotherapy benefit neurotic patients? A re-analysis of the Smith, Glass, & Miller data. *Archives of General Psychiatry*, 38: 1203–8.

Andrews, G., & Peters, L. (1998). The psychometric properties of the Composite International Diagnostic Interview. *Social Psychiatry and Psychiatric Epidemiology*, 29: 124–32.

Andrews, G., Creamer, M., Crino, R., Hunt, C., Lampe, L., & Page, A. (2003). *The treatment of anxiety disorders: Clinician guides and patient manuals* (2nd edn.). Cambridge University Press.

Andrews, G., Crino, R., Hunt, C., Lampe, L., & Page, A. (1999). A list of essential psychotherapies. In J. J. Lopez-Ibor, F. Lieh-Mak, H. M., Visotsky, & M. Maj (eds.), *One world, one language: Paving the way to better perspectives for mental health* (pp. 240–6). Göttingen: Hogrefe & Huber.

Andrews, G., Cuijpers, P., Craske, M. G., McEvoy, P., & Titov, N. (2010). Computer therapy for the anxiety and depressive disorders is effective, acceptable and practical health care: A meta-analysis. *PloS one*, 5(10): e13196.

Andrews, G., Davies, M., & Titov, N. (2011). Effectiveness randomized controlled trial of face to face versus Internet cognitive behaviour therapy for social phobia. *Australian and New Zealand Journal of Psychiatry*, 45(4): 337–40.

Angold, A., & Costello, E. J. (2000). The Child and Adolescent Psychiatric Assessment (CAPA). *Journal of the American Academy of Child and Adolescent Psychiatry*, 39: 39–48.

Angold, A., Prendagast, M., Cox, A., Harrington, R., Smirnoff, E., & Rutter, M. (1995). The Child and Adolescent Psychiatric Assessment (CAPA). *Psychological Medicine*, 25(4): 739–53.

Arkowitz, H., Westra, H. A., Miller, W. R., & Rollnick, S. (eds.) (2007). *Motivational interviewing in the treatment of psychological problems*. New York: Guilford Press.

Asay, T. P., Lambert, M. J., Gregerson, A. T., & Goates, M. K. (2002). Using patient-focused research in evaluating treatment outcome in private practice. *Journal of Clinical Psychology*, 58(10): 1213–25.

Australian Bureau of Statistics (2001). *1216.0 Australian Standard Geographical Classification (ASGC) 2001*. www.abs.gov.au/Ausstats/abs@.nsf/0/a3658d8f0ad7a9b6ca256ad4007f1c42?OpenDocument [accessed 20 March 2005].

(2011). Australian Social Trends March 2011: Health outside major cities. www.ausstats.abs.gov.au/ausstats/subscriber.nsf/LookupAttach/4102.0Publication25.03.114/$File/41020_HealthOMC_Mar2011.pdf [accessed 28 April 2014].

Australian Government Department of Health (2013). *Better Access to Psychiatrists, Psychologists and General Practitioners through the MBS (Better Access) Initiative*. www.health.gov.au/mentalhealth-betteraccess

Australian Psychological Society (2003). Code of ethics. www.psychology.org.au/aps/ethics/code_of_ethics.pdf [accessed 30 March 2005].

Aveyard, P., Begh, R., Parsons, A., & West, R. (2011). Brief opportunistic smoking cessation interventions: A systematic review and meta-analysis to compare advice to quit and offer of assistance. *Addiction*, 107(6): 1066–73.

Azrin, N. H., & Foxx, R. M. (1974). *Toilet training in less than a day*. New York: Simon & Schuster.

Azrin, N. H., & Nunn, R. (1973). Habit reversal: A method of eliminating nervous habits and tics. *Behaviour Research and Therapy*, 11(4): 619–28.

Babor, T. F., & Higgens-Biddle, J. C. (2001). *Brief intervention for hazardous and harmful drinking: A manual for use in primary care*. Geneva: World Health Organization.

Baddeley, A. D. (1986). *Working memory*. Oxford University Press.

(1990). *Human memory: Theory and practice*. Hove, UK: Erlbaum.

Bandura, A. (1977). *Social learning theory*. Englewood Cliffs, NJ: Prentice Hall.

Barber, J. P., Muran, J. C., McCarthy, K. S., & Keefe, R. J. (2013). Research on psychodynamic therapies. In M. J. Lambert (ed.), *Bergin and Garfield's handbook of psychotherapy and behavior change* (6th edn.) (pp. 443–94). Hoboken, NJ: John Wiley.

Barbopolous, A., & Clark, J. M. (2003). Practising psychology in rural settings: Issues and guidelines. *Canadian Psychology*, 44(4): 410–24.

Barkham, M., Bewick, B., Mullin, T., Gilbody, S., Connell, J., Cahill, J., Mellor-Clark, J., Richards, D., Unsworth, G., & Evans, C. (2013). The CORE-10: A short measure of psychological distress for routine use in the psychological therapies. *Counselling & Psychotherapy Research*, 13(1): 3–13.

Barkham, M., Hardy, G. E., & Mellor-Clark, J. (2010a). *Developing and delivering practice-based evidence*. Chichester: Wiley.

Barkham, M., Mellor-Clark, J., Connell, J., Evans, C., Evans, R., & Margison, F. (2010b). Clinical Outcomes in Routine Evaluation (CORE) – the CORE measures and system: Measuring, monitoring and managing quality evaluation in the psychological therapies. In M. Barkham, G. E. Hardy, & J. Mellor-Clark (eds.), *Developing and delivering practice-based evidence: A guide for the psychological therapies* (pp. 175–219). New York: Wiley-Blackwell.

Barlow, D. H. (1988). *Anxiety and its disorders: The nature and treatment of anxiety and panic*. New York: Guilford Press.
  (2002). *Anxiety and its disorders: The nature and treatment of anxiety and panic* (2nd edn.). New York: Guilford Press.
  (2010). Negative effects from psychological treatments: A perspective. *American Psychologist*, 65(1): 13–20.

Barlow, D. H., & Durand, V. M. (2015). *Abnormal psychology: An integrative approach* (7th edn.). Stamford, CT: Cengage.

Barnett, J. E. (2008). Online 'sharing' demands caution. *The National Psychologist*, 17: 10–11.

Barnhill, J. W. (2013). *DSM-5 Clinical Cases*. Washington, DC: American Psychiatric Publishing.

Baumeister, R. F., Campbell, J. D., Krueger, J. I., & Vohs, K. D. (2003). Does high self-esteem cause better performance, interpersonal success, happiness, or healthier lifestyles? *Psychological Science in the Public Interest*, 4(1): 1–44.

Bech, P., Gudex, C., & Johansen, K. S. (1996). The WHO (Ten) Well-being Index: Validation in diabetes. *Psychotherapy and Psychosomatics*, 65(4): 183–90.

Beck, A. T. (1967). *Depression: Causes and treatment*. Philadelphia: University of Pennsylvania Press.

Beck, A. T., & Dozois, D. J. (2011). Cognitive therapy: Current status and future directions. *Annual Review of Medicine*, 62: 397–409.

Beck, A. T., Steer, R. A., & Brown, G. K. (1996). *Manual for the Beck Depression Inventory* (2nd edn.). San Antonio, TX: The Psychological Corporation.

Beck, A. T., Steer, R. A., & Garbin, M. A. (1988). Psychometric properties of the Beck Depression Inventory: Twenty-five years of evaluation. *Clinical Psychology Review*, 8(1): 77–100.

Beck, A. T., Ward, C. H., Mendelson, M., Mock, J., & Erbaugh, J. (1961). An inventory for measuring depression. *Archives of General Psychiatry*, 4(6): 561–71.

Beck, J. S. (1995). *Cognitive therapy: Basics and beyond*. New York: Guilford Press.
  (2011). *Cognitive behavior therapy: Basics and beyond*. New York: Guilford Press.

Bedics, J. D., Atkins, D. C., Comtois, K. A., & Linehan, M. M. (2012). Treatment differences in the therapeutic relationship and introject during a 2-year randomized controlled trial of dialectical behavior therapy versus nonbehavioral psychotherapy experts for borderline personality disorder. *Journal of Consulting and Clinical Psychology*, 80(1), 66–77.

Belar, C. D. (2012). Reflections on the future: Psychology as a health profession. *Professional Psychology: Research and Practice*, 43: 545–50.

Bellack, A. S., & Hersen, M. (eds.) (1998). *Behavioral assessment: A practical handbook* (4th edn.). New York: Pergamon.

Bennett-Levy, J., Butler, G., Fennell, M. J. V., Hackmann, A., Mueller, M., & Westbrook, D. (eds.) (2004). *The Oxford guide to behavioural experiments in cognitive therapy*. Oxford University Press.

Bernard, J. M., & Goodyear, R. K. (2004). *Fundamentals of clinical supervision* (3rd edn.). Boston, MA: Pearson.

Bernstein, D. A., & Borkovec, T. D. (1973). *Progressive relaxation training: A manual for the helping professions*. Champaign, IL: Research Press.

Berwick, D. M. (2003). Disseminating innovations in health care. *Journal of the American Medical Association*, 289(15): 1969–75.

Beutler, L. E., & Clarkin, J. F. (1990). *Systematic treatment selection: Towards targeted therapeutic interventions*. New York: Brunner/Mazel.

Beutler, L. E., & Harwood, M. T. (2000). *Prescriptive therapy: A practical guide to systematic treatment selection*. New York: Oxford University Press.

Beutler, L. E., Malik, M., Alimohamed, S., Harwood, T. M., Talebi, H., Noble, S., & Wong, E. (2004). Therapist variables. In M. J. Lambert (ed.), *Bergin and Garfield's handbook of psychotherapy and behavior change* (5th edn.) (pp. 227–306). New York: John Wiley.

Beutler, L. E., Moliero, C., & Talebi, H. (2002). How practitioners can systematically use empirical evidence in treatment selection. *Journal of Clinical Psychology*, 58(10): 1199–212.

Bickman, L., Kelley, S. D., Breda, C., de Andrade, A. R., & Riemer, M. (2011). Effects of routine feedback to clinicians on mental health outcomes of youths: Results of a randomized trial. *Psychiatric Services*, 62(12): 1423–29.

Birchler, G. R. (1988). Handling resistance to change. In I. R. H. Falloon (ed.), *Handbook of behavioural marital therapy* (pp. 128–55). London: Hutchinson.

Blashfield, R. K. (1998). Diagnostic models and systems. In A. S. Bellack & M. Hersen (eds.), *Comprehensive clinical psychology: Assessment* (pp. 57–80). New York: Pergamon.

Blumenthal, J. A., Sherwood, A., Gullette, E. C. D., Georgiades, A., & Tweedy, D. (2002). Biobehavioral approaches to the treatment of essential hypertension. *Journal of Consulting and Clinical Psychology*, 70: 569–89.

Bohart, A. C., & Wade, A. G. (2013). The client in psychotherapy. In M. J. Lambert (ed.), *Bergin and Garfield's handbook of psychotherapy and behavior change* (6th edn.) (pp. 219–57). Hoboken, NJ: John Wiley.

Bongar, B., & Sullivan, G. (2013). *The suicidal patient: Clinical and legal standards of care* (3rd edn.). Washington, DC: American Psychological Association.

Bordin, E. S. (1979). The generalizability of the psychoanalytic concept of the working alliance. *Psychotherapy: Theory, Research, and Practice*, 16(3): 252–60.

Borgeat, F., Stravynski, A., & Chalou, H. L. (1983). The influence of two different sets of information and suggestions on the subjective effects of relaxation. *Journal of Human Stress*, 9: 40–5.

Borkovec, T. D. (2004). Research in training clinics and practice research networks: A route to the integration of science and practice. *Clinical Psychology: Science and Practice*, 11(2): 211–15.

Borkovec, T. D., & Sides, J. K. (1979). Critical procedural variables related to the physiological effects of progressive relaxation: A review. *Behaviour Research and Therapy*, 17(2): 119–25.

Borkovec, T. D., Echemendia, R. J., Ragusea, S. A., & Ruiz, M. (2001). The Pennsylvania Practice Research Network and future possibilities for clinically meaningful and scientifically rigorous psychotherapy research. *Clinical Psychology: Science and Practice*, 8(2): 155–68.

Borkovec, T. D., Grayson, J. B., & Cooper, K. M. (1978). Treatment of general tension: Subjective and physiological effects of progressive relaxation. *Journal of Consulting and Clinical Psychology*, 46(3): 518–28.

Bornat, J. (1994). *Reminiscence reviewed: Perspectives, evaluations, achievements*. Buckingham: Open University Press.

Bouton, M. E. (1991). A contextual analysis of fear extinction. In P. R. Martin (ed.), *Handbook of behavior therapy and psychological science: An integrative*

approach (pp. 435–53). New York:
Pergamon Press.

Bouton, M. E., & Todd, T. P. (2014). A
fundamental role for context in
instrumental learning and extinction.
Behavioural Processes, 104: 13–19.

Boyd, C. P., Hayes, L., Sewell, J., Caldwell, K.,
Kemp, E., Harvie, L., Aisbett, D. L., &
Nurse, S. (2008). Mental health
problems in rural contexts: A broader
perspective. *Australian Psychologist*,
43(1): 2–6.

Brauer, A. P., Horlick, L., Nelson, E., Farquhar,
J. W., Agras, W. S., & Farquhar, J.
(1979). Relaxation therapy for essential
hypertension: A Veterans Administration
Outpatient study. *Journal of Behavioral
Medicine*, 2(1): 21–9.

Breiner, M. J., Stritzke, W. G. K., & Lang, A. R.
(1999). Approaching avoidance: A step
essential to the understanding of craving.
Alcohol Research and Health, 23(3):
197–206.

Bridge, P., & Bascue, L. O. (1990).
Documentation of psychotherapy
supervision. *Psychotherapy in Private
Practice*, 8(1): 79–86.

British Psychological Society (2005). *Code of
conduct, ethical principles and guidelines*.
Leicester, UK: British Psychological
Society.

Broadhead, W. E., Leon, A. C., Weissman, M.
M., Barrett, J. E., Blackllow, R. S., Gilbert,
T. T., Keller, M. B., Olfson, M., & Higgins,
E. S. (1995). Development and validation
of the SDSS-PC screen for multiple
mental disorders in primary care.
Archives of Family Medicine, 4(3):
211–19.

Broggs, K. M., Griffin, R. S., & Gross, A M.
(2002). Children. In M. Hersen, & S. M.
Turner (eds.), *Diagnostic interviewing*
(3rd edn.) (pp. 393–413). New York:
Kluwer Academic/Plenum Press.

Brown, R. A. (2003). Intensive behavioral
treatment. In D. B. Abrams, R. Niaura,
R. A. Brown, K. M. Emmons, M. G.
Goldstein, & P. M. Monti (eds.), *The
tobacco dependence treatment handbook:
A guide to best practice* (pp. 118–77). New
York: Guilford Press.

Brown, T. A., & Barlow, D. H. (1995). Long-
term outcome in cognitive-behavioral

treatment of panic disorder: Clinical
predictors of alternative strategies for
assessment. *Journal of Consulting and
Clinical Psychology*, 63(5): 754–65.

Brown, T. A., Di Nardo, P. A., & Barlow,
D. H. (1994). *Anxiety Disorders
Interview Schedule for DSM-IV (ADIS-
IV)*. San Antonio, TX: Psychological
Corporation.

Bryant, M. J., Simons, A. D., & Thase, M. E.
(1999). Therapist skill and patient
variables in homework compliance:
Controlling an uncontrolled variable
in cognitive therapy outcome.
Cognitive Therapy and Research,
23(4): 381–99.

Burian, B. K., & Slimp, A. O. (2000). Social
dual-role relationships during internship:
A decision-making model. *Professional
Psychology: Research and Practice*, 31(3):
332–8.

Burlingame, G., Strauss, B., & Joyce, A. (2013).
Change mechanisms and effectiveness of
small group treatments. In M. J. Lambert
(ed.), *Bergin and Garfield's handbook
of psychotherapy and behavior change*
(pp. 640–89). Hoboken, NJ: John
Wiley.

Burns, D. (1980). *Feeling good: The new mood
therapy*. Melbourne: Information
Australia.

  (1999). *The feeling good handbook*. New
York: Plume.

Burns, D. D., & Auerbach, A. H. (1992). Does
homework compliance enhance recovery
from depression? *Psychiatric Annals*, 22:
464–9.

Butler, A. C., Chapman, J. E., Forman, E. M., &
Beck, A. T. (2006). The empirical status
of cognitive-behavioral therapy: A review
of meta-analyses. *Clinical Psychology
Review*, 26(1): 17–31.

Byrne, S. L., Hooke, G. R., Newnham, E. A., &
Page, A. C. (2012). The effects of progress
monitoring on subsequent readmission to
psychiatric care: A six-month follow-up.
Journal of Affective Disorders, 137(1–3):
113–16.

Campbell, C. D., & Gordon, M. C. (2003).
Acknowledging the inevitable:
Understanding multiple relationships in
rural practice. *Professional Psychology:
Research and Practice*, 34(4): 430–4.

Canadian Psychological Association (2000). *Canadian code of ethics for psychologists* (3rd edn.). Ottawa: CPA Publications.

Canadian Psychological Association Task Force on Prescriptive Authority for Psychologists in Canada (2010). *Report to the Canadian Psychological Association Board of Directors.* www.cpa.ca/docs/file/Task_Forces/CPA_RxPTaskForce_FinalReport_Dec2010_RevJ17.pdf [accessed 28 April 2014].

Cannon, J. A., Warren, J. S., Nelson, P. L., & Burlingame, G. M. (2010). Change trajectories for the Youth Outcome Questionnaire Self-Report: Identifying youth at risk for treatment failure. *Journal of Clinical Child and Adolescent Psychology*, 39(3): 289–301.

Carey, K. B., Scott-Sheldon, L. A. J., Elliott, J. C., Garey, L., & Carey, M. P. (2012). Face-to-face versus computer-delivered alcohol interventions for college drinkers: a meta-analytic review, 1998 to 2010. *Clinical Psychology Review*, 32(8): 690–703.

Carlbring, P., Apelstrand, M., Sehlin, H., Amir, N., Rousseau, A., Hofmann, S. G., & Andersson, G. (2012). Internet-delivered attention bias modification training in individuals with social anxiety disorder-a double blind randomized controlled trial. *BMC Psychiatry*, 12(1): 66.

Carr, E. G. (1977). The motivation of self-injurious behavior: A review of some hypotheses. *Psychological Bulletin*, 84(4): 800–16.

Carr, E. G., Robinson, S., & Palumbo, L. W. (1990). The wrong issue: Aversive versus nonaversive treatment. The right issue: Functional versus non-functional treatment. In A. C. Repp & N. Singh (eds.), *Perspectives on the use of nonaversive and aversive interventions for persons with developmental disabilities* (pp. 361–379). Sycamore, IL: Sycamore Publishing.

Castonguay, L. G. (2011). Psychotherapy, psychopathology, research and practice: Pathways of connections and integration. *Psychotherapy Research*, 21(2): 125–40.

Castonguay, L. G., & Beutler, L. E. (eds.) (2006). *Principles of therapeutic change that work.* Oxford University Press

Castonguay, L. G., Barkham, M., Lutz, W., & McAleavey, A. (2013). Practice-oriented research: Approaches and applications. In M. J. Lambert (ed.), *Bergin and Garfield's handbook of psychotherapy and behavior change* (6th edn.) (pp. 85–133). Hoboken, NJ: John Wiley.

Chadwick, P., Williams, C., & Mackenzie, J. (2003). Impact of case formulation in cognitive behaviour therapy for psychosis. *Behaviour Research and Therapy*, 41(6): 671–80.

Chambless, D. L., & Hollon, S. D. (1998). Defining empirically supported psychological interventions. *Journal of Consulting and Clinical Psychology*, 66: 7–18.

Charney, D. S., Barlow, D. H., Botteron, K., Cohen, J. D., Goldman, D., Gur, R. E., Lin, K-M., López, J. F., Meador-Woodruff, J. H., Moldin, S. O., Nestler, E. J., Watson, S. J., & Zulcman, S. J. (2002). Neuroscience research agenda to guide development of a pathophysiologically based classification system. In D. J. Kupfer, M. B. First, & D. A. Regier (eds.), *A research agenda for DSM-V* (pp. 31–83). Washington, DC: American Psychiatric Association.

Chiles, J. A., Lambert, M. J., & Hatch, A. L. (1999). The impact of psychological interventions on medical cost offset: A meta-analytic review. *Clinical Psychology: Science and Practice*, 6(2): 204–20.

Christensen, A. J., & Nezu, A. M. (2013). Behavioral medicine and clinical health psychology: Introduction to the special issue. *Journal of Consulting and Clinical Psychology*, 81(2): 193–5.

Clark, D. M. (1986). A cognitive approach to panic. *Behaviour Research and Therapy*, 24(4): 461–70.

(2011). Implementing NICE guidelines for the psychological treatment of depression and anxiety disorders: The IAPT experience. *International Review of Psychiatry*, 23: 318–27.

Clark, D. M., & Salkovskis, P. M. (1996). *Cognitive therapy for panic attacks: Therapist's manual.* Department of Psychiatry, University of Oxford.

Clum, G. A., & Knowles, S. L. (1991). Why do some people with panic disorders become avoidant? A review. *Clinical Psychology Review*, 11(3): 295–313.

Clum, G. A., Clum, G., & Surls, R. (1993). A meta-analysis of treatments for panic disorder. *Journal of Consulting and Clinical Psychology*, 61(2): 317–26.

Comer, J. S., & Barlow, D. H. (2014). The occasional case against broad dissemination and implementation: Retaining a role for specialty care in the delivery of psychological treatments. *American Psychologist*, 69: 1–18.

Commission on Chronic Illness (1957). *Chronic illness in the United States*, Vol. 1. Cambridge, MA: Commonwealth Fund/Harvard University Press.

Compare, A., Zarbo, C., Manzoni. G. M., Castelnuovo, G., Baldassari, E., Bonardi, A., Callus, E., & Romagnoni, C. (2013). Social support, depression, and heart disease: A ten year literature review. *Frontiers in Psychology*, 4, Article 384: 1–7.

Connell, J., Barkham, M., Stiles, W. B., Twigg, E., Singleton, N., Evans, O., & Miles, J. N. (2007). Distribution of CORE-OM scores in a general population, clinical cut-off points and comparison with the CIS-R. *British Journal of Psychiatry*, 190(1): 69–74.

Conoley, J. C., & Impara, J. C. (eds.) (1995). *The twelfth measurements yearbook*. Lincoln, NE: Buros Institute of Mental Measurements.

Cooper, Z., Fairburn, C. G., & Hawker, D. M. (2003). *Cognitive-behavioral treatment of obesity: A clinician's guide*. New York: Guilford Press.

Copeland, J. R., Kelleher, M. J., Kellett, J. M., Gourlay, A. J., Gurland, B. J., Fleiss, J. L., & Sharpe, L. (1976). A semistructured clinical interview for the assessment and diagnosis and mental state in the elderly: The Geriatric Mental State Schedule: 1. Development and reliability. *Psychological Medicine*, 6(3): 439–49.

Costa, P. T., & McCrae, R. R. (1992). *Revised NEO Personality Inventory (NEO PI-R) and NEO Five-Factor Inventory (NEO FFI): Professional manual*. Lutz, FL: Psychological Assessment Resources Inc.

Cox, B. J., Endler, N. S., Lee, P. S., & Swinson, R. P. (1992). A meta-analysis of treatments for panic disorder with agoraphobia: Imipramine, alprazolam, and in vivo exposure. *Journal of Behavior Therapy and Experimental Psychiatry*, 23: 175–82.

Coyne, J. C., Thompson, R., Klinkman, M. S., & Nease, D. E. (2002). Emotional disorders in primary care. *Journal of Consulting and Clinical Psychology*, 70(3): 798–809.

Craik, F. I., & Salthouse, T. A. (2007). *The handbook of aging and cognition* (3rd edn.). New York: Psychological Press.

Craske, M. G. (1999). *Anxiety disorders: Psychological approaches to theory and treatment*. Boulder, CO: Westview Press.
    (2003). *Origins of phobias and anxiety disorders: Why more women than men?* Amsterdam: Elsevier.

Craske, M. G., & Barlow, D. H. (2008). Panic disorder and agoraphobia. In D. H. Barlow (ed.), *Clinical handbook of psychological disorders: A step-by-step manual* (4th edn.) (pp. 1–64). New York: Guilford Press.

Crawford, J., Cayley, C., Lovibond, P. F., Wilson, P. H., & Hartley, C. (2011). Percentile norms and accompanying interval estimates from an Australian general adult population sample for self-report mood scales (BAI, BDI, CRSD, CES-D, DASS, DASS-21, STAI-X, STAI-Y, SRDS, and SRAS). *Australian Psychologist*, 46(1): 3–14.

Cubic, B., Mance, J., Turgesen, J. N., & Lamanna, J. D. (2012). Interprofessional education: Preparing psychologists for success in integrated primary care. *Journal of Clinical Psychology in Medical Settings*, 19(1): 84–92.

Cuijpers, P., Donker, T., Van Straten, A., Li, J., & Andersson, G. (2010). Is guided self-help as effective as face-to-face psychotherapy for depression and anxiety disorders? A systematic review and meta-analysis of comparative outcome studies. *Psychological Medicine*, 40(12): 1943–57.

Cuijpers, P., Geraedts, A. S., van Oppen, P., Andersson, G., Markowitz, J. C., & van Straten, A. (2011). Interpersonal psychotherapy for depression: A meta-analysis. *American Journal of Psychiatry*, 168(6): 581–92.

Cuijpers, P., van Straten, A., & Andersson, G. (2008). Internet-administered cognitive behavior therapy for health problems: A systematic review. *Journal of Behavioral Medicine*, 31(2): 169–77.

Cummings, N. A. (1999). Medical cost offset, meta-analysis, and implications for future research and practice. *Clinical Psychology: Science and Practice*, 6(2): 221–4.

Daniel, M. S., & Crider, C. J. (2003). Mental status examination. In M. Hersen & S. M. Turner (eds.), *Diagnostic interviewing* (3rd edn.). New York: Kluwer Academic/ Plenum Press.

Davison, G. C. (2000). Stepped care: Doing more with less? *Journal of Consulting and Clinical Psychology*, 68(4): 580–5.

de Jong, K., Nugter, A., Polak, M., Wagenborg, H., Spinhoven, P., & Heiser, W. (2008). The Dutch version of the Outcome Questionnaire (OQ-45): A cross-cultural validation. *Psychologie & Gezondheid*, 36(1): 35–45.

de Jong, K., van Sluis, P., Nugter, M., Heiser, W. J., & Spinhoven, P. (2012). Understanding the differential impact of outcome monitoring: Therapist variables that moderate feedback effects in a randomized clinical trial. *Psychotherapy Research*, 22(4): 464–74.

Deacon, B. J. (2013). The biomedical model of mental disorder: A critical analysis of its validity, utility, and effects on psychotherapy research. *Clinical Psychology Review*, 33(7): 846–61.

DeLeon, P. H., Fox, R. E., & Graham, S. R. (1991). Prescription privileges: Psychology's next frontier? *American Psychologist*, 46: 384–93.

DeLeon, P. H., Wakefield, M., & Hagglund, K. J. (2003). The behavioral health care needs of rural communities in the 21st century. In B. H. Stamm (ed.), *Rural behavioral health care: An interdisciplinary guide* (pp. 23–31). Washington, DC: American Psychological Association.

DeNelsky, G. Y. (1991). Prescription privileges for psychologists: The case against. *Professional Psychology: Research and Practice*, 22: 188–93.

Derogatis, L. R. (1994). *The SCL-90-R: Administration, scoring, and procedures manual* (3rd edn.). Baltimore, MD: Clinical Psychometric Research.

Derogatis, L. R., & Spencer, P. (1982). *The Brief Symptom Inventory: Administration, scoring and procedures manual*. Baltimore, MD: Clinical Psychometric Research.

Dies, R. R. (1992). The future of group therapy. *Psychotherapy*, 29: 58–64.

Dixon, R. A. (2003). *Themes in the aging of intelligence: Robust decline with intriguing possibilities*. Washington, DC: American Psychological Association.

Druss, B. G., Ji, X., Glick, G., & von Esenwein, S. A. (2014). Randomized trial of an electronic personal health record for patients with serious mental illness. *American Journal of Psychiatry*, 171(3): 360–8.

Dunbar, E. (1982). Educating social workers for rural mental health settings. In H. A. Dengerink & H. J. Cross (eds.), *Training professionals for rural mental health* (pp. 54–69). Lincoln, NE: University of Nebraska Press.

Durand, V. M., & Crimmins, D. B. (1988). Identifying the variables maintaining self-injurious behavior. *Journal of Autism and Developmental Disorders*, 18(1): 99–117.

Dyckman, J. M., & Cowan, E. A. (1978). Imagining vividness and the outcome of in vivo and imagined scene desensitization. *Journal of Consulting and Clinical Psychology*, 48: 1155–6.

Dyer, K., Hooke, G., & Page, A. C. (2014). Development and psychometrics of the five item daily index in a psychiatric sample. *Journal of Affective Disorders*, 152: 409–15.

D'Zurilla, T. J. (1986). *Problem-solving therapy*. New York: Springer.

Eberlein, L. (1987). Introducing ethics to beginning psychologists: A problem-solving approach. *Professional Psychology: Research and Practice*, 18(4): 353–9.

Edelstein, B. (ed.) (1998). *Comprehensive clinical psychology*, Vol. 7: *Clinical geropsychology* (pp. 193–229). Oxford: Elsevier.

Edelstein, B., Koven, L., Spira, A., & Shreve-Neiger, A. (2002). Older adults. In A. S. Bellack & M. Hersen (eds.), *Behavioral* assessment: A practice handbook (4th edn.) (pp. 433–54). Boston, MA: Allyn & Bacon.

Edwards, R. (1987). Implementing the scientist-practitioner model: The school psychologist as data-based problem solver. Professional School Psychology, 2: 155–61.

Eells, T. D. (1997a). Psychotherapy case formulation: History and current status. In T. D. Eells (ed.), Handbook of psychotherapy case formulation. New York: Guilford Press.

(ed.) (1997b). Handbook of psychotherapy case formulation. New York: Guilford Press.

(2007a). Psychotherapy case formulation: History and current status. In T. D. Eells (ed.), Handbook of psychotherapy case formulation (2nd edn.) (pp. 3–32). New York: Guilford Press.

(ed.) (2007b). Handbook of psychotherapy case formulation (2nd edn.). New York: Guilford Press.

Egan, G. (2002). The skilled helper: A problem management and opportunity development approach to helping. Pacific Grove, CA: Brooks/Cole.

Eisen, S. V., & Grob, M. C. (1989). Substance abuse in an inpatient population. McLean Hospital Journal, 14: 1–22.

Elkin, I., Shea, T., Watkins, J. T., Imber, S. D., Sotsky, S. M., Collins, J. F., Glass, D. R., Pilkonis, P. A., Leber, W. R., Docherty, J. P., Fiester, S. J., & Parloff, M. B. (1989). National Institute of Mental Health Treatment of Depression Collaborative Research Program: General effectiveness of treatments. Archives of General Psychiatry, 46(11): 971–82.

Elliott, R., Watson, J. C., Goldman, R. N., & Greenberg, L. S. (2004). Learning emotion-focused therapy: The process-experiential approach to change. Washington, DC: American Psychological Association.

Ellis, A. (1962). Reason and emotion in psychotherapy. New York: Lyle Stuart.

Ellis, A., & Harper, R. A. (1975). A new guide to rational living. Englewood Cliffs, NJ: Prentice Hall.

Ellis, M. V., Krengel, M., & Beck, M. (2002). Testing self-focused attention theory in clinical supervision: Effects on supervisee

anxiety and performance. Journal of Counseling Psychology, 49: 101–16.

Emmons, K. M. (2003). Increasing motivation to stop smoking. In D. B. Abrams, R. Niaura, R. A. Brown, K. M. Emmons, M. G. Goldstein, & P. M. Monti (eds.), The tobacco dependence treatment handbook: A guide to best practice (pp. 73–100). New York: Guilford Press.

Enidcott, J., & Spitzer, R. L. (1978). A diagnostic interview: The Schedule for Affective Disorders and Schizophrenia. Archives of General Psychiatry, 35(7): 837–44.

Eysenck, H. J. (1949). Training in clinical psychology: An English point of view. American Psychologist, 4: 173–6.

(1950). Function and training of the clinical psychologist. Journal of Mental Science, 96: 710–25.

(1952). The effects of psychotherapy: An evaluation. Journal of Consulting Psychology, 16: 319–24.

Fairburn, C. G. (1995). Overcoming binge eating. New York: Guilford Press.

Falender, C. A., & Shafranske, E. P. (2004). Clinical supervision: A competency-based approach. Washington, DC: American Psychological Association.

(2012). The importance of competency-based clinical supervision and training in the twenty-first century: Why bother? Journal of Contemporary Psychotherapy, 42(3): 129–37.

Falvey, J. E., & Cohen, C. R. (2003). The buck stops here: Documenting clinical supervision. The Clinical Supervisor, 22(2): 63–80.

Farrell, S. P., & McKinnon, C. R. (2003). Technology and rural mental health. Archives of Psychiatric Nursing, 17: 20–6.

Faust, D., & Fogel, B. (1989). The development and initial validation of a sensitive bedside cognitive screening test. Journal of Nervous and Mental Disease, 177(1): 25–31.

Fava, G. A. (2003). Can long-term treatment with antidepressant drugs worsen the course of depression? Journal of Clinical Psychiatry, 64: 123–33.

Fava, G. A., & Offidani, E. (2011). The mechanisms of tolerance in antidepressant action. Progress in Neuro-Psychopharmacology & Biological Psychiatry, 35: 1593–602.

Fiori, M. C., Bailey, W. C., Cohen, S. J., Dorfman, S. F., Goldstein, M. G., Gritz, E. R., Heyman, R. B., Jaen, C. R., Kottke, T. E., Lando, H. A., Mecklenburg, R., E., Mullen, P. D., Nett, L. M., Robinson, L., Stitzer, M. L., Tommasello, A. C., Villejo, L., & Wewers, M. E. (2000). *Treating tobacco use and dependence: Clinical practice guideline*, 20 June. Rockville, MD: US Department of Health and Human Services, Public Health Service.

First, M. B., Bell, C. C., Cuthbert, B., Krystal, J. H., Malison, R., Offord, D. R., Reiss, D., Shea, T., Widiger, T., & Wisner, K. L. (2002). Personality disorders and relational disorders. In D. J., Kupfer, M. B. First, & D. A. Regier (eds.), *A research agenda for DSM-V* (pp. 123–99). Washington, DC: American Psychiatric Association.

First, M. B., Spitzer, R. L., Gibbon, M., & Williams, J. B. W. (1996). *Structured Clinical Interview for DSM-IV Axis-I Disorders Research Version – Patient Version (SCID-I/P)*. New York: New York State Psychiatric Institute, Biometrics Research Department.
(1997). *Structured Clinical Interview for DSM-IV Axis-I Disorders (SCID-I) – Clinical Version*. Washington, DC: American Psychiatric Publishing.

Fishman, D. B. (1999). *The case for pragmatic psychology*. New York University Press.
(2000). Transcending the efficacy versus effectiveness research debate: Proposal for a new, electronic 'Journal of Pragmatic Case Studies'. Prevention & Treatment, 3, Article 8, 3 May. http://journals.apa.org/prevention/volume3/pre0030008a.html

Fiske, A., Kasl-Godley, J. E., & Gatz, M. (1998). Mood disorders in late life. In B. Edelstein (ed.), *Comprehensive clinical psychology*, Vol. 7: *Clinical geropsychology* (pp. 193–229). Oxford: Elsevier.

Fiske, A., Wetherell, J. L., & Gatz, M. (2009). Depression in older adults. *Annual Review of Clinical Psychology*, 5(1): 363–89.

Flavell, J. E. (1977). *The power of positive reinforcement*. Springfield, IL: Charles Thomas.

Fleischmann, A., Bertolote, J. M., Wasserman, D., De Leo, D., Bolhari, J., Botega, N. J., De Silva, D., Phillips, M., Vijayakumar, L., Värnik, A., Schlebusch, L., & Thanh, H. T. T. (2008). Effectiveness of brief intervention and contact for suicide attempters: A randomized controlled trial in five countries. *Bulletin of the World Health Organization*, 86: 703–9.

Folstein, M. F., Folstein, S. E., & McHugh, P. R. (1975). Mini-mental state: A practical method for grading the cognitive state for the clinician. *Journal of Psychiatry Research*, 12(3): 189–98.

Forsyth, J. P., Fusé, T., & Acheson, D. T. (2009). Interoceptive exposure for panic disorder. In W. T. O'Donohue & J. E. Fisher (eds.), *General principles and empirically supported techniques of cognitive behavior therapy* (pp. 394–406). New York: John Wiley.

Fowler, J. C. (2012). Suicide risk assessment in clinical practice: Pragmatic guidelines for imperfect assessments. *Psychotherapy*, 49(1): 81–90.

Fox, J. C., Blank, M., Rovnyak, V. G., & Barnett, R. Y. (2001). Barriers to help seeking for mental disorders in a rural impoverished population. *Community Mental Health Journal*, 37(5): 421–36.

Fox, R. E., DeLeon, P. H., Newman, R., Sammons, M. T., Dunivin, D. L., & Baker, D. C. (2009). Prescriptive authority and psychology: A status report. *American Psychologist*, 64: 257–68.

Foxhall, K. (2000). How would your practice records look to the FBI? *Monitor on Psychology*, 31(1): 50–1.

France, C. R., Masters, K. S., Belar, C. D., Kerns, R. D., Klonoff, E. A., Larkin, K. T., Smith, T. W., Suchday, S., & Thorn, B. E. (2008). Application of the competency model to clinical health psychology. *Professional Psychology: Research and Practice*, 39(6): 573–80.

Frances, A. (2013). *Saving normal: An insider's look at what caused the epidemic of mental illness and how to cure it*. New York: HarperCollins.

Frank, J. D. (1973). *Persuasion and healing: A comparative study of psychotherapy* (rev. edn.) Baltimore, MD: Johns Hopkins University Press.

Freeman, A. (1992). Developing treatment conceptualizations in cognitive therapy. In A. Freeman & F. Dattilio (eds.), *Casebook of cognitive-behavior therapy* (pp. 13–23). New York: Plenum Press.

Frith, C. D., & Frith, U. (2012). Mechanisms of social cognition. *Annual Review of Psychology*, 63: 287–313.

Garcia, J., & Koelling, R. A. (1966). Relation of cue to consequence in avoidance learning. *Psychonomic Science*, 4(3): 123–4.

Garfield, S. L. (1966). Clinical psychology and the search for identity. *American Psychologist*, 21: 353–62.

Gatchel, R. J. (2005). *Clinical essentials of pain management*. Washington, DC: American Psychological Association.

Gatchel, R. J., & Oordt, M. S. (2003). *Clinical health psychology and primary care: Practical advice and clinical guidance for successful collaboration*. Washington, DC: American Psychological Association.

Gibb, H., Livesey, L., & Zyla, W. (2003). At 3 am who the hell do you call? Case management issues in sole practice as a rural community mental health nurse. *Australasian Psychiatry*, 11(S1): S127–S130.

Gibson, F. (2004). *The past in the present: Using reminiscence in health and social care*. London: Health Professions Press.

Gil, A. G., Wagner, E. F., & Vega, W. A. (2000). Acculturation, familism, and alcohol use among Latino adolescent males: Longitudinal relations. *Journal of Community Psychology*, 28(4): 442–58.

Goldberg, D. (1972). *The detection of psychiatric illness by questionnaire*. Oxford University Press.

Goldstein, M. G. (2003). Pharmacotherapy for smoking cessation. In D. B. Abrams, R. Niaura, R. A. Brown, K. M. Emmons, M. G. Goldstein, & P. M. Monti (eds.), *The tobacco dependence treatment handbook: A guide to best practice* (pp. 230–48). New York: Guilford Press.

Goldstein, N. E. S., Kemp, K. A., Leff, S. S., & Lochman, J. E. (2012). Guidelines for adapting manualized interventions for new target populations: A step-wise approach using anger management as a model. *Clinical Psychology: Science and Practice*, 19(4): 385–401.

Gonsalvez, C. J., & Milne, D. L. (2010). Clinical supervisor training in Australia: A review of current problems and possible solutions. *Australian Psychologist*, 45(4): 233–42.

Gonsalvez, C. J., Oades, L. G., & Freestone, J. (2002). The objectives approach to clinical supervision: Towards integration and empirical evaluation. *Australian Psychologist*, 37(1): 68–77.

Gould, R. A., Otto, G. A., & Pollack, M. H. (1995). A meta-analysis of treatment outcome for panic disorder. *Clinical Psychology Review*, 15(8): 819–44.

Gray, G. V., Brody, D. S., Johnson, D. (2005). The evolution of behavioral primary care. *Professional Psychology: Research and Practice*, 36(2): 123–9.

Greenberg, G. (2013). *The book of woe: The DSM and the unmaking of psychiatry*. New York: Blue Rider Press.

Greysen, S. R., Chretien, K. C., Kind, T., Young, A., & Gross, C. P. (2012). Physician violations of online professionalism and disciplinary actions: A national survey of state medical boards. *Journal of the American Medical Association*, 307(11): 1141–2.

Grove, W. M., Zald, D. H., Lebow, B. S., Snitz, B. E., & Nelson, C. (2000). Clinical versus mechanical prediction: A meta-analysis. *Psychological Assessment*, 12(1): 19–30.

Gunlicks-Stoessel, M. and Weissman, M. M. (2010). Interpersonal Psychotherapy (IPT). In L. M. Horowitz and S. Strack (eds.), *Handbook of Interpersonal Psychology* (pp. 533–44). Hoboken, NJ: John Wiley.

Gurland, J., Goldon, R. R., Teresi, J. A., & Challop, J. (1984). The SHORT-CARE: An efficient instrument for the assessment of depression, dementia, and disability. *Journal of Gerontology*, 39(2): 166–9.

Gurland, B. J., Kuriansky, J., Sharpe, L., Simon, R., Stiller, P., & Birkelt, P. (1977). The Comprehensive Assessment and Referral Evaluation (CARE): Rationale, development, and reliability. *International Journal of Ageing and Human Development*, 8(1): 9–42.

Haaga, D. A. F. (2000). Introduction to the special section on stepped care models in psychotherapy. *Journal of Consulting and Clinical Psychology*, 68: 547–8.

Hadjistavropoulos, H., Kehler, M., & Hadjistavropoulos, T. (2010). Training graduate students to be clinical supervisors: A survey of Canadian professional psychology programs. *Canadian Psychology*, 51(3): 206–12.

Haley, W. E., McDaniel, S. H., Bray, J. H., Frank, R. G., Heldring, M., Johnson, S. B., Lu, E. G., Reed, G. M., & Wiggins, J. G. (1998). Psychological practice in primary care settings: Practical tips for clinicians. *Professional Psychology: Research and Practice*, 29(3): 237–44.

Hamilton, M. (1959). The assessment of anxiety states by rating. *British Journal of Medical Psychology*, 32(1): 50–5.

(1967). Development of a rating scale for primary depressive illness. *Journal of Social and Clinical Psychology*, 6(4): 278–96.

Hannan, C., Lambert, M. J., Harmon, C., Nielsen, S. L., Smart, D. W., Shimokawa, K., & Sutton, S. W. (2005). A lab test and algorithms for identifying clients at risk for treatment failure. *Journal of Clinical Psychology*, 61(2): 155–63.

Hargrove, D. S. (1982). An overview of professional considerations in the rural community. In P. A. Keller & J. D. Murray (eds.), *Handbook of rural community health* (pp. 169–82). New York: Human Sciences Press.

Harlow, H. F. (1949). The formation of learning sets. *Psychological Review*, 56: 51–65.

Harmon, C., Hawkins, E. J., Lambert, M. J., Slade, K., & Whipple, J. L. (2005). Improving outcomes for poorly desponding clients: The use of clinical support tools and feedback to clients. *Journal of Clinical Psychology*, 61(2): 175–85.

Harrison, D. P., Stritzke, W. G. K., Fay, N., Ellison, T. M., & Hudaib, A. R. (2014). Probing the implicit suicidal mind: Does the Death/Suicide Implicit Association Test reveal a desire to die, or a diminished desire to live? *Psychological Assessment*. www.researchgate.net/publication/260680995 [accessed 28 April 2014].

Hawkins, E. J., Lambert, M. J., Vermeersch, D. A., Slade, K. L., & Tuttle, K. C. (2004). The therapeutic effects of providing patient progress information to therapists and patients. *Psychotherapy Research*, 14(3): 308–27.

Hawton, K., & Kirk, J. (1989). Problem-solving. In K. Hawton, P. Salkovskis, J. Kirk, & D. M. Clark (eds.), *Cognitive behaviour therapy for psychiatric problems* (pp. 406–49). Oxford University Press.

Hayes, S. C., & Strosahl, K. D. (2004). *A practical guide to acceptance and commitment therapy*. New York: Springer-Verlag.

Hayes, S. C., Barlow, D. H., & Nelson-Gray, R. O. (1999a). *The scientist-practitioner: Research and accountability in the age of managed care* (2nd edn.). Boston, MA: Allyn & Bacon.

Hayes, S. C., Strosahl, K. D., & Wilson, K. G. (1999b). *Acceptance and commitment therapy: An experimental approach to behavior change*. New York: Guilford Press.

(2011). *Acceptance and commitment therapy: The process and practice of mindful change*. New York: Guilford Press.

Haynes, S. N., & O'Brien, W. H. (1990). Functional analysis in behavior therapy. *Clinical Psychology Review*, 10(6): 649–68.

Haynes, S. N., Lemsky, C., & Sexton-Radek, K. (1987). Why clinicians infrequently do research. *Professional Psychology: Research and Practice*, 18: 515–19.

Hazlett-Stevens, H., & Craske, M. G. (2009). Breathing retraining and diaphragmatic breathing techniques. In W. T. O'Donohue & J. E. Fisher (eds.), *General principles and empirically supported techniques of cognitive behavior therapy* (pp. 166–72). New York: John Wiley.

Health Service Psychology Education Collaborative (2013). Professional psychology in health care services: A blueprint for education and training. *American Psychologist*, 68(6): 411–26.

Health Workforce Australia (2011). National Health Workforce Innovation and Reform Strategic Framework for Action 2011–2015. Adelaide, Australia.

www.hwa.gov.au/sites/uploads/hwa-wir-strategic-framework-for-action-201110.pdf [accessed 28 April 2014].

Hendricks, M. (1994). Making a splash: Reporting evaluation results effectively. In J. S. Wholey, H. P. Hatry, & K. E. Newcomer (eds.), *Handbook of practical program evaluation* (pp. 549–75). San Francisco, CA: Jossey-Bass.

Hershenberg, R., Drabick, D. A., & Vivian, D. (2012). An opportunity to bridge the gap between clinical research and clinical practice: Implications for clinical training. *Psychotherapy*, 49(2): 123–34.

Heyman, S. R., & VandenBos, G. R. (1989). Developing local resources to enrich the practice of rural community psychology. *Hospital and Community Psychiatry*, 40(1): 21–3.

Hickie, I. B., Groom, G. L., McGorry, P. D., Davenport, T. A., & Luscombe, G. M. (2005). Australian mental health reform: Time for real outcomes. *Medical Journal of Australia*, 182(8): 401–6.

Hillenberg, J. B., & Colins, F. L. (1982). The importance of home practice for progressive relaxation training. *Behaviour Research and Therapy*, 21(6): 633–42.

HM Department of Health (2012). *IAPT three-year report: The first million patients.* London: HM Department of Health. www.iapt.nhs.uk/silo/files/iapt-3-year-report.pdf [accessed 28 April 2014].

HM Government (2011). *No health without mental health: A cross-government mental health outcomes strategy for people of all ages.* London: HM Government. www.gov.uk/government/uploads/system/uploads/attachment_data/file/213761/dh_124058.pdf [accessed 28 April 2014].

Hodges, K., Kline, J., Stern, L., Cytyrn, L., & McKnew, D. (1982). The development of a child assessment interview for research and clinical use. *Journal of Abnormal Child Psychology*, 10(2): 173–89.

Hofmann, S. G., Asnaani, A., Vonk, I. J., Sawyer, A. T., & Fang, A. (2012). The efficacy of cognitive behavioral therapy: A review of meta-analyses. *Cognitive Therapy and Research*, 36(5): 427–40.

Horvath, A. O., & Bedi, R. P. (2002). The alliance. In J. C. Norcross (ed.), *Psychotherapy relationships that work* (pp. 37–70). New York: Oxford University Press.

Horvath, A. O., & Greenberg, L. S. (1989). Development and validation of the Working Alliance Inventory. *Journal of Consulting and Clinical Psychology*, 36(2): 223–33.

Hoshmand, L. T., & Polkinghorne, D. E. (1992). Redefining the science–practice relationship and professional training. *American Psychologist*, 47(1): 55–66.

Howard, K. I., Brill, P. L., Lueger, R. J., O'Mahoney, M. T., & Grissom, G. R. (1995). *Integra outcome tracking system.* Philadelphia, PA: Integra Inc.

Howard, K. I., Kopta, S. M., Krause, M. S., & Orlinsky, D. E. (1986). The dose–response relationship in psychotherapy. *American Psychologist*, 41(2): 159–64.

Howard, K. I., Moras, K., Brill, P. L., Martinovich, Z., & Lutz, W. (1996). Evaluation of psychotherapy: Efficacy, effectiveness, and patient progress. *American Psychologist*, 51(10): 1059–64.

Hughes, J. R. (2000). Reduced smoking: An introduction and review of the evidence. *Addiction*, 95(Suppl. 1): 3–7.

Ito, L. M., de Araujo, L. A., Tess, V. L. C., de Barros-Neto, T. P., Asbahr, F. R., & Marks, I. (2001). Self-exposure for panic disorder with agoraphobia. *British Journal of Psychiatry*, 178: 331–6.

Ivey, L. C., & Doenges, T. (2013). Resolving the dilemma of multiple relationships for primary care behavioural health providers. *Professional Psychology: Research and Practice*, 44: 218–24.

Iwata, B. A., Dorsey, M. F., Slifer, K. J., Bauman, K. E., & Richman, G. S. (1982). Toward a functional analysis of self-injury. *Analysis and intervention in developmental disabilities*, 2(1): 3–20.

(1990a). Experimental analysis and extinction of self-injurious escape behavior. *Journal of Applied Behavior Analysis*, 23(1): 11–27.

Iwata, B. A., Vollmer, T. R., & Zarcone, J. H. (1990b). The experimental (functional) analysis of behavior disorders: Methodology, applications, and limitations. In A. C. Repp & N. Singh (eds.), *Perspectives on the use of* nonaversive and aversive interventions for persons with developmental disabilities (pp. 301–30). Sycamore, IL: Sycamore Publishing.

Jacobs, J., Berhard, M., Delgado, A., & Strain, J. (1977). Screening for organic mental syndromes in the medically mentally ill. *Annals of Internal Medicine*, 86(1): 40–6.

Jacobs, W. J., & Nadel, L. (1985). Stress-induced recovery of fears and phobias. *Psychological Review*, 92(4): 512–31.

Jacobson, N. S. (1984). The modification of cognitive processes in behavioral marital therapy: Integrating cognitive and behavioral intervention strategies. In K. Hahlweg & N. S. Jacobson (eds.), *Marital interaction: Analysis and modification* (pp. 285–308). New York: Guilford Press.

Jacobson, N. S., & Truax, P. (1991). Clinical significance: A statistical approach to defining meaningful change in psychotherapy research. *Journal of Consulting and Clinical Psychology*, 59(1): 12–19.

Jacobson, N. S., Follette, W. C., & Revenstorf, D. (1984). Psychotherapy outcome research: Methods for reporting variability and evaluating clinical significance. *Behavior Therapy*, 15(4): 336–52.

Johnson, E. A., & Stewart, D. W. (2000). Clinical supervision in Canadian academic and service settings: The importance of education, training, and workplace support for supervisor development. *Canadian Psychology*, 41: 124–30.

Johnson, J., Wood, A. M., Gooding, P., Taylor, P. J., & Tarrier, N. (2011). Resilience to suicidality: The buffering hypothesis. *Clinical Psychology Review*, 31(4): 563–91.

Johnson, N. G. (2003). Psychology and health: Research, practice, and policy. *American Psychologist*, 58: 670–7.

Johnstone, K., & Page, A. C. (2004). Attention to phobic stimuli during exposure: The effect of distraction on anxiety reduction, self-efficacy, and perceived control. *Behaviour Research and Therapy*, 42(3): 249–75.

Joiner, T. E., Walker, R. L., Rudd, M. D., & Jobes, D. A. (1999). Scientizing and routinizing the assessment of suicidality in outpatient practice. *Professional Psychology: Research and Practice*, 30(5): 447–53.

Joint Task Force for the Development of Telepsychology Guidelines for Psychologists (2013). Guidelines for the practice of telepsychology. *American Psychologist*, 68(9): 791–800.

Kahn, R., Goldfarb, A., Pollack, M., & Peck, A. (1960). Brief objective measures for the determination of mental status in the aged. *American Journal of Psychiatry*, 117: 326–8.

Kaner, E., Newbury-Birch, D., & Heather, N. (2009). Brief intervention. In P. M. Miller (ed.), *Evidence-based addiction treatment* (pp. 189–213). New York: Academic Press.

Kanfer, F. H., & Gaelick-Buys, L. (1991). Self-management methods. In F. H. Kanfer & A. P. Goldstein (eds.), *Helping people change: A textbook of methods* (pp. 305–60). New York: Pergamon.

Kaplan, H. I., & Sadock, B. J. (2004). *Comprehensive textbook of psychiatry/VIII* (8th edn.). Baltimore, MD: Williams and Wilkins.

Kaplan, R. M., & Groessl, E. J. (2002). Applications of cost-effectiveness methodologies in behavioral medicine. *Journal of Consulting and Clinical Psychology*, 70: 482–93.

Karel, M. J., Gatz, M., & Smyer, M. A. (2012). Aging and mental health in the decade ahead: What psychologists need to know. *American Psychologist*, 67(3): 184–98.

Karlin, B. E., & Cross, G. (2014). From the laboratory to the therapy room: National dissemination and implementation of evidence-based psychotherapies in the U.S. Department of Veterans Affairs Health Care System. *American Psychologist*, 69(1): 19–33.

Kaslow, F. W., Patterson, T., & Gottlieb, M. (2011). Ethical dilemmas in psychologists accessing internet data: Is it justified? *Professional Psychology: Research and Practice*, 42(2): 105–12.

Kaszniak, A. W., & Christenson, G. D. (1994). Differential diagnosis of dementia and depression. In M. Storandt & G. R. Vanden (eds.), *Neuropsychological assessment of dementia and depression in older adults: A clinician's guide* (pp. 81–118). Washington, DC: American Psychological Association.

Kazantzis, N., & L'Abate, L. (eds.) (2007). *Handbook of homework assignments in psychotherapy: Research, practice, and prevention.* New York: Springer.

Kazantzis, N., Deane, F. P., & Ronan, K. R. (2000). Homework assignments in cognitive and behavioural therapy: A meta-analysis. *Clinical Psychology: Science and Practice*, 7: 189–202.

Kazantzis, N., Deane, F. P., Ronan, K. R., & L'Abate, L. (eds.) (2005). *Using homework assignments in cognitive behavioral therapy.* New York: Routledge.

Kazarian, S. S., & Evans, D. R. (eds.) (1998). *Cultural clinical psychology: Theory, research, and practice.* New York: Oxford University Press.

Kazdin, A. E. (2011). Evidence-based treatment research: Advances, limitations, and next steps. *American Psychologist*, 66(8): 685–98.

Kazdin, A. E., & Blase, S. L. (2011). Rebooting psychotherapy research and practice to reduce the burden of mental illness. *Perspectives on Psychological Science*, 6(1): 21–37.

Keith-Spiegel, P., & Koocher, G. P. (1985). *Ethics in psychology: Professional standards and cases.* New York: Random House.

Keller, P. A., & Prutsman, T. D. (1982). Training for professional psychology in the rural community. In P. A. Keller & J. D. Murray (eds.), *Handbook of rural community health* (pp. 190–9). New York: Human Sciences Press.

Kelley, S. D., & Bickman, L. (2009). Beyond outcomes monitoring: Measurement feedback systems in child and adolescent clinical practice. *Current Opinion in Psychiatry*, 22(4): 363–8.

Kelley, S. D., Bickman, L., & Norwood, E. (2010). Evidence-based treatments and common factors in youth psychotherapy. In B. L. Duncan, S. D. Miller, B. E. Wampold, and M. A. Hubble (eds.), *The heart and soul of change: Delivering what works in therapy* (2nd edn.) (pp. 325–55). Washington, DC: American Psychological Association.

Kelly, J. F., & Coons, H. L. (2012). Integrated health care and professional psychology: Is the setting right for you? *Professional Psychology: Research and Practice*, 43: 586–95.

Kennedy, A., Maple, M. J., McKay, & Brumby, S. A. (2014). Suicide and accidental death in Australia's rural farming communities: A review of the literature. *Rural and Remote Health*, 14: 2517.

Khoury, B., Lecomte, T., Fortin, G., Masse, M., Therien, P., Bouchard, V., Chapleau, M. A., Paquin, K., & Hofmann, S. G. (2013). Mindfulness-based therapy: A comprehensive meta-analysis. *Clinical Psychology Review*, 33(6): 763–71.

Kiesler, C. A. (2000). The next wave of change for psychology and mental health services in the health care revolution. *American Psychologist*, 55: 481–7.

Kirkley, A., Birmingham, T. B., Litchfield, R. B., Giffin, J. R., Willits, K. R., Wong, C. J., Feagan, B. G., Donner, A., Griffin, S. H., D'Ascanio, L. M., Pope, J. E., & Fowler, P. J. (2008). A randomized trial of arthroscopic surgery for osteoarthritis of the knee. *New England Journal of Medicine*, 359(11): 1097–107.

Kleiman, E. M., & Beaver, J. K. (2013). A meaningful life is worth living: Meaning in life as a suicide resiliency factor. *Psychiatry Research*, 210(3): 934–9.

Klein, R. H. (1993). Short-term group psychotherapy. In H. I. Kaplan & B. J. Sadock (eds.), *Comprehensive group psychotherapy* (3rd edn.) (pp. 256–70). Baltimore, MD: Williams & Wilkins.

Klerman, G. L., & Weissman, M. M. (1993). *New applications of interpersonal psychotherapy.* Washington, DC: American Psychiatric Press.

Klerman, G. L., Weissman, M. M., Rounsaville, & Chevron, E. S. (1984). *Interpersonal psychotherapy for depression: A brief, focused, specific strategy.* New York: Aronson.

Kliem, S., Kröger, C., & Kosfelder, J. (2010). Dialectical behavior therapy for borderline personality disorder: A meta-analysis using mixed-effects modeling. *Journal of Consulting and Clinical Psychology*, 78(6): 936–51.

Kluckhohn, F. R., & Stodtbeck, F. L. (1961). *Variations in value orientations*. Evanston, IL: Row, Peterson.

Knight, B. G. (2004). *Psychotherapy with older adults* (3rd edn.). Thousand Oaks, CA: Sage Publications.

Knight, B. G., & Poon, C. Y. (2008). Contextual adult life span theory for adapting psychotherapy with older adults. *Journal of Rational-Emotive & Cognitive-Behavior Therapy*, 26(4): 232–49.

Kolmes, K. (2012). Social media in the future of professional psychology. *Professional Psychology: Research and Practice*, 43: 606–12.

Kovacs, M. (1997). *The Interview Schedule for Children and Adolescents (ISCA): Current and lifetime (ISCA-C & L) and current interim (ISCA – C & I) versions*. Pittsburgh: Western Psychiatric Institute and Clinic.

Kraus, D. R., Castonguay, L., Boswell, J. F., Nordberg, S. S., & Hayes, J. A. (2011). Therapist effectiveness: Implications for accountability and patient care. *Psychotherapy Research*, 21(3): 267–76.

Kreitman, N. (1986). Alcohol consumption and the preventive paradox. *British Journal of Addictions*, 81(3): 353–63.

Kutash, I. L., & Wolf, A. (1993). Psychoanalysis in groups. In H. I. Kaplan & B. J. Sadock (eds.), *Comprehensive group psychotherapy* (3rd edn.) (pp. 126–38). Baltimore, MD: Williams & Wilkins.

Lambert, M. J. (1976). Spontaneous remission in adult neurotic disorders: A revision and summary. *Psychological Bulletin*, 83(1): 107–19.

(2010). *Prevention of treatment failure: The use of measuring, monitoring, & feedback in clinical practice*. Washington, DC: American Psychological Association.

(ed.) (2013). *Bergin and Garfield's handbook of psychotherapy and behavior change* (6th edn.). Hoboken, NJ: John Wiley.

Lambert, M. J., & Finch, A. E. (1999). The Outcome Questionnaire. In M. E. Maruish (ed.), *The use of psychological testing for treatment planning and outcomes assessment* (2nd edn.) (pp. 831–69). Mahwah, NJ: Lawrence Erlbaum Associates.

Lambert, M. J., & Hawkins, E. J. (2001). Using information about patient progress in supervision: Are outcomes enhanced? *Australian Psychologist*, 36(2): 131–8.

Lambert, M. J., Gregersen, A. T., & Burlingame, G. M. (2004). The Outcome Questionnaire-45. In M. E. Maruish (ed.), *The use of psychological testing for treatment planning and outcomes assessment*, Vol. 3: *Instruments for adults* (3rd edn.) (pp. 191–234). Mahwah, NJ: Lawrence Erlbaum Associates.

Lambert, M. J., Hansen, N. B., & Bauer, S. (2008). Assessing the clinical significance of outcome results. In A. M. Nezu & C. M. Nezu (eds.), *Evidence-based outcome research: A practical guide to conducting randomized controlled trials for psychosocial interventions* (pp. 359–78). New York: Oxford University Press.

Lambert, M. J., Harmon, C., Slade, K. L., Whipple, J. L., & Hawkins, E. J. (2005). Providing feedback to psychotherapists on their patients' progress: Clinical results and practice suggestions. *Journal of Clinical Psychology*, 61(2): 165–74.

Lambert, M. J., Whipple, J. L., Smart, D. W., Vermeersch, D. A., Nielsen, S. L., & Hawkins, E. J. (2001). The effects of providing therapists with feedback on patient progress during psychotherapy: Are outcomes enhanced? *Psychotherapy Research*, 11: 49–68.

Lambert, M. J., Whipple, J. L., Vermeersch, D. A., Smart, D. W., Hawkins, E. J., Nielsen, S. L., & Goates, M. (2002). Enhancing psychotherapy outcomes via providing feedback on patient progress: A replication. *Clinical Psychology and Psychotherapy*, 9(2): 91–103.

Lancee, J., Sorbi, M. J., Eisma, M. C., van Straten, A., & van den Bout, J. (2014). The effect of support on Internet-delivered treatment for insomnia: Does baseline depression severity matter? *Behavior Therapy*, 45(4): 507–16.

Lauderdale, S. A., Cassidy-Eagle, E. L., Nguyen, C., & Sheikh, J. I. (2011). Late life anxiety disorders. In M. E. Agronin & G. J. Maletta (eds.), *Principles and Practice of Geriatric Psychiatry* (2nd edn.) (pp. 493–514). Philadelphia, PA: Williams & Wilkins.

Lavoie, K. L., & Barone, S. (2006). Prescription privileges for psychologists: A comprehensive review and critical analysis of current issues and controversies. *CNS Drugs*, 20(1): 51–66.

Lazarus, A. A., & Fay, A. (1982). Resistance or rationalization? A cognitive-behavioural perspective. In P. L. Wachtel (ed.), *Resistance: Psychodynamic and behavioural approaches* (pp. 115–32). New York: Plenum Press.

Lewinsohn, P. M., & Graf, M. (1973). Pleasant activities and depression. *Journal of Consulting and Clinical Psychology*, 41: 261–8.

Lewis, B. L. (2001). Health psychology specialty practice opportunities in a rural community hospital: Practicing local clinical science. *Professional Psychology: Research and Practice*, 32(1): 59–64.

Lezak, M. D., Howieson, D. B., & Loring, D. W. (2004). *Neuropsychological assessment* (4th edn.). New York: Oxford University Press.

Lichte, C. (1996). The delivery of psychology services in rural and remote Australia. In R. Griffiths, P. Dunn, & S. Ramanathan (eds.), *Psychology services in rural and remote Australia* (pp. 37–41). Wagga Wagga, NSW: Australian Rural Health Research Institute.

Lichtenberg, P. A. (2010). *Handbook of assessment in clinical gerontology* (2nd edn.). New York: John Wiley.

Lichtenstein, E., Zhu, S., & Tedeschi, G. J. (2010). Smoking cessation quitlines: An underrecognized intervention success story. *American Psychologist*, 65(4): 252–61.

Liese, B. S., & Beck, J. S. (1997). Cognitive therapy supervision. In C. E. Watkins (ed.), *Handbook of psychotherapy supervision* (pp. 114–33). New York: John Wiley.

Lilienfeld, S. O. (2012). Public skepticism of psychology: Why many people perceive the study of human behavior as unscientific. *American Psychologist*, 67(2): 111–29.

Lilienfeld, S. O., Ammirati, R., & David, M. (2012). Distinguishing science from pseudoscience in school psychology: Science and scientific thinking as safeguards against human error. *Journal of School Psychology*, 50(1): 7–36.

Linehan, M. M. (1993a). *Cognitive behavioral treatment of borderline personality disorder*. New York: Guilford Press.

(1993b). *Skills training manual for treating borderline personality disorder*. New York: Guilford Press.

Linehan, M. M., Goodstein, J. L., Nielsen, S. L., & Chiles, J. A. (1983). Reasons for staying alive when you are thinking of killing yourself: The Reasons for Living Inventory. *Journal of Consulting and Clinical Psychology*, 51: 276–86.

Lipsitz, J. D., & Markowitz, J. C. (2013). Mechanisms of change in interpersonal therapy (IPT). *Clinical Psychology Review*, 33(8): 1134–47.

Litrownik, A. J., Franzini, L. R., & Turner, G. L. (1976). Acquisition of concepts by TMR children as a function of type of modeling, rule verbalization, and observer gender. *American Journal of Mental Deficiency*, 80: 620–8.

Littlefield, L. (2012). New APS model of psychology education under consideration. *InPsych*, 34: 6–9.

López, S. R. (1997). Cultural competencies in psychotherapy: A guide for clinicians and their supervisors. In C. E. Watkins Jr. (ed.), *Handbook of psychotherapy supervision* (pp. 570–88). New York: John Wiley.

Lovibond, S. H. (1964). *Conditioning and enuresis*. Oxford: Pergamon Press.

Löwe, B., Spitzer, R. L., Gräfe, K., Kroenke, K., Quenter, A., Zipfel, S., Buchholz, C., Witte, S., & Herzog, W. (2004). Comparative validity of three screening questionnaires for DSM-IV depressive disorders and physicians' diagnoses. *Journal of Affective Disorders*, 78(2): 131–40.

Luepker, E. T. (2003). *Record keeping in psychotherapy and counseling: Protecting confidentiality and the professional relationship*. New York: Brunner-Routledge.

Lundahl, B., & Burke, B. L. (2009). The effectiveness and applicability of motivational interviewing: A practice-friendly review of four metaanalyses. *Journal of Clinical Psychology*, 65(11): 1232–45.

Lustria, M. L. A., Noar, S. M., Cortese, J., Van Stee, S. K., Glueckauf, R. L., & Lee, J. (2013). A meta-analysis of web-delivered tailored health behavior change interventions. *Journal of Health Communication*, 18(9): 1039–69.

Lutz, W., Martinovich, Z., & Howard, K. I. (1999). Patient profiling: An application of random coefficient regression models to depicting the response of a patient to outpatient psychotherapy. *Journal of Consulting and Clinical Psychology*, 67(4): 571–7.

Lutz, W., Martinovich, Z., Howard, K. I., & Leon, S. C. (2002). Outcomes management, expected treatment response, and severity-adjusted provider profiling in outpatient psychotherapy. *Journal of Clinical Psychology*, 58(10): 1291–304.

Lutz, W., Stulz, N., & Kock, K. (2009). Patterns of early change and their relationship to outcome and follow-up among patients with major depressive disorders. *Journal of Affective Disorders*, 118(1–3): 60–8.

Lyons, J. S., Howard, K. I., O'Mahoney, M. T., & Lish, J. D. (1996). *The measurement and management of clinical outcomes in mental health*. New York: John Wiley.

MacIntyre, S. (2001). *Socio-economic inequalities in health in Scotland: Social Justice Annual Report Scotland 2001*. www.scotland.gov.uk/library3/sjar-41.asp [accessed 28 April 2014].

MacIntyre, S., & Petticrew, M. (2000). Good intentions and received wisdom are not enough. *Journal of Epidemiology and Community Health*, 54(11): 802–3.

Maheu, M. M., Pulier, M. L., McMenamin, J. P., & Posen, L. (2012). Future of telepsychology, telehealth, and various technologies in psychological research and practice. *Professional Psychology: Research and Practice*, 43(6): 613–21.

Malone, J. I. (2012). Ethical professional practice: exploring the issues for health services to rural Aboriginal communities. *Rural and Remote Health*, 12: 1891.

Malone, K. M., Oquendo, M. A., Haas, G. L., Ellis, S. P., Li, S., & Mann, J. J. (2000). Protective factors against suicidal acts in major depression: Reasons for living.

American Journal of Psychiatry, 157(7): 1084–8.

Markowitz, J. C., & Swartz, H. A. (1997). Case formulation in interpersonal psychotherapy for depression. In T. D. Eells (ed.), *Handbook of psychotherapy case formulation* (pp. 192–222). New York: Guilford Press.

Marmar, C. R., Weiss, D. S., & Gaston, L. (1989). Toward the validation of the California Therapeutic Alliance Rating System. *Psychological Assessment*, 1(1): 46–52.

Martin, D. J., Garske, J. P., & Davis, M. K. (2000). Relation of the therapeutic alliance with outcome and other variables: A meta-analytic review. *Journal of Consulting and Clinical Psychology*, 68(3): 438–50.

Martin, P. (2004). President's report. In Annual Report of the Australian Psychological Society (pp. 4–6). www.psychology.org.au/aps/annualreport2004part2.pdf [accessed 28 April 2005].

Martin, P. R. (1989). The scientist-practitioner model and clinical psychology: Is it time for a change? *Australian Psychologist*, 24: 71–92.

Matarazzo, J. D. (1980). Behavioral health and behavioral medicine: Frontiers for a new health psychology. *American Psychologist*, 35: 807–17.

Mathews (2011). Profile of the regional, rural and remote psychology workforce. *InPsych*, October. www.psychology.org.au/Content.aspx?ID=3961 [accessed 28 April 2014].

Mattick, R. P., Andrews, G., Hadzi-Pavlovic, D., & Christinesen, H. (1990). Treatment of panic disorder and agoraphobia. *Journal of Nervous and Mental Disease*, 178(9): 567–76.

McCambridge, J., & Cunningham, J. A. (2013). The early history of ideas on brief interventions for alcohol. *Addiction*, 109(4): 538–46.

McClellan, A. T., Woody, G. E., Luborsky, L., O'Brien, C. P., & Druley, K. A. (1983). Increased effectiveness of substance abuse treatment: A prospective study of patient-treatment 'matching'. *Journal of Nervous and Mental Disease*, 171(10): 597–605.

McClendon, D. T., Warren, J. S., Green, K. M., Burlingame, G. M., Eggett, D. L.,

& McClendon, R. J. (2011). Sensitivity to change of youth treatment outcome measures: A comparison of the CBCL, BASC-2, and Y-OQ. *Journal of Clinical Psychology*, 67(1): 111–25.

McFall, R. M. (1991). Manifesto for a science of clinical psychology. *The Clinical Psychologist*, 44(6): 75–88.

McHugh, R. K., & Barlow, D. H. (2010). The dissemination and implementation of evidence-based psychological treatments: A review of current efforts. *American Psychologist*, 65(2): 73–84.

McHugh, R. K., Whitton, S. W., Peckham, A. D., Welge, J. A., & Otto, M. W. (2013). Patient preference for psychological vs pharmacologic treatment of psychiatric disorders: A meta-analytic review. *Journal of Clinical Psychiatry*, 74(6): 595–602.

Medco Health Solutions (2011). America's state of mind. http://apps.who.int/medicinedocs/documents/s19032en/s19032en.pdf

Meighan, M., Davis, M. W., Thomas, S. P., & Droppleman, P. G. (1999). Living with postpartum depression: The father's experience. *American Journal of Maternal Child Nursing*, 24(4): 202–8.

Meltzoff, J., & Kornreich, M. (1970). *Research in psychotherapy*. New York: Atherton Press.

Menzies, R. G., & Clarke, J. C. (1994). Retrospective studies of the origins of phobias: A review. *Anxiety, Stress, and Coping*, 7(4): 305–18.

(1995). The etiology of phobias: A non-associative account. *Clinical Psychology Review*, 15: 23–48.

Meuret, A. E., Wolitzky-Taylor, K. B., Twohig, M. P., & Craske, M. G. (2012). Coping skills and exposure therapy in panic disorder and agoraphobia: Latest advances and future directions. *Behavior Therapy*, 43(2): 271–84.

Meyer, R. G. & Weaver, C. M. (2012). *Case studies in abnormal behavior* (9th edn.). Boston, MA: Allyn & Bacon.

Michelson, L. K., Marchione, K. E., Greenwald, M., Testa, S., & Marchione, N. J. (1996). A comparative outcome and follow-up investigation of panic disorder with agoraphobia: The relative and combined efficacy of cognitive therapy relaxation training and therapist-assisted exposure. *Journal of Anxiety Disorders*, 10(5): 297–330.

Miller, G. (1969). Psychology as a means of promoting human welfare. *American Psychologist*, 24(12): 1063–75.

Miller, M., & Wood, L. (2002). *Smoking cessation interventions: Review of evidence and implications for best practice in health care settings*. Canberra, Australia: Commonwealth Department of Health and Ageing.

Miller, S. D., Duncan, B. L., & Hubble, M. A. (2005a). Outcome-informed clinical work. In J. C. Norcross & M. R. Goldfried (eds.), *Handbook of psychotherapy integration* (2nd edn.) (pp. 84–102). New York: Oxford University Press.

Miller, S. D., Duncan, B. L., Sorrell, R., & Brown, G. S. (2005b). The partners for change outcome management system. *Journal of Clinical Psychology*, 61(2): 199–208.

Miller, T. W. (ed.) (1996). *Theory and assessment of stressful life events*. Madison, CT: International Universities Press.

Miller, T. W., Miller, J. M., Kraus, R. F., Kaak, O., Sprang, R., & Veltkamp, L. J. (2003). Telehealth: A clinical application model for rural consultation. *Consulting Psychology Journal: Practice and Research*, 55: 119–127.

Miller, W. R., & Baca, L. M. (1983). Two-year follow-up of bibliotherapy and therapist-directed controlled drinking training for alcohol problems. *Behavior Therapy*, 14(3), 441–8.

Miller, W. R., & Heather, N. (eds.) (1998). *Treating addictive behaviors* (2nd edn.). New York: Plenum Press.

Miller, W. R., & Page, A. C. (1991). Warm turkey: Other routes to abstinence. *Journal of Substance Abuse Treatment*, 8(4): 227–32.

Miller, W. R., & Rollnick, S. (eds.) (2012). *Motivational interviewing: Helping people change* (3rd edn.). New York: Guilford Press.

Miller, W. R., Taylor, C. A., & West, J. C. (1980). Focused versus broad spectrum behavior therapy for problem drinkers. *Journal of Consulting and Clinical Psychology*, 48: 590–601.

Miller, W. R., Wilbourne, P. L., & Hettema, J. E. (2003). What works? A summary of alcohol treatment outcome research. In R. K. Hester & W. R. Miller (eds.), *Handbook of alcoholism treatment approaches: Effective alternatives* (3rd edn.) (pp. 13–63). Boston, MA: Allyn & Bacon.

Milne, D. & Oliver, V. (2000). Flexible formats of clinical supervision: Description, evaluation and implementation. *Journal of Mental Health*, 9(3): 291–304.

Mintz, J., & Kiesler, D. J. (1982). Individualized measures of psychotherapy outcome. In P. C. Kendall & J. N. Butcher (eds.), *Handbook of research methods in clinical psychology* (pp. 491–534). New York: John Wiley.

Mitchell, P. F. (2011). Evidence-based practice in real-world services for young people with complex needs: New opportunities suggested by recent implementation science. *Children and Youth Services Review*, 33(2): 207–16.

Moseley, J. B., O'Malley, K., Petersen, N. J., Menke, T. J., Brody, B. A., Kuykendall, D. H., Hollingsworth, J. C., Ashton, C. M., & Wray, N. P. (2002). A controlled trial of arthroscopic surgery for osteoarthritis of the knee. *New England Journal of Medicine*, 347: 81–8.

Mowrer, O. H., & Mowrer, W. M. (1938). Enuresis: A method for its study and treatment. *American Journal of Orthopsychiatry*, 8(3): 436–59.

Moye, J. & Marson, D. C. (2007). Assessment of decision making capacity in older adults: An emerging area of research and practice. *Journal of Gerontology*, 62(1): 3–11.

Munder, T., Wilmers, F., Leonhart, R., Linster, H. W., & Barth, J. (2010). Working Alliance Inventory-Short Revised (WAI-SR): Psychometric properties in outpatients and inpatients. *Clinical Psychology & Psychotherapy*, 17(3): 231–9.

Muran, J. C., & Segal, Z. V. (1992). The development of an idiographic measure of self-schemas: An illustration of the construction and use of scenarios. *Psychotherapy*, 29: 524–35.

Nathan, P. E. (2000). The Boulder model: A dream deferred – or lost? *American Psychologist*, 55(2): 250–2.

Nathan, P. E., & Gorman, J. M. (eds.) (2002). *A guide to treatments that work* (2nd edn.). New York: Oxford University Press.

(2007). *A guide to treatments that work* (3rd edn.). New York: Oxford University Press.

Nelson, P. L., Warren, J. S., Gleave, R. L., & Burlingame, G. M. (2013). Youth psychotherapy change trajectories and early warning system accuracy in a managed care setting. *Journal of Clinical Psychology*, 69(9): 880–95.

Neufeldt, S. A. (1999). *Supervision strategies for the first practicum* (2nd edn.). Alexandria, VA: American Counseling Association.

Neufeldt, S. A. (2003). Becoming a clinical supervisor. In M. J. Prinstein & M. D. Patterson (eds.), *The portable mentor: Expert guide to a successful career in psychology* (pp. 209–18). New York: Kluwer Academic/Plenum Press.

Neufeldt, S. A., & Nelson, M. L. (1998). Research in training clinics: A bridge between science and practice. *Journal of Clinical Psychology*, 54(3): 315–27.

Neufeldt, S. A., Karno, M. P., & Nelson, M. L. (1996). A qualitative study of experts' conceptualization of supervisee reflectivity. *Journal of Counseling Psychology*, 43(1): 3–9.

Newnham, E. A., & Page, A. C. (2007). Client-focused research: New directions in outcome assessment. *Behaviour Change*, 24: 1–6.

(2010). Bridging the gap between best evidence and best practice in mental health. *Clinical Psychology Review*, 30(1): 127–42.

Newnham, E. A., Harwood, K. E., & Page, A. C. (2007). Evaluating the clinical significance of responses by psychiatric inpatients to the mental health subscales of the SF-36. *Journal of Affective Disorders*, 98(1–2): 91–7.

(2009). The subscale structure and clinical utility of the Health of the Nation Outcome Scale. *Journal of Mental Health*, 18: 326–34.

Newnham, E. A., Hooke, G. R., & Page, A. C. (2010a). Monitoring treatment response and outcomes using the World Health Organization's Wellbeing Index in psychiatric care. *Journal of Affective Disorders*, 122(1–2): 133–8.

(2010b). Progress monitoring and feedback in psychiatric care reduces depressive symptoms. *Journal of Affective Disorders*, 127(1–3): 139–46.

Nezu, A. M., & Nezu, C. M. (eds.) (1989). *Clinical decision making in behavior therapy: A problem-solving perspective*. Champaign, IL: Research Press.

Niaura, W. G., & Shadal, W. G. (2003). Assessment to inform smoking cessation treatment. In D. B. Abrams, R. Niaura, R. A. Brown, K. M. Emmons, M. G. Goldstein, & P. M. Monti (eds.), *The tobacco dependence treatment handbook: A guide to best practice* (pp. 27–72). New York: Guilford Press.

Nicassio, P. M., Meyerowitz, B. E., & Kerns, R. D. (2004). The future of health psychology interventions. *Health Psychology*, 23(2): 132–7.

Nicholson, I. R. (2011). New technology, old issues: Demonstrating the relevance of the *Canadian Code of Ethics for Psychologists* to the ever-sharper cutting edge of technology. *Canadian Psychology/ Psychologie canadienne*, 52(3): 215–24.

Nisbett, R. E., & Wilson, T. D. (1977). Telling more than we can know: Verbal reports on mental processes. *Psychological Review*, 84(3): 231–59.

Norcross, J. C. (ed.) (2000). *Psychotherapy relationships that work: Therapist contributions and responsiveness to patients*. Oxford University Press.

(ed.) (2002). *Psychotherapy relationships that work: Therapist contributions and responsiveness to patient needs*. New York: Oxford University Press.

(2010). The therapeutic relationship. In B. L. Duncan, S. D. Miller, B. E. Wampold, & M. A. Hubble (eds.), *The heart and soul of change: Delivering what works in therapy* (2nd edn.) (pp. 113–42). Washington, DC: American Psychological Association.

Norcross, J. C., & Karpiak, C. P. (2012). Clinical psychologists in the 2010s: 50 years of the APA Division of Clinical Psychology. *Clinical Psychology: Science and Practice*, 19(1): 1–12.

Norcross, J. C., & Wampold, B. E. (2011). Evidence-based therapy relationships:

Research conclusions and clinical practices. *Psychotherapy*, 48(1): 98–102.

Nordberg, S. S., Castonguay, L. G., Fisher, A. J., Boswell, J. F., & Kraus, D. (2014). Validating the rapid responder construct within a Practice Research Network. *Journal of Clinical Psychology*. doi: 10.1002/jclp.22077

O'Donnell, A., Anderson, P., Newbury-Birch, D., Schulte, B., Schmidt, C., Reimer, J., & Kaner, E. (2014). The impact of brief alcohol interventions in primary healthcare: A systematic review of reviews. *Alcohol and Alcoholism*, 49(1): 66–78.

O'Donohue, W., & Krasner, L. (eds.) (1995). *Theories of behavior therapy: Exploring behavior change*. Washington, DC: American Psychological Association.

O'Leary, K. D., Curley, A., Rosenbaum, A., & Clarke, C. (1986). Assertion training for abused wives: A potentially hazardous treatment. *Journal of Marital and Family Therapy*, 11(3): 319–22.

O'Neill, R. E., Horner, R. H., Albin, R. W., Storey, K., & Sprague, J. R. (1990). *Functional analysis of problem behavior: A practical assessment guide*. Sycamore, IL: Sycamore Publishing.

O'Rourke, N., Cappeliez, P., & Claxton, A. (2011). Functions of reminiscence and the psychological well-being of young-old and older adults over time. *Aging & Mental Health*, 15(2): 272–81.

Ogles, B. M., Lunnen, K. M., & Bonesteel, K. (2001). Clinical significance: History, application, and current practice. *Clinical Psychology Review*, 21(3): 421–46.

Olfson, M., Marcus, S. C., Druss, B., Elinson, L., Tanielian, T., & Pincus, H. A. (2002). National trends in the outpatient treatment of depression. *Journal of the American Medical Association*, 287(2): 203–9.

Olfson, M., Marcus, S. C., Tedeschi, M., & Wan, G. J. (2006). Continuity of antidepressant treatment for adults with depression in the United States. *American Journal of Psychiatry*, 163(1): 101–8.

Oliver, N. S., & Page, A. C. (2003). Fear reduction during in vivo exposure to blood-injection stimuli: Distraction vs. attentional focus. *British Journal of Clinical Psychology*, 42: 13–25.

Oltmans, T. F., Neale, J. M., & Davison, G. C. (2003). *Case studies in abnormal psychology* (6th edn.). New York: John Wiley.

Oltmans, T. F., Martin, M. T., Neale, J. M., & Davison, G. C. (2012).*Case studies in abnormal psychology* (9th edn.). New York: John Wiley.

Oordt, M. S., Jobes, D. A., Rudd, M. D., Fonseca, V. P., Runyan, C. N., Stea, J. B., Campise, R. L., & Talcott, G. W. (2005). Development of a clinical guide to enhance care for suicidal patients. *Professional Psychology: Research and Practice*, 36: 208–18.

Organisation for Economic Co-operation and Development (OECD) (2013). *OECD Health Data 2013*. www.oecd.org/health/health-systems/oecdhealthdata.htm [accessed 28 April 2014].

Orlinsky, D. E., Botermans, J.-F., & Rønnestad, M. H. (2001). Towards an empirically grounded model of psychotherapy training: Four thousand therapists rate influences on their development. *Australian Psychologist*, 36(2): 139–48.

Orlinsky, D. E., Grawe, K., & Parks, B. K. (1994). Process and outcome in psychotherapy – Noch Einmal. In A. E. Bergin & S. L. Garfield (eds.), *Handbook of psychotherapy and behavior change* (4th edn.) (pp. 270–376). New York: John Wiley.

Orlinsky, D. E., Rønnestad, M. H., & Willutzki, U. (2004). Fifty years of psychotherapy process-outcome research: Continuity and change. In M. J. Lambert (ed.), *Bergin and Garfield's handbook of psychotherapy and behavior change* (5th edn.) (pp. 307–89). New York: John Wiley.

Öst, L. G., & Westling, B. E. (1995). Applied relaxation vs cognitive behavior therapy in the treatment of panic disorder. *Behaviour Research and Therapy*, 33(2): 145–58.

Otis, J. D., Reid, M. C., & Kerns, R. D. (2005). Multidisciplinary approaches to pain management in primary care settings. In L. C. James & R. A. Folen (eds.), *The primary care consultant: The next frontier for psychologists in hospitals and clinics* (pp. 41–59). Washington, DC: American Psychological Association.

Owen, J. M., & Rogers, P. J. (1999). *Program evaluation: Forms and approaches* (2nd edn.). St. Leonards, NSW: Allen & Unwin.

Pachana, N. A., Sofronoff, K., Scott, T., & Helmes, E. (2011). Attainment of competencies in clinical psychology training: Ways forward in the Australian context. *Australian Psychologist*, 46(2): 67–76.

Page, A. C. (1991a). An assessment of structured diagnostic interviews for adult anxiety disorders. *International Review of Psychiatry*, 3(2): 265–78.

(1991b). Teaching developmentally disabled people self-regulation in sexual behaviour. *Australian and New Zealand Journal of Developmental Disabilities*, 17(1): 81–88.

(2002a). *Don't panic: Anxiety, phobias and tension*. Sydney: ACP & Media 21.

(2002b). Nature and treatment of panic disorder. *Current Opinion in Psychiatry*, 15(2): 149–55.

Page, A. C., & Hooke, G. R. (2009). Increased attendance in inpatient group psychotherapy improves patient outcomes. *Psychiatric Services*, 60(4): 426–8.

Panos, P. T., Jackson, J. W., Hasan, O., & Panos, A. (2013). Meta-analysis and systematic review assessing the efficacy of Dialectical Behavior Therapy (DBT). *Research on Social Work Practice*, 24(2): 213–23.

Parsons, T. (1951). Illness and the role of the physician: A sociological perspective. *American Journal of Orthopsychiatry*, 21(3): 452–60.

Patterson, C. H. (1997). Client-centered supervision. In C. E. Watkins (ed.), *Handbook of psychotherapy supervision* (pp. 134–46). New York: John Wiley.

Pavlov, I. P. (1927). *Conditioned reflexes: An investigation of the physiological activity of the cerebral cortex*. New York: Dover.

Pearce, J. M., & Bouton, M. E. (2001). Theories of associative learning in animals. *Annual Review of Psychology*, 52: 111–13.

Pearson, Q. M. (2004). Getting the most out of clinical supervision: Strategies for mental health counseling students. *Journal of Mental Health Counseling*, 26(4): 361–73.

Penfold, K., & Page, A. C. (1999). Distraction enhances within-session fear reduction during in vivo exposure. *Behavior Therapy*, 30: 607–21.

Persons, J. B., & Tompkins, M. A. (1989). Cognitive-behavioral case formulation. In J. B. Persons (ed.), *Cognitive therapy in practice: A case formulation approach* (pp. 314–39). New York: W. W. Norton.

(2007). Cognitive-behavioral case formulation. In T. D. Eells (ed.), *Handbook of psychotherapy case formulation* (2nd edn.) (pp. 290–316). New York: Guilford Press.

Peterson, A., & Halstead, T. (1998). Group cognitive behavior therapy for depression in a community setting: A clinical replication series. *Behavior Therapy*, 29(1): 3–18.

Peterson, D. R. (1968). *The clinical study of social behavior*. New York: Appleton-Century-Crofts.

(1976a). Is psychology a profession? *American Psychologist*, 31: 572–81.

(1976b). Need for a Doctor of Psychology degree in professional psychology. *American Psychologist*, 31: 792–8.

(1991). Connection and disconnection of research and practice in the education of professional psychologists. *American Psychologist*, 46: 422–9.

(1997). *Educating professional psychologists: History and guiding conception*. Washington, DC: American Psychological Association.

(2004). Science, scientism, and professional responsibility. *Clinical Psychology: Science and Practice*, 11(2): 196–210.

Pettit, J. W., Voelz, Z. R., & Joiner, T. E. (2001). Combined treatments for depression. In M. T. Sammons, & N. B. Schmidt (eds.), *Combined treatments for mental disorders: A guide to psychological and pharmacological interventions* (pp. 131–59). Washington, DC: American Psychological Association.

Pfeiffer, E. (1975). A short portable mental status questionnaire for the assessment of organic deficit in elderly patients. *Journal of the American Geriatrics Society*, 23: 433–41.

Pilecki, B., Arentoft, A., & McKay, D. (2011). An evidence-based causal model of panic disorder. *Journal of Anxiety Disorders*, 25(3): 381–8.

Pilgrim, D., & Treacher, A. (1992). *Clinical psychology observed*. London: Tavistock/Routledge.

Premack, D. (1959). Toward empirical behavior laws: I. Positive reinforcement. *Psychological Review*, 66(4): 219–33.

Prince, M., Patel, V., Saxena, S., Maj, M., Maselko, J., Phillips, M. R., & Rahman, A. (2007). No health without mental health. *Lancet*, 370(9590): 859–77.

Prioleau, L., Murdock, M., & Brody, N. (1983). An analysis of psychotherapy versus placebo studies. *Behavioral and Brain Sciences*, 6(2): 275–85.

Prochaska, J. O., & Norcross, J. C. (1998). *Systems of psychotherapy: A transtheoretical analysis* (4th edn.). Pacific Grove, CA: Brooks/Cole.

Prochaska, J. O., Norcross, J. C., & DiClemente, C. C. (1995). *Changing for good*. New York: Avon.

Radloff, L. S. (1977). The CES-D scale: A self report depression scale for research in the general population. *Applied Psychological Measurement*, 1(3): 385–401.

Raimy, V. C. (ed.) (1950). *Training in clinical psychology (Boulder Conference)*. New York: Prentice Hall.

Rapee, R. (1991). The conceptual overlap between cognition and conditioning in clinical psychology. *Clinical Psychology Review*, 11(2): 193–203.

Rapee, R. M., & Heimberg, R. G. (1997). A cognitive-behavioral model of anxiety in social phobia. *Behaviour Research and Therapy*, 35(8): 741–56.

Rapee, R. M., Brown, T. A., Antony, M. M., & Barlow, D. H. (1992). Response to hyperventilation and inhalation of 5.5% carbon dioxide-enriched air across the DSM-III-R anxiety disorders. *Journal of Abnormal Psychology*, 101: 538–52.

Rapee, R., Mattick, R. P., & Murrell, E. (1986). Cognitive mediation in the affective component of spontaneous panic attacks. *Journal of Behavior Therapy and*

Experimental Psychiatry, 17(4): 245–53.

Ravindran, A. V., Welburn, K., & Hardesty, J. R. M. (1994). Semistructured depression scale sensitive to change with treatment for use in the elderly. *British Journal of Psychiatry*, 164: 522–7.

Raw, M., McNeill, A., & West, R. (1998). Smoking cessation guidelines for health professionals: A guide to effective smoking cessation interventions for the health care system. *Thorax*, 53(Suppl. 5): 1–19.

Redlich, F., & Pope, K. (1980). Ethics of mental health training. *Journal of Nervous and Mental Disease*, 168(12): 709–14.

Repp, A. C., Karsh, K. G., Munk, D., & Dahlquist, C. M. (1995). Hypothesis-based interventions: A theory of clinical decision making. In W. O'Donohue & L. Krasner (eds.), *Theories of behavior therapy: Exploring behavior change* (pp. 585–608). Washington, DC: American Psychological Association.

Rescorla, R. A. (1988). Pavlovian conditioning: It's not what you think it is. *American Psychologist*, 43(3): 151–60.

Rescorla, R. A., & Wagner, A. R. (1972). A theory of Pavlovian conditioning: Variations in the effectiveness of reinforcement and nonreinforcement. In A. H. Black & W. F. Prokasy (eds.), *Classical conditioning II: Current research and theory* (pp. 64–99). New York: Appleton-Century-Crofts.

Resnicow, K., DiIorio, C., Soet, J. E., Borrelli, B., Ernst, D., Hecht, J., & Thevos, A. K. (2002). Motivational interviewing in medical and public health settings. In W. R. Miller & S. Rollnick (eds.), *Motivational interviewing: Preparing people for change* (2nd edn.) (pp. 251–69). New York: Guilford Press.

Ribeiro, J. D., Bodell, L. P., Hames, J. L., Hagan, C. R., & Joiner, T. E. (2013). An empirically based approach to the assessment and management of suicidal behaviour. *Journal of Psychotherapy Integration*, 23: 207–21.

Richards, D., & Richardson, T. (2012). Computer-based psychological treatments for depression: A systematic review and meta-analysis. *Clinical Psychology Review*, 32(4): 329–42.

Rieger, E., Van Buren, D. J., Bishop, M., Tanofsky-Kraff, M., Welch, R., & Wilfley, D. E. (2010). An eating disorder-specific model of interpersonal psychotherapy (IPT-ED): Causal pathways and treatment implications. *Clinical Psychology Review*, 30(4): 400–10.

Rincover, A. (1978). Sensory extinction: A procedure for eliminating self-stimulatory behavior in developmentally disabled children. *Journal of Abnormal Child Psychology*, 6(3): 299–310.

Robiner, W. N., Tumlin, T. R., & Tompkins, T. L. (2013). Psychologists and medications in the era of interprofessional care: Collaboration is less problematic and costly than prescribing. *Clinical Psychology: Science and Practice*, 20(4): 489–507.

Robins, L. N., Cottler, L., Bucholz, K., & Compton, W. (1995). *The Diagnostic Interview Schedule Version IV*. St Louis, MO: Washington University Medical School.

Robins, L. N., Wing, J., Wittchen, H.-U., Helzer, J. E., Babor, T. F., Burke, J., Farmer, A., Jablensky, A., Pickens, R., Regier, D. A., Sartorius, N., & Towle, L. H. (1988). The Composite International Diagnostic Interview: An epidemiological instrument suitable for use in conjunction with different diagnostic systems in different cultures. *Archives of General Psychiatry*, 45(12): 1069–77.

Robinson, J. D., & James, L. C. (2005). Assessing the patient's need for medical evaluation: A psychologist's guide. In L. C. James & R. A. Folen (eds.), *The primary care consultant: The next frontier for psychologists in hospitals and clinics* (pp. 29–37). Washington, DC: American Psychological Association.

Rogers, R. (1995). *Diagnostic and structured interviewing: A handbook for psychologists*. Odessa, FL: Psychological Assessment Resources.

(2001). *Handbook of diagnostic and structured interviewing*. New York: Guilford Press.

Ronk, F. R., Hooke, G. R., & Page, A. C. (2012). How consistent are clinical significance classifications when calculation methods and outcome measures differ? *Clinical Psychology: Science and Practice*, 19(2): 167–79.

Rosas, J. M., Todd, T. P., & Bouton, M. E. (2013). Context change and associative learning. *Wiley Interdisciplinary Reviews: Cognitive Science*, 4(3): 237–44.

Rose, S. D. (1993). Cognitive-behavioral group psychotherapy. In H. I. Kaplan & B. J. Sadock (eds.), *Comprehensive group psychotherapy* (3rd edn.) (pp. 205–14). Baltimore, MD: Williams & Wilkins.

Rosenthal, T. L., & Steffek, B. D. (1991). Modeling methods. In F. H. Kanfer & A. P. Goldstein (eds.), *Helping people change: A textbook of methods* (pp. 70–121). New York: Pergamon.

Roth, A., & Fonagy, P. (2004). *What works for whom? A critical review of psychotherapy research* (2nd edn.). New York: Guilford Press.

Roth, M., Tym, E., Mountjoy, C. Q., Huppert, F. A., Hendie, F. A., Verma, S., & Goddard, R. (1986). CAMDEX: A standardized instrument for the diagnosis of mental disorders in the elderly with special reference to the early detection of dementia. *British Journal of Psychiatry*, 149: 698–709.

Rounsaville, B. J., Alarcón, R. D., Andrews, G., Jackson, J. S., Kendell, R. E., & Kendler, K. (2002). Basic nomenclature for DSM-V. In D. J. Kupfer, M. B. First, & D. A. Regier (eds.), *A research agenda for DSM-V* (pp. 1–30). Washington, DC: American Psychiatric Association.

Rowan, A. B., & Runyan, C. N. (2005). A primer on the consultation model of primary care behavioral health integration. In L. C. James & R. A. Folen (eds.), *The primary care consultant: The next frontier for psychologists in hospitals and clinics* (pp. 9–27). Washington, DC: American Psychological Association.

Rudd, M. D. (2008). The fluid nature of suicide risk: Implications for clinical practice. *Professional Psychology: Research and Practice*, 39: 409–10.

Rudd, M. D., Cukrowicz, K. C., & Bryan, C. J. (2008). Core competencies in suicide risk assessment and management: Implications for supervision. *Training and Education in Professional Psychology*, 2(4): 219–28.

Rudd, M. D., Joiner, T. E., Jobes, D. A., & King, C. A. (1999). The outpatient treatment of suicidality: An integration of science and recognition of its limitations. *Professional Psychology: Research and Practice*, 30(5): 437–46.

Rudd, M. D., Mandrusiak, M., & Joiner, T. E. (2006). The case against no-suicide contracts: The commitment to treatment statement as a practice alternative. *Journal of Clinical Psychology*, 62(2): 243–51.

Rutan, S. (1993). Psychoanalytic group psychotherapy. In H. I. Kaplan & B. J. Sadock (eds.), *Comprehensive Group Psychotherapy* (3rd edn.) (pp. 138–46). Baltimore, MD: Williams & Wilkins.

Ryder, A. G., Ban, L. M., & Chentsova-Dutton, Y. E. (2011). Towards a cultural-clinical psychology. *Social and Personality Psychology Compass*, 5(12): 960–75.

Safran, J. D., & Muran, J. C. (2006). Has the concept of the alliance outlived its usefulness? *Psychotherapy*, 43(3): 286–91.

Safran, J. D., Abreu, I., Ogilvie, J., & DeMaria, A. (2011a). Does psychotherapy research influence the clinical practice of researcher–clinicians? *Clinical Psychology: Science and Practice*, 18(4): 357–71.

Safran, J. D., Eubanks-Carter, C., & Muran, J. C. (2010). Emotion-focused/interpersonal cognitive therapy. In N. Kazantzis, M. A. Reinecke, & A. Freeman (eds.), *Cognitive and behavioral theories in clinical practice* (pp. 332–62). New York: Guilford Press.

Safran, J. D., Muran, J. C., & Eubanks-Carter, C. (2011b). Repairing alliance ruptures. *Psychotherapy*, 48(1): 80–87.

Safran, J., Muran, J. C., Demaria, A., Boutwell, C., Eubanks-Carter, C., & Winston, A. (2014). Investigating the impact of alliance-focused training on interpersonal process and therapists' capacity for experiential reflection. *Psychotherapy Research* (ahead of print): 1–17.

Saitz, R. (2010). Alcohol screening and brief intervention in primary care: Absence of evidence for efficacy in people with dependence or very heavy drinking. *Drug and Alcohol Review*, 29(6): 631–40.

Salkovskis, P. M., Clark, D. M., & Hackman, A. (1991). Treatment of panic attacks using cognitive therapy without exposure or breathing retraining. *Behaviour Research and Therapy*, 29(2): 161–6.

Salovey, P., Rothman, A. J., Detweiler, J. B., & Steward, W. T. (2000). Emotional states and physical health. *American Psychologist*, 55(1): 110–21.

Salvendy, J. T. (1993). Selection and preparation of patients and organization of the group. In H. I. Kaplan & B. J. Sadock (eds.), *Comprehensive Group Psychotherapy* (3rd edn.) (pp. 72–84). Baltimore, MD: Williams & Wilkins.

SAMHSA (2014). *Screening, Brief Intervention, and Referral to Treatment (SBIRT)*. www.integration.samhsa.gov/clinical-practice/sbirt [accessed 28 April 2014].

Sanchez, L. M., & Turner, S. M. (2003). Practicing psychology in the era of managed care: Implications for practice and training. *American Psychologist*, 58(2): 116–29.

Sánchez-Meca, J., Rosa-Alcázar, A. I., Marín-Martínez, F., & Gómez-Conesa, A. (2010). Psychological treatment of panic disorder with or without agoraphobia: A meta-analysis. *Clinical Psychology Review*, 30(1): 37–50.

Santucci, L. C., McHugh, R. K., & Barlow, D. H. (2012). Direct-to-consumer marketing of evidence-based psychological interventions. *Behavior Therapy*, 43(2): 231–5.

Sapyta, J., Riemer, M., & Bickman, L. (2005). Feedback to clinicians: Theory, research, and practice. *Journal of Clinical Psychology*, 61(2): 145–53.

Sattler, D. N., Shabatay, V., & Kramer, G. P. (1998). *Abnormal psychology in context: Voices and perspectives*. New York: Houghton Mifflin.

Sattler, J. E. (2008). *Assessment of children: Cognitive foundations* (5th edn.). La Mesa, CA: Jerome M. Sattler Publishers.
(2014). *Foundations of behavioral, social, and clinical assessment of children* (6th edn.). La Mesa, CA: Jerome M. Sattler Publishers.

Schaie, K. W., & Willis, S. (eds.) (2011). *Handbook of the psychology of aging* (7th edn.). New York: Academic Press.

Schank, J. A., & Skovholt, T. M. (1997). Dual-relationship dilemmas of rural and small-community psychologists. *Professional Psychology: Research and Practice*, 28(1): 44–9.

Scheidlinger, S. (2004). Group psychotherapy and related helping groups today: An overview. *American Journal of Psychotherapy*, 58(3): 265–80.

Schein, L. A., Bernard, H. S., Spitz, H. I., & Muskin, P. R. (eds.) (2003). *Psychosocial treatment for medical conditions: Principles and techniques*. New York: Brunner-Routledge.

Schoenwald, S. K., Hoagwood, K. E., Atkins, M. S., Evans, M. E., & Ringeisen, H. (2010). Workforce development and the organization of work: The science we need. *Administration and Policy in Mental Health and Mental Health Services Research*, 37(1–2): 71–80.

Schön, D. A. (1983). *The reflective practitioner: Toward a new design for teaching and learning in the professions*. San Francisco, CA: Jossey-Bass.

Schou, L., & Wight, C. (1994). Mothers' educational level, dental health behaviours and response to a dental health campaign in relation to their 5 year old children's caries experience. *Health Bulletin*, 52: 232–9.

Schulte, D. (1997). Behavioural analysis: Does it matter? *Behavioural & Cognitive Psychotherapy*, 25: 231–49.

Schulte, D., & Eifert, G. H. (2002). What to do when manuals fail? The dual model of psychotherapy. *Clinical Psychology: Science and Practice*, 9(3): 312–28.

Scogin, F., & Shah, A. (2012). *Making evidence-based psychological treatment work with older adults*. Washington, DC: American Psychological Association.

Scott, K., & Lewis, C. C. (2014). Using measurement-based care to enhance any treatment. *Cognitive and Behavioral Practice* (ahead of print).

Sears, S. F., Evans, G. D., & Kuper, B. D. (2003). Rural social service systems as behavioral health delivery systems. In B. H. Stamm (ed.), *Rural behavioral health care: An interdisciplinary guide* (pp. 109–20). Washington, DC: American Psychological Association.

Segal, D. L., & Falk, S. B. (1997). Structured interviews and rating scales. In A. S. Bellack & M. Hersen (eds.), *Behavioral assessment: A practical handbook* (4th edn.) (pp. 24–57). Boston, MA: Allyn & Bacon.

Segal, D. L., Hersen, M., & van Hasselt, V. B. (1994). Reliability of the Structured Clinical Interview for DSM-III-R: An evaluative review. *Comprehensive Psychiatry*, 35(4): 316–27.

Segal, Z. V., Williams, J. M. G., & Teasdale, J. D. (2002). *Mindfulness-based cognitive therapy for depression: A new approach to preventing relapse*. New York: Guilford Press.

Seligman, M. E. P. (1975). *Helplessness*. San Francisco, CA: W. H. Freeman.
   (1995). The effectiveness of psychotherapy: The Consumer Reports study. *American Psychologist*, 50: 965–74.
   (1996a). Science as an ally of practice. *American Psychologist*, 51: 1072–9.
   (1996b). A creditable beginning. *American Psychologist*, 51: 1086–8.

Shaffer, D., Fisher, P. W., Lucas, C. P., Dulcan, M., & Schwab-Stone, M. E., (2000). NIMH Diagnostic Interview Schedule for Children, Version IV (NIMH DISC-IV): Description, differences from previous versions, and reliability of some common diagnoses. *Journal of the American Academy of Child and Adolescent Psychiatry*, 39(1): 28–38.

Shakow, D. (1976). What *is* clinical psychology? *American Psychologist*, 31: 553–60.

Shakow, D., Hilgard, E. R., Kelly, E. L., Luckey, B., Sanford, R. N., & Shaffer, L. F. (1947). Recommended graduate training program in clinical psychology. *American Psychologist*, 2: 539–58.

Shapiro, D. (2002). Renewing the scientist-practitioner model. *The Psychologist*, 15(5): 232–4.

Shapiro, D. A., Barkham, M., Rees, A., Hardy, G. E., Reynolds, S., & Startup, M. (1994). Effects of treatment duration and severity of depression on the effectiveness of cognitive-behavioral and psychodynamic-interpersonal psychotherapy. *Journal of Consulting and Clinical Psychology*, 63: 378–87.

Sheehan, D. V., Janavus, R., Baker, R., Harnett-Sheehan, K., Knapp, E., & Sheehan, M. (1999). *Mini-International Neuropsychiatric Interview*. Tampa, FL: University of South Florida Press.

Sheehan, D. V., Lecrubier, Y., Harnett-Sheehan, K., Amorim, P., Janavus, R., Weiller, E., Hergueta, T., Baker, R., & Dunbar, G. C. (1998). The Mini-International Neuropsychiatric Interview (MINI): The development and validation of a structured diagnostic psychiatric interview for DSM-IV and ICD-10. *Journal of Clinical Psychiatry*, 59(Suppl. 20): 22–33.

Shelton, J. L., & Levy, R. L. (1979). Home practice activities and compliance: Two sources of error variance in behavioral research. *Journal of Applied Behavior Analysis*, 12: 325–33.
   (1981a). A survey of reported use of assigned homework activities in contemporary behavior therapy literature. *The Behavior Therapist*, 4: 13–14.
   (1981b). *Behavioral assignments and treatment compliance: A handbook of clinical strategies*. Champaign, IL: Research Press.

Sheridan, C. L., & Radmacher, S. A. (2003). Significance of psychosocial factors to health and disease. In L. A. Schein, H. S. Bernard, H. I. Spitz, & P. R. Muskin (eds.), *Psychosocial treatment for medical conditions: Principles and techniques* (pp. 3–25). New York: Brunner-Routledge.

Sherrill, J. T., & Kovacs, M. (2000). Interview schedule for children and adolescents (ISCA). *Journal of the American Academy of Child and Adolescent Psychiatry*, 39(1): 67–75.

Shimokawa, K., Lambert, M. J., & Smart, D. W. (2010). Enhancing treatment outcome of patients at risk of treatment failure: Meta-analytic and mega-analytic review of a psychotherapy quality assurance system. *Journal of Consulting and Clinical Psychology*, 78(3): 298–311.

Smith, D. (2002). Psychologists now eligible for reimbursement under six new health and behavior codes. *Monitor on Psychology*, 33. www.apa.org/monitor/jan02/medicare.html [accessed 28 April 2005].

Smith, M. L., Glass, G. W. V., & Miller, T. L. (1980). *The benefits of psychotherapy*. Baltimore, MD: Johns Hopkins University Press.

Smith, T. W., & Hopkins, P. N. (2003). Psychosocial considerations in essential hypertension, coronary heart disease, and end-stage renal disease. In L. A. Schein, H. S. Bernard, H. I. Spitz, & P. R. Muskin (eds.), *Psychosocial treatment for medical conditions: Principles and techniques* (pp. 133–79). New York: Brunner-Routledge.

Sonnichsen, R. C. (1994). Evaluators as change agents. In J. S. Wholey, H. P. Hatry, & K. E. Newcomer (eds.), *Handbook of practical program evaluation* (pp. 534–48). San Francisco, CA: Jossey-Bass.

Soucy Chartier, I., & Provencher, M. D. (2013). Behavioural activation for depression: Efficacy, effectiveness and dissemination. *Journal of Affective Disorders*, 145(3): 292–9.

Spence, S. H., Wilson, J., Kavanagh, D., Strong, J., & Worrall, L. (2001). Clinical supervision in four mental health professions: A review of the evidence. *Behaviour Change*, 18: 135–55.

Spencer, T. D., Detrich, R., & Slocum, T. A. (2012). Evidence-based practice: A framework for making effective decisions. *Education and Treatment of Children*, 35(2): 127–51.

Sperry, L., Brill, P. L., Howard, K. I., & Grissom, G. R. (1996). *Treatment outcomes in psychotherapy and psychiatric interventions*. New York: Brunner/Mazel.

Spitzer, R. L., & Williams, J. B. W. (1987). Revising DSM-III: The process and major issues. In G. L. Tischler (ed.), *Diagnosis and classification in psychiatry* (pp. 425–34). New York: Cambridge University Press.

Spitzer, R. L., Gibbon, M., Skodol, A. E., Williams, J. B.W., & First, M. B. (2001). *DSM-IV-TR Casebook: A Learning Companion to the Diagnostic and Statistical Manual of Mental Disorders, Fourth Edition, Text Revision*. Washington, DC: American Psychiatric Association.

Spitzer, R. L., Kroenke, K., & Williams, J. B. (1999). Validation and utility of a self-report version of PRIME-MD: The PHQ primary care study. Primary Care Evaluation of Mental Disorders Patient Health Questionnaire. *Journal of the American Medical Association*, 282: 1737–44.

Spitzer, R. L., Kroenke, K., Linzer, M., Hahn, S. R., Williams, J. B., deGruy, F. V., Brody, D., & Davies, M. (1995). Health-related quality of life in primary care patients with mental disorder: Results from the PRIME-MD study. *Journal of the American Medical Association*, 274: 1511–17.

Spurling, M. C., & Vinson, D. C. (2005). Alcohol-related injuries: Evidence for the prevention paradox. *Annals of Family Medicine*, 3(1): 47–52.

Stamm, B. H. (2003). Bridging the rural–urban divide with telehealth and telemedicine. In B. H. Stamm (ed.), *Rural behavioral health care: An interdisciplinary guide* (pp. 145–55). Washington, DC: American Psychological Association.

Stamm, B. H., Metrick, S. L., Kenkel, M. B., Davenport, J. A., Davenport III, J., Hudnall, A. C., Ruth, A. W., Higson-Smith, C., & Markstrom, C. A. (2003). Introduction. In B. H. Stamm (ed.), *Rural behavioral health care: An interdisciplinary guide* (pp. 3–10). Washington, DC: American Psychological Association.

Stanley, B., & Brown, G. K. (2012). Safety planning intervention: A brief intervention to mitigate suicide risk. *Cognitive and Behavioral Practice*, 19(2): 256–64.

Stanley, M. A., & Mouton, S. G. (1996). Trichotillomania treatment manual. In V. B. Van Hasselt & M. Hersen (eds.), *Sourcebook of psychological treatment manuals for adult disorders* (pp. 657–87). New York: Plenum Press.

Sterns, H. L., & Dawson, N. T. (2012). Emerging perspectives on resilience in adulthood and later life: Work, retirement, and resilience. *Annual Review of Gerontology and Geriatrics*, 32(1): 211–30.

Stewart, R. E., Stirman, S. W., & Chambless, D. L. (2012). A qualitative investigation of practicing psychologists' attitudes toward research-informed practice: Implications for dissemination strategies. *Professional Psychology: Research and Practice*, 43(2): 100–9.

Stokes, D., Li, B., & Collins, L. (2012). *The Australian Psychological Society's Response to Health Workforce Australia's Consultation Paper on a Health Professional Prescribing Pathway in Australia*. www.hwa.gov.au/sites/uploads/HPPP-Australian-Psychological-Society-45-20121019.pdf [accessed 28 April 2014].

Stoltenberg, C. D., & McNeill, B. W. (1997). Clinical supervision from a developmental perspective: Research and practice. In C. E. Watkins (ed.), *Handbook of psychotherapy supervision* (pp. 184–202). New York: John Wiley.

Stowell, J. R., McGuire, L., Robles, T., Glaser, R., & Kiecolt-Glaser, J. K. (2003). Psychoneuroimmunology. In A. M. Nezu & P. A. Geller (eds.), *Handbook of Psychology*, Vol. 9: *Health Psychology* (pp. 75–95). New York: John Wiley.

Strauss, J. L., Hayes, A. M., Johnson, S. L., Newman, C. F., Brown, G. K., Barber, J. P., Laurenceau, J-P., & Beck, A. T. (2006). Early alliance, alliance ruptures, and symptom change in a nonrandomized trial of cognitive therapy for avoidant and obsessive-compulsive personality disorders. *Journal of Consulting and Clinical Psychology*, 74(2): 337–45.

Stricker, G. (2002). What is a scientist-practitioner anyway? *Journal of Clinical Psychology*, 58(10): 1277–83.

Stricker, G., & Trierweiler, S. J. (1995). The local clinical scientist: A bridge between science and practice. *American Psychologist*, 50(12): 995–1002.

Stritzke, W. G. K., Chong, J. L. Y., & Ferguson, D. (2009). *Treatment manual for smoking cessation groups: A guide for therapists*. Cambridge University Press.

Strong, J., Kavanagh, D., Wilson, J., Spence, S. H., Worrall, L., & Crow, N. (2003).

Supervision practice for allied health professionals within a large mental health service: Exploring the phenomenon. *The Clinical Supervisor*, 22: 191–210.

Strub, R. L., & Black, F. W. (2000). *The mental status examination in neurology* (4th edn.). Philadelphia, PA: F. A. Davis Company.

Sue, D. W., & Sue, D. (2012). *Counseling the culturally diverse: Theory and practice*. New York: John Wiley.

Summerfeldt, L. J., & Antony, M. M. (2002). Structured and semistructured diagnostic interviews. In M. M. Antony & D. H. Barlow (eds.), *Handbook of assessment and treatment planning for psychological disorders* (pp. 3–37). New York: Guilford Press.

Sundberg, N. D. (1987). Review of the Beck Depression Inventory (revised edition). In J. J. Kramer & J. C. Conoley (eds.), *Mental measurements yearbook* (11th edn.) (pp. 79–81). Lincoln, NE: University of Nebraska Press.

Task Force on Promotion and Dissemination of Psychological Procedures (1995). Training in and dissemination of empirically validated psychologist treatments: Report and recommendations. *Clinical Psychologist*, 48: 3–23.

Tate, D. F., & Zabinski, M. F. (2003). Computer and Internet applications for psychological treatment: Update for clinicians. *Journal of Clinical Psychology*, 60(2): 209–20.

Taylor, S. (2000). *Understanding and treating panic disorder: Cognitive-behavioral approaches*. New York: John Wiley.

Teachman, B. A., Marker, C. D., & Smith-Janik, S. B. (2008). Automatic associations and panic disorder: trajectories of change over the course of treatment. *Journal of Consulting and Clinical Psychology*, 76(6): 988–1002.

Thorne, F. C. (1947). The clinical method in science. *American Psychologist*, 2: 161–6.

Tolin, D. F. (2010). Is cognitive-behavioral therapy more effective than other therapies? A meta-analytic review. *Clinical Psychology Review*, 30(6): 710–20.

Toukmanian, S. G., & Brouwers, M. C. (1998). Cultural aspects of self-disclosure and psychotherapy. In S. S. Kazarian & D. R. Evans (eds.), *Cultural clinical psychology: Theory, research, and practice* (pp. 106–24). New York: Oxford University Press.

Tovian, S. M. (2004). Health services and health care economics: The health psychology market place. *Health Psychology*, 23: 138–41.

Townend, M., Iannetta, L., & Freeston, M. H. (2002). Clinical supervision in practice: A survey of UK cognitive behavioural psychotherapists accredited by the BABCP. *Behavioural and Cognitive Psychotherapy*, 30(4): 485–500.

Treatment Protocol Project (1997). *Management of mental disorders* (2nd edn.). Sydney, NSW: World Health Organization Collaborating Centre for Mental Health and Substance Abuse.

Trierweiler, S. J., & Stricker, G. (1998). *The scientific practice of professional psychology*. New York: Plenum Press.

Truscott, D., & Crook, K. H. (2013). *Ethics for the practice of psychology in Canada*. Alberta: University of Alberta Press.

Turkat, I. D. (1985). *Behavioral case formulation*. New York: Plenum Press.

Turkat, I. D., & Maisto, S. A. (1985). Application of the experimental method to the formulation and modification of personality disorders. In D. H. Barlow (ed.), *Clinical handbook of psychological disorders* (pp. 502–70). New York: Guilford Press.

Urry, H. L., & Gross, J. J. (2010). Emotion regulation in older age. *Current Directions in Psychological Science*, 19(6): 352–7.

US Census Bureau (2002). *Census 2000 urban and rural classification*. www.census.gov/geo/www/ua/ua_2k.html [accessed 20 March 2005].

US Department of Health & Human Services (2010). *Affordable Care Act*. www.hhs.gov/healthcare/rights/law/index.html [accessed 28 April 2014].

Van Brunt, D. L., Riedel, B. B. W., & Lichstein, K. L. (1996). Insomnia. In V. B. Van Hasselt & M. Hersen (eds.), *Sourcebook of psychological treatment manuals for adult disorders* (pp. 539–66). New York: Plenum Press.

Veehof, M. M., Oskam, M. J., Schreurs, K. M., & Bohlmeijer, E. T. (2011). Acceptance-based interventions for the treatment of chronic pain: A systematic review and meta-analysis. *Pain*, 152(3): 533–42.

Wachtel, P. (1982). *Resistance: Psychodynamic and behavioral approaches*. New York: Plenum Press.

Wampold, R. E. (2001). *The great psychotherapy debate: Models, methods, and findings*. Mahwah, NJ: Lawrence Erlbaum Associates.

Ward, T., Nathan, P., Drake, C. R., Lee, J. K. P., & Pathé, M. (2000). The role of formulation-based treatment for sexual offenders. *Behaviour Change*, 17(4): 251–64.

Watkins, C. E. (ed.) (1997). *Handbook of psychotherapy supervision*. New York: John Wiley.

Watson, J. B. (1924). *Behaviorism*. University of Chicago Press.

Weisz, J. R., & Kazdin, A. E. (eds.) (2010). *Evidence-based psychotherapies for children and adolescents* (2nd edn.). New York: Guilford Press.

Weller, E. B., Weller, R. A., Fristead, M. A., Rooney, M. T., & Schechter, J. (2000). Children's Interview for Psychiatric Syndromes (ChIPS). *Journal of the American Academy of Child and Adolescent Psychiatry*, 39: 76–84.

Weller, E. B., Weller, R. A., Teare, M., & Fristead, M. A. (1999). *Children's Interview for Psychiatric Syndromes (ChIPS)*. Washington, DC: American Psychiatric Press.

Wennberg, P., Philips, B., & de Jong, K. (2010). The Swedish version of the Outcome Questionnaire (OQ-45): Reliability and factor structure in a substance abuse sample. *Psychology and Psychotherapy: Theory, Research and Practice*, 83(3): 325–9.

West, R., McNeill, A., & Raw, M. (2000). Smoking cessation guidelines for health professionals: An update. *Thorax*, 55(12): 987–99.

Whipple, J. L., Lambert, M. J., Vermeersch, D. A., Smart, D. W., Nielsen, S. L., & Hawkins, E. J. (2003). Improving the effects of psychotherapy: The use of early identification of treatment failure and problem solving strategies in routine practice. *Journal of Counseling Psychology*, 50(1): 59–68.

Wholey, J. S., Hatry, H. P., & Newcomer, K. E. (1994). *Handbook of practical program evaluation*. San Francisco, CA: Jossey-Bass.

Williams, J. M. G., Watts, F. N., MacLeod, C., & Mathews, A. (1997). *Cognitive psychology and the emotional disorders* (2nd edn.). New York: John Wiley.

Williams, S. L., & Falbo, J. (1996). Cognitive and performance-based treatments for panic attacks in people with varying degrees of agoraphobic disability. *Behaviour Research and Therapy*, 34(3): 253–64.

Wilson, G. T. (1996a). Treatment of bulimia nervosa: When CBT fails. *Behaviour Research and Therapy*, 34(3): 197–212.

(1996b). Manual-based treatments: The clinical application of research findings. *Behaviour Research and Therapy*, 34(4): 295–314.

Witmer, L. (1907). Clinical psychology. *Psychological Clinic*, 1: 1–9. http:// psychclassics.yorku.ca/Witmer/clinical. htm.

Wolfenden, K. (1996). Enhancing opportunities: Recruitment and retention. In R. Griffiths, P. Dunn, & S. Ramanathan (eds.), *Psychology services in rural and remote Australia* (pp. 25–9). Wagga Wagga, NSW: Australian Rural Health Research Institute.

Wolpe, J., & Turkat, I. D. (1985). Behavioral case formulation of clinical cases. In I. D. Turkat (ed.), *Behavioral case formulation* (pp. 5–36). New York: Plenum Press.

Wood, J. A. V., Miller, T. W., & Hargrove, D. S. (2005). Clinical supervision in rural settings: A telehealth model. *Professional Psychology: Research and Practice*, 36: 173–9.

Woods, B., Spector, A., Jones, C., Orrell, M., & Davies, S. (2005). Reminiscence therapy for dementia. *Cochrane Database of Systematic Reviews 2005*, Issue 2. Article no. CD001120.

Woody, S. R., Detweiler-Bedell, J., Teachman, B. A., & O'Hearn, T. (2003). *Treatment planning in psychotherapy: Taking the guesswork out of clinical care*. New York: Guilford Press.

World Health Organization (1992). *The ICD-10 classification of mental and behavioral disorders: Clinical descriptions and diagnostic guidelines*. Geneva: World Health Organization.

(1993). *The ICD-10 classification of mental and behavioral disorders: Research diagnostic criteria*. Geneva: World Health Organization.

(1998). *Schedules for clinical assessment in neuropsychiatry, Version 2.1*. Geneva: World Health Organization.

(2010). *International classification of diseases and related health problems (ICD-10)* (10th rev.). Geneva: World Health Organization.

(2013). *Mental health action plan 2013–2020*. Geneva: World Health Organization.

Wrzus, C., Hänel, M., Wagner, J., & Neyer, F. J. (2013). Social network changes and life events across the life span: A meta-analysis. *Psychological Bulletin*, 139(1): 53–80.

Yalom, I. D. (1995). *The theory and practice of group psychotherapy* (4th edn.). New York: Basic Books.

Yates, B. T. (1995). Cost-effectiveness analysis, cost-benefit analysis, and beyond: Evolving models for scientist-practitioner-manager. *Clinical Psychology: Science and Practice*, 2(4): 385–98.

Index

Locators in **bold** refer to figures and tables

Lightning Source UK Ltd.
Milton Keynes UK
UKHW021624080119
335187UK00013BA/399/P